SPORTS-RELATED CONCUSSIONS IN YOUTH

Improving the Science, Changing the Culture

Committee on Sports-Related Concussions in Youth

Board on Children, Youth, and Families

Robert Graham, Frederick P. Rivara, Morgan A. Ford,
and Carol Mason Spicer, *Editors*

INSTITUTE OF MEDICINE *AND*
NATIONAL RESEARCH COUNCIL
OF THE NATIONAL ACADEMIES

THE NATIONAL ACADEMIES PRESS
Washington, D.C.
www.nap.edu

THE NATIONAL ACADEMIES PRESS   500 Fifth Street, NW   Washington, DC 20001

NOTICE: The project that is the subject of this report was approved by the Governing Board of the National Research Council, whose members are drawn from the councils of the National Academy of Sciences, the National Academy of Engineering, and the Institute of Medicine. The members of the committee responsible for the report were chosen for their special competences and with regard for appropriate balance.

This study was supported by contracts between the National Academy of Sciences and the Centers for Disease Control and Prevention (CDC) (200-2011-38807); the CDC Foundation (Unnumbered Award) with support from the National Football League; the Department of Defense (HT0011-12-C-0023); the Department of Education (ED-OSE-12-P-0049); the Health Resources and Services Administration (HHSH250200976014I); the National Athletic Trainers' Association Research and Education Foundation (0512SETGRANT); and the National Institutes of Health (HHSN263201200074I). Any opinions, findings, conclusions, or recommendations expressed in this publication are those of the author(s) and do not necessarily reflect the views of the organizations or agencies that provided support for the project.

International Standard Book Number-13: 978-0-309-28800-2
International Standard Book Number-10: 0-309-28800-2

Additional copies of this report are available for sale from the National Academies Press, 500 Fifth Street, NW, Keck 360, Washington, DC 20001; (800) 624-6242 or (202) 334-3313; http://www.nap.edu.

For more information about the Institute of Medicine, visit the IOM home page at: **www.iom.edu.**

Printed in the United States of America

The serpent has been a symbol of long life, healing, and knowledge among almost all cultures and religions since the beginning of recorded history. The serpent adopted as a logotype by the Institute of Medicine is a relief carving from ancient Greece, now held by the Staatliche Museen in Berlin.

Suggested citation: Institute of Medicine (IOM) and National Research Council (NRC). 2014. *Sports-related concussions in youth: Improving the science, changing the culture.* Washington, DC: The National Academies Press.

THE NATIONAL ACADEMIES
Advisers to the Nation on Science, Engineering, and Medicine

The **National Academy of Sciences** is a private, nonprofit, self-perpetuating society of distinguished scholars engaged in scientific and engineering research, dedicated to the furtherance of science and technology and to their use for the general welfare. Upon the authority of the charter granted to it by the Congress in 1863, the Academy has a mandate that requires it to advise the federal government on scientific and technical matters. Dr. Ralph J. Cicerone is president of the National Academy of Sciences.

The **National Academy of Engineering** was established in 1964, under the charter of the National Academy of Sciences, as a parallel organization of outstanding engineers. It is autonomous in its administration and in the selection of its members, sharing with the National Academy of Sciences the responsibility for advising the federal government. The National Academy of Engineering also sponsors engineering programs aimed at meeting national needs, encourages education and research, and recognizes the superior achievements of engineers. Dr. C. D. Mote, Jr., is president of the National Academy of Engineering.

The **Institute of Medicine** was established in 1970 by the National Academy of Sciences to secure the services of eminent members of appropriate professions in the examination of policy matters pertaining to the health of the public. The Institute acts under the responsibility given to the National Academy of Sciences by its congressional charter to be an adviser to the federal government and, upon its own initiative, to identify issues of medical care, research, and education. Dr. Harvey V. Fineberg is president of the Institute of Medicine.

The **National Research Council** was organized by the National Academy of Sciences in 1916 to associate the broad community of science and technology with the Academy's purposes of furthering knowledge and advising the federal government. Functioning in accordance with general policies determined by the Academy, the Council has become the principal operating agency of both the National Academy of Sciences and the National Academy of Engineering in providing services to the government, the public, and the scientific and engineering communities. The Council is administered jointly by both Academies and the Institute of Medicine. Dr. Ralph J. Cicerone and Dr. C. D. Mote, Jr., are chair and vice chair, respectively, of the National Research Council.

www.national-academies.org

COMMITTEE ON SPORTS-RELATED CONCUSSIONS IN YOUTH

NEHA P. RAUKAR, Assistant Professor of Emergency Medicine, and Director, Division of Sports Medicine, Warren Alpert School of Medicine, Brown University, Providence, Rhode Island

NANCY R. TEMKIN, Professor, Departments of Biostatistics and Neurological Surgery, University of Washington, Seattle

KASISOMAYAJULA VISWANATH, Associate Professor of Social and Behavioral Sciences, Harvard School of Public Health, and Director, Health Communication Core, Dana-Farber/Harvard Cancer Center, Boston, Massachusetts

KEVIN D. WALTER, Associate Professor, Departments of Orthopaedic Surgery and Pediatrics, Medical College of Wisconsin, Milwaukee

JOSEPH L. WRIGHT, Senior Vice President, Community Affairs, Children's National Medical Center, and Professor of Pediatrics (Vice Chair), Emergency Medicine and Health Policy, George Washington University, Washington, DC

Study Staff

MORGAN A. FORD, Study Director
CAROL MASON SPICER, Associate Program Officer
WENDY KEENAN, Program Associate (through April 2013)
SAMANTHA ROBOTHAM, Senior Program Assistant
PAMELLA ATAYI, Administrative Assistant
KIMBER BOGARD, Director, Board on Children, Youth, and Families

Reviewers

This report has been reviewed in draft form by individuals chosen for their diverse perspectives and technical expertise, in accordance with procedures approved by the National Research Council's Report Review Committee. The purpose of this independent review is to provide candid and critical comments that will assist the institution in making its published report as sound as possible and to ensure that the report meets institutional standards for objectivity, evidence, and responsiveness to the study charge. The review comments and draft manuscript remain confidential to protect the integrity of the deliberative process. We wish to thank the following individuals for their review of this report:

Gordon Bloom, McGill University
R. Dawn Comstock, University of Colorado, Denver
Joseph J. Trey Crisco, Brown University
John DiFiori, University of California, Los Angeles
Corey S. Goodman, venBio LLC
Michael V. Johnston, Johns Hopkins University
Matthew W. Kreuter, Washington University
Brad G. Kurowski, University of Cincinnati
Karen McAvoy, Rocky Mountain Youth Sports Medicine Institute
Tamara C. Valovich McLeod, A.T. Still University
Barclay Morrison, Columbia University
Cara Camiolo Reddy, University of Pittsburgh
Thomas L. Schwenk, University of Nevada

CAPT Jack W. Tsao, Uniformed Services University of the Health Sciences
Keith O. Yeates, Nationwide Children's Hospital

Although the reviewers listed above have provided many constructive comments and suggestions, they were not asked to endorse the conclusions or recommendations nor did they see the final draft of the report before its release. The review of this report was overseen by **Bradford H. Gray,** The Urban Institute, and **Floyd E. Bloom,** The Scripps Research Institute. Appointed by the National Research Council and the Institute of Medicine, they were responsible for making certain that an independent examination of this report was carried out in accordance with institutional procedures and that all review comments were carefully considered. Responsibility for the final content of this report rests entirely with the authoring committee and the institution.

Acknowledgments

The Institute of Medicine-National Research Council (IOM-NRC) Committee on Sports-Related Concussions in Youth and its supporting staff thank the colleagues, organizations, and agencies that shared their expertise and information during the committee's information-gathering meetings (see Appendix A for the names of the speakers). Their contributions informed the committee's deliberations and enhanced the quality of this report. The study sponsors gladly provided information and responded to questions. The committee also thanks the National Collegiate Athletic Association and the Datalys Center for Sports Injury Research and Prevention, Inc., and Dawn Comstock (University of Colorado, Denver) for responding to questions and providing concussion incidence data for use in the committee's report. The IOM-NRC staff, including board director Kimber Bogard, study director Morgan Ford, associate program officer Carol Mason Spicer, as well as Wendy Keenan, Samantha Robotham, Pamella Atayi, Colin Fink, and Daniel Bearss, were central in shepherding the report though all its stages. The committee would also like to thank study consultant Stefan Duma (Virginia Tech–Wake Forest University), for preparing a background paper to inform the committee's deliberations on the effectiveness of helmets to reduce sports-related concussions in youth. The committee and staff extend their gratitude to Laura DeStefano, Nicole Joy, and Abbey Meltzer, IOM Office of Reports and Communications, and Jennifer Walsh, Office of News and Public Information, for their assistance with report release and communication activities. Last but not least, the committee and staff thank Clyde Behney, Interim Leonard D. Schaeffer Executive Officer of the IOM, for the guidance he provided throughout this important study.

Contents

APPENDIXES

Boxes, Figures, and Tables

BOXES

FIGURES

TABLES

Abbreviations and Acronyms

ACE	Acute Concussion Evaluation
AE	athletic exposure
AIS	Abbreviated Injury Scale
ALS	amyotrophic lateral sclerosis
ANAM	Automated Neuropsychological Assessment Metrics
APOE	apolipoprotein E
APP	amyloid precursor protein
ATD	anthropomorphic test device
ATP	adenosine triphosphate
BESS	Balance Error Scoring System
CBF	cerebral blood flow
CBT	cognitive behavioral therapy
CCAT	Computerized Cognitive Assessment Tool
CCI	controlled cortical impact
CDC	Centers for Disease Control and Prevention
CI	confidence interval
CMRglc	cerebral metabolic rate of glucose consumption
CNS	central nervous system
CPSC	Consumer Product Safety Commission
CRI	Concussion Resolution Index
CSI	Concussion Symptom Inventory
CT	computed tomography
CTE	chronic traumatic encephalopathy

CTP   cleaved tau protein

DNA   deoxyribonucleic acid
DTI   diffusion tensor imaging

ED   emergency department
EE   enriched environment
EEG   electroencephalogram
ERP   event-related potential

FA   fractional anisotropy
fMRI   functional magnetic resonance imaging
FTLD   frontotemporal lobar degeneration

GCS   Glasgow Coma Scale
GSC/GSS   Graded Symptom Checklist/Scale

HBI   Health and Behavior Inventory
HIT   Head Impact Telemetry

ICC   intraclass correlation coefficient
IEP   individualized educational plan
ImPACT   Immediate Post-Concussion Assessment and Cognitive
               Testing
iNOS   inducible isoform of nitric oxide synthase
IOM   Institute of Medicine

MACE   Military Acute Concussion Evaluation
MD   mean diffusivity
MRI   magnetic resonance imaging
MRS   magnetic resonance spectroscopy
mTBI   mild traumatic brain injury
MWM   Morris water maze

NAA   N-Acetylaspartic acid
NC   non-concussed
NCAA   National Collegiate Athletic Association
NCAA ISS   National Collegiate Athletic Association Injury
               Surveillance System
NEISS-AIP   National Electronic Injury Surveillance System—All Injury
               Program
NFHS   National Federation of State High School Associations

NFL	National Football League
NFT	neurofibrillary tangle
NHIS	National Health Interview Survey
NHL	National Hockey League
NMDA	N-methyl-D-aspartate
NOCSAE	National Operating Committee on Standards for Athletic Equipment
NOR	novel object recognition
NSE	neuron-specific enolase
OR	odds ratio
OSSAA	Oklahoma Secondary School Activities Association
PARP	poly-ADP ribose polymerase
PCS	post-concussion syndrome
PCSI	Post-Concussion Symptom Inventory
PCSS	Post-Concussion Symptom Scale
PET	positron emission tomography
PR	prolonged recovery
PTSD	posttraumatic stress disorder
QEEG	quantitative EEG
RCT	randomized controlled trial
RIO	Reporting Information Online
ROS	reactive oxygen species
RPCSQ	Rivermead Post-Concussion Symptoms Questionnaire
SAC	Standardized Assessment of Concussion
SAT	Scholastic Aptitude Test
SCAT	Sport Concussion Assessment Tool
SLAM	Sports as a Laboratory Assessment Model
SOT	Sensory Organization Test
TBI	traumatic brain injury
TR	typical recovery
VA	Department of Veterans Affairs

Summary

In the past decade, few issues at the intersection of medicine and sports have had as high a profile or have generated as much public interest as sports-related concussions. In recent years there has been a growing awareness and understanding that all concussions involve some level of injury to the brain and that athletes suspected of having a concussion should be removed from play for further evaluation (CDC, 2013; Halstead et al., 2010). Despite the increased attention, however, confusion and controversy persist in many areas, from how to define a concussion and how multiple concussions affect the vulnerability of athletes to future injury, to when it is safe for a player to return to sports and the effectiveness of protective devices and other interventions in reducing the incidence and severity of concussive injuries (Wilde et al., 2012). Parents worry about choosing sports that are safe for their children to play, about finding the equipment that can best protect their children, and about when, if a child does receive a concussion, it will be safe for him or her to return to play or if it might be time to quit a much-loved sport entirely.

It is within this context that the Institute of Medicine (IOM) and National Research Council (NRC), in October 2012, convened the Committee on Sports-Related Concussions in Youth to review the science of sports-related concussions in youth from elementary school through young adulthood, including military personnel and their dependents, and to prepare a report on that topic based on that review. The committee was charged with reviewing the available literature on concussions within the context of developmental neurobiology, specifically relating to the causes of concussions, their relationship to impacts to the head or body during sports, the effectiveness of protective devices and equipment, screening for and diagnosis of concussions, their treatment and management, and their long-term consequences. Specific topics of interest included

- the acute, subacute, and chronic effects of single and repetitive concussive and non-concussive head impacts on the brain;
- risk factors for sports concussions, post-concussion syndrome, and chronic traumatic encephalopathy;
- the spectrum of cognitive, affective, and behavioral alterations that can occur during acute, subacute, and chronic posttraumatic phases;
- physical and biological triggers and thresholds for injury;
- the effectiveness of equipment and sports regulations in preventing injury;
- hospital- and non-hospital-based diagnostic tools; and
- treatments for sports concussions.

Based on its review of the available evidence, the committee was asked to identify findings in each of the above topic areas and to make recommendations geared toward research funding agencies, legislatures, state and school superintendents and athletic directors, athletic personnel, military personnel, parents, and equipment manufacturers.

The study was sponsored by the Centers for Disease Control and Prevention (CDC), the CDC Foundation with support from the National Football League, the Department of Defense, the Department of Education, the Health Resources and Services Administration, the National Athletic Trainers' Association Research and Education Foundation, and the National Institutes of Health.

EPIDEMIOLOGY

As this report discusses, there is currently a lack of data to accurately estimate the incidence of sports-related concussions across a variety of sports and for youth across the pediatric age spectrum. Nevertheless, existing data suggest that sports-related concussions represent a significant public health concern. It has been estimated that as many as 1.6 million to 3.8 million sports- and recreation-related traumatic brain injuries (TBIs), including concussions and other head injuries, occur in the United States each year (Langlois et al., 2006). Because many concussions go unreported, this figure likely represents a conservative estimate. Data also suggest that an increase in reported sports-related concussions has occurred in recent years, a trend that may have been caused by a greater awareness of concussions. For example, a review of National Collegiate Athletic Association data for 15 sports showed that the overall reported concussion rate doubled from 1.7 to 3.4 concussions per 1,000 athletic exposures[1] between the 1988-1989 and 2003-2004 academic years (Hootman et al., 2007). Among youth ages 19 and under, the reported number of individuals treated for concussions and other nonfatal, sports- and recreation-related TBIs increased from 150,000 to 250,000 between 2001 and 2009. The rate of emergency department visits for such injuries increased 57 percent over the same time period (Gilchrist et al., 2011).

The incidence of reported concussions varies substantially by sport (see Table S-1). Available data show that among male athletes in the United States at the high school and collegiate levels, football, ice hockey, lacrosse, wrestling, and soccer consistently are associated with the highest rates of reported concussions (Datalys Center, 2013a,b; Gessel et al., 2007; Hootman et al., 2007; Lincoln et al., 2011; Marar et al., 2012). For female athletes, the high school and college sports associated with the highest rates of reported concussions are soccer, lacrosse, and basketball (Datalys Center, 2013a,b; Gessel et al., 2007; Hootman et al., 2007; Lincoln et al., 2011; Marar et al., 2012). Women's ice hockey has one of the highest rates of reported concussions at the collegiate level (Agel and Harvey, 2010; Datalys Center, 2013b; Hootman et al., 2007), but data on the incidence of concussions for female ice hockey players at the high school level are currently unavailable. A major limitation to existing data on sports-related concussions in youth is a lack of research on the incidence of such injuries in nonacademic settings, such as in intramural and club sports, and for athletes younger than high school age.

Part of the committee's charge was to examine sports-related concussions among military dependents as well as concussions in military personnel ages 18 to 21 that result from sports and physical training at military service academies or during recruit training. There is no evidence about whether the risks for concussion are different for these youth than for youth in general, although there is no reason to think that they would be (Goldman, 2013; Tsao, 2013). The committee also found that among military personnel, mild traumatic brain injuries (mTBIs)—of which concussions are one category—represent the majority (about 85 percent in 2012) of all TBIs and that most mTBIs (about 80 percent in 2012) do not occur in the deployed setting. These TBIs are instead most commonly caused by motor vehicle crashes (privately owned and military vehicles), falls, sports and recreation activities, and military training (DVBIC, 2013). However, it is unknown what proportion of these injuries are concussions and, among those, what proportions occur during sports and recreation activities or

---

[1]Athletic exposures are the number of practices and competitions in which an individual actively participates (i.e., in which he or she is exposed to the possibility of athletic injury).

TABLE S-1 Reported Concussion Rates by Sport, Sex, and Competition Level (High School and College) (Rates per 10,000 Athletic Exposures)

| Sport | High School | | | |
	Lincoln et al. (1997-2008)	Gessel et al. (2005-2006)	Marar et al. (2008-2010)	Datalys Center[a] (2010-2012)
Football	6.0	4.7	6.4	11.2
Ice Hockey (W)	—	—	—	—
Ice Hockey (M)	—	—	5.4	—
Lacrosse (W)	2.0	—	3.5	5.2
Lacrosse (M)	3.0	—	4.0	6.9
Soccer (W)	3.5	3.6	3.4	6.7
Soccer (M)	1.7	2.2	1.9	4.2
Wrestling	1.7	1.8	2.2	6.2
Field Hockey	1.0	—	2.2	4.2
Basketball (W)	1.6	2.1	2.1	5.6
Basketball (M)	1.0	0.7	1.6	2.8
Softball	1.1	0.7	1.6	1.6
Baseball	0.6	0.5	0.5	1.2
Volleyball	—	0.5	0.6	2.4

[a]Reported rates are based on preliminary data from NATA NATION reported by athletic trainers in participating high schools. Data collection began with 25 schools in 2010-2011 and currently has more than 100 participants in the 2013-2014 academic year.

[b]The data from Hootman and colleagues (2007) represent 16 years (1988-2004), except in the case of women's ice hockey for which data collection began in 2000.

during military training. Concerning concussions sustained by military personnel ages 18 to 21 who play intramural or service academy sports, there is no reason to suspect that the concussion risks are different from those for nonmilitary athletes of the same age, although military service academies require certain physical training activities, such as combatives and ropes courses, and offer other activities, such as boxing, that may pose a high risk of concussion (Kelly, 2013; Wolfe, 2013). Although the committee found anecdotal evidence that military personnel sustain concussions during hand-to-hand combatives training courses (Sapien and Zwerdling, 2012), there are no published data on the occurrence of concussions during such training.

COMMITTEE'S APPROACH

In approaching its task, the committee performed a review of the peer-reviewed scientific literature that was relevant to the various aspects of the

College				
Hootman et al. (1988-2004)	Gessel et al. (2005-2006)	Agel and Harvey (2000-2007)	Datalys Center[c] (2004-2009)	Datalys Center[c] (2009-2013)
3.7	6.1	—	6.0	6.3
9.1[b]	—	8.2	7.0	5.0
4.1	—	7.2	6.0	8.2
2.5	—	—	6.2	5.5
2.6	—	—	6.0	3.1
4.1	6.3	—	6.7	6.5
2.8	4.9	—	4.2	3.1
2.5	4.2	—	4.9	12.4
1.8	—	—	4.0	14.5[d]
2.2	4.3	—	4.8	6.1
1.6	2.7	—	3.4	3.5
1.4	1.9	—	2.3	3.5
0.7	0.9	—	1.1	0.7[e]
0.9	1.8	—	1.8	3.3

[c]Data for the period 2004-2009 are from the NCAA Injury Surveillance System. The Datalys Center for Sports Injury Research and Prevention, Inc., assumed management of the NCAA injury surveillance program in 2009.

[d]Rate calculated with fewer than 30 raw frequencies.

[e]Average of participating teams over the time period.

SOURCES: Agel and Harvey, 2010; Datalys Center, 2013a,b; Gessel et al., 2007; Hootman et al., 2007; Lincoln et al., 2011; Marar et al., 2012.

statement of task. In doing so the committee identified several limitations to the current scientific evidence base. One such limitation is the use of terminology that is poorly defined and applied inconsistently across studies (e.g., "concussion" versus "mild traumatic brain injury"), which made it challenging for the committee to determine the applicability of many studies to concussions in youth. The committee acknowledges that there is no single, universally used definition of "concussion." A concussion may be described as a brain injury that has been induced by biomechanical forces and that may be identified by a constellation of physical, cognitive, behavioral, and emotional symptoms and may also be associated with physiological changes. Of the many existing definitions of "concussion," the committee found that the one that is currently most widely used is the definition set forth at the Fourth International Conference on Concussion in Sport held in Zurich in November 2012, which states, in part, "Concussion is a brain injury and is defined as a complex pathophysiological process affecting the brain, induced by biomechanical forces" (McCrory et al., 2013, p. 1).

Other limitations to the existing evidence base include the fact that relatively little research has focused specifically on concussions versus the more severe forms of TBI, particularly in youth ages 5 to 12; that there are few published studies on the effectiveness of protective devices and other interventions to reduce the occurrence of sports-related concussions in youth; and that there are relatively few data on the psychometric properties of sideline screening tools. Furthermore, many studies have small sample sizes and methodological weaknesses that limit the validity of their findings. However, the committee determined that even studies of limited strength could provide some useful information and inform future research needs.

As a supplement to its literature review, the committee hosted two public workshops with presentations and panel discussions on the various elements of the committee's statement of task. Speakers included experts in: the diagnosis, management, and rehabilitation of concussed youth athletes, including their reintegration into academic and athletic settings; the genetic and neurogenetic sources of increased risk; the development of biomarkers and imaging technologies for concussion diagnosis and evaluation; protective equipment safety standards and effectiveness; and the role of sports rules and training in the prevention of sports-related concussions. To help address the portion of its charge concerning concussions among military personnel and their dependents, an area for which there is little published research, the committee heard from experts on concussions in military and service academy training programs. In addition, the committee heard the perspectives of stakeholder representatives, including athletes, parents, coaches, officials, and youth sports organizations. The committee's information gathering also included reviews of previous IOM and NRC reports such as *Is Soccer Bad for Children's Heads?: Summary of the IOM Workshop on Neuropsychological Consequences of Head Impact in Youth Soccer* (IOM, 2002), *From Neurons to Neighborhoods: The Science of Early Childhood Development* (IOM and NRC, 2000), and *Gulf War and Health: Volume 7: Long-Term Consequences of Traumatic Brain Injury* (IOM, 2008). Finally, the committee took into consideration current consensus and position statements on the diagnosis and management of sports-related concussions developed by the international Concussion in Sport Group (McCrory et al., 2013), the American Academy of Neurology (Giza et al., 2013), the American Academy of Pediatrics (Halstead et al., 2010), and the American Medical Society for Sports Medicine (Harmon et al., 2013).

A central part of the committee's responsibility in preparing this report was to carefully review the science and evidence related to the causes, incidence, and biophysiology of concussions in youth. The findings, conclusions, and recommendations presented in this report reflect this approach. Yet, as we did our research, listened to public testimony, and reflected on our own experiences, we came to have a growing appreciation for the role of "culture" in the current recognition and management of concussions in young athletes. Culture is created by the sum of beliefs and behaviors within a group. And it is clear to us that currently, in many settings, the seriousness of the threat to the health of an athlete, both acute and long term, from suffering a concussion is not fully appreciated or acted upon. Too many times the committee read or heard first-person accounts of young athletes being encouraged by coaches or peers to "play through it." This attitude is an insidious influence that can cause athletes to feel that they should jeopardize their own individual health as a sign of commitment to their teams.

COMMITTEE'S FINDINGS[2]

Culture of Resistance in Sports Concussion

Despite increased knowledge about concussions and a growing rec-ognition in recent years that concussions involve some level of injury to the brain and therefore need to be diagnosed promptly and managed ap-propriately, there is still a culture among athletes and military personnel that resists both the self-reporting of concussions and compliance with ap-propriate concussion management plans. In surveys, youth profess that the game and the team are more important than their individual health and that they may play through a concussion to avoid letting down their teammates, coaches, schools, and parents.

Concussion Definition and Surveillance Needs

The National Collegiate Athletic Association Injury Surveillance Sys-tem and High School RIO[TM] (Reporting Information Online) data systems are the only ongoing, comprehensive sources of sports-related injury data, including data on concussions, in youth athletes. Such data are not avail-able for athletes younger than high-school age, nor are they available for participants in club sports and other youth engaging in competitive and recreational sports outside of an academic setting. There is currently no comprehensive system for acquiring accurate data on the incidence of sports and recreation-related concussions across all youth age groups and sports. Furthermore, studies of sports-related concussions in youth do not routinely include information on the race, ethnicity, or socioeconomic

---

[2]This section does not include references. Citations to support the committee's findings are given in the body of the report.

status of the participants.[3] There are no published data on the incidence of reported concussions during basic training for military recruits. More complete epidemiologic data would help researchers identify possible differences in the rates of sports-related concussions across subpopulations of youth and help them assess the effectiveness of interventions in reducing the incidence of such injuries.

The published literature includes numerous working definitions of "concussion" and exhibits an inconsistent use of terminology (e.g., confounding "concussion" and "mild TBI" even though the latter includes more severe brain injuries). These differences pose challenges for interpreting and comparing findings across studies on concussion.

Effects of Single and Multiple Concussive and Non-Concussive Head Impacts

Research primarily involving animals and individuals with more severe head injury has provided a limited framework for understanding the neuroscience of concussions. This research indicates that there is a series of molecular and functional changes that take place in the brain following a head injury, some of which may serve as important biomarkers for the pathophysiology of concussion. However, little research has been conducted specifically on changes in the brain following concussions in youth, and little research has attempted to evaluate differences in such changes between female and male youth. Research using newer noninvasive imaging techniques in the first hours and days following injury may help to improve understanding of the neurobiology of concussion.

Findings of studies of repetitive head impacts (sometimes called "subconcussive" impacts) have been mixed, with some showing an association between such impacts and functional impairments, and others not. Preliminary imaging research suggests that changes in brain white matter may appear after repetitive head impacts; this preliminary finding is supported by the animal literature.

Although the findings of studies on the effects of multiple concussions on cognitive function and symptom presentation have been mixed, more studies report unfavorable changes than do not. The most commonly observed neuropsychological impairments have been in the areas of memory and processing speed. Some studies have found that symptom load (i.e., the

---

[3]Racial and ethnic differences in rates of reported injury may reflect a number of factors. These include cultural and psychosocial factors, real or perceived experiences of discrimination in the health care system that can affect how and whether individuals seek care and the quality of the care that they receive, socioeconomic status, education, and access to care. Such differences, if they are found to exist, will suggest areas for future investigation.

number and severity of symptoms) is increased in athletes with a history of two or more concussions, but the strongest studies show no differences. There is some evidence from surveys of retired professional football players of a positive association between the number of concussions an individual has sustained and risk for depression. Athletes who have already had one or more concussions may subsequently have more severe concussions and may take longer to recover. Preliminary evidence indicates that, in addition to the number of concussions an individual has sustained, the time interval between concussions may be an important factor in the risk for and severity of subsequent concussions.

Risk Factors for Sports-Related Concussions, Post-Concussion Syndrome, and Chronic Traumatic Encephalopathy

There are normal changes in brain structure, blood flow, and metabolism that occur with brain development that may influence the susceptibility to and prognosis following concussions in youth. Available data indicate that female youth athletes and youth with a history of prior concussions have higher rates of reported sports-related concussions. The extent to which these findings are due to physiological, biomechanical, and other factors (e.g., possible differences between males and females in the reporting of concussion symptoms, player aggressiveness) is not yet well understood. Concussion rates appear to be higher among college athletes than among high school athletes, higher during competition than during practice (except for cheerleading), and higher in certain sports than in others. While it has been suggested that the physiological and biomechanical risks for concussion may differ between younger children and older youth and adults, there are not yet sufficient epidemiologic data from various sports to calculate and compare rates of sports-related concussions across the age spectrum. The findings of studies examining associations between genetic factors and the risk of concussion have been mixed, and their validity is limited by their small sample sizes.

Short-term predictors of prolonged recovery and post-concussion syndrome vary across studies but appear to include older age (adolescent versus child), high initial symptom load, and initial presenting symptoms of amnesia and loss of consciousness. Some evidence supports premorbid conditions (e.g., previous concussions, learning difficulties, psychiatric difficulties) as contributing to symptom persistence.

Whether repetitive head impacts and multiple concussions sustained in youth lead to long-term neurodegenerative diseases, such as chronic traumatic encephalopathy (CTE), remains unclear. Additional research is needed to determine whether CTE represents a unique disease entity and, if so, to develop diagnostic criteria for it. There is preliminary evidence that a genetic variant (e4) of apolipoprotein E (APOE) is associated with neuropathological features of CTE in individuals with a history of head injury.

Cognitive, Affective, and Behavioral Changes Following Concussion

The signs and symptoms of concussions typically fall into four categories—physical, cognitive, emotional, and sleep—with patients experiencing one or more symptoms from one or more categories. Very few studies—and none that included pre-high-school-age athletes—have tracked the course of recovery for youth from sports concussion over time in order to elucidate the typical cognitive, affective, and behavioral changes that occur following a concussion.

Thresholds for Concussive Injury

Available studies of head injury biomechanics have identified the importance of linear and rotational movements of the head in injury causation. However, they are based on models that have limited applicability to concussions in youth or to concussions that occur in sports environments. Thus there are currently inadequate data to define the direction- and age-related thresholds for linear and rotational acceleration specifically associated with concussions in youth. In addition, it is unclear if or when the threshold of injury for a second concussion might be lower than for an initial concussive injury.

Effectiveness of Equipment and Sports Regulations for the Prevention of Sports-Related Concussions

There is limited evidence from epidemiological and biomechanical studies that current helmet designs reduce the risk of sports-related concussions. However, there is evidence that helmets reduce the risk of other injuries, such as skull fracture, and thus the use of properly fitted helmets should be promoted. There is currently no evidence that mouthguards or facial protection, such as facemasks worn in ice hockey, reduce concussion risk, although their use should be promoted to prevent other sports-related injuries, such as those to the eyes, face, mouth, and teeth. The marketing of some protective devices designed specifically for youth athletes, such as mouthguards and soccer head gear, has included statements that these devices reduce concussion risk without sufficient scientific foundation to support such claims.

Because of the nonlinear relationship between the mechanical input and injury risk, reductions in a specific biomechanical parameter, such as head acceleration, by a particular protective device do not correspond to an equivalent reduction in concussion risk. Furthermore, current testing standards and rating systems for protective devices do not incorporate measures of rotational head acceleration or velocity and therefore do not comprehensively evaluate a particular device's ability to mitigate concussion risk.

Although additional research across a variety of sports is needed, some studies involving youth ice hockey and soccer players have shown that the enforcement of rules and fair play policies contributes to reductions in the incidence of sports-related injuries, including concussions. In response to concerns about the long-term consequences of repetitive head impacts, several organizations have called for a "hit count" in youth sports, which is defined as a limit on the amount of head contact a particular player experiences over a given amount of time. While the concept of limiting the number of head impacts is fundamentally sound, the committee found that, based on the evidence available at this time, implementing a specific threshold for the number of impacts or the magnitude of impacts per week or per season is without scientific basis.

Research indicates that concussion education programs are effective in improving concussion knowledge and awareness, although there is limited evidence concerning the effect of these programs on behavior. Preliminary evidence suggests a need for additional research to evaluate the effectiveness of educational programs that emphasize improving attitudes and beliefs about concussions among athletes, coaches, and parents in order to improve concussion reporting among youth athletes.

Most state concussion laws include requirements for concussion education, criteria for removal from play, and standards for health care providers who make return-to-play decisions. There is variation across states in the specific educational requirements for coaches, student athletes, and parents; in the qualifications of providers who are permitted to make return-to-play decisions; and in the populations to which the legislation applies. Given that most states are still in the early stages of implementing these laws, there is so far very little evidence of their efficacy.

Hospital- and Non-Hospital-Based Assessment Tools

Currently concussion diagnosis is based primarily on the symptoms reported by the individual rather than on objective diagnostic markers, which might also serve as objective markers of recovery. The use of multiple evaluation tools—such as symptom scales and checklists, balance testing, and neurocognitive testing—may increase the sensitivity and specificity of concussion identification, although there is currently insufficient evidence to determine the best combination of measures. Such traditional neuroimaging techniques as computerized tomography and magnetic resonance imaging (MRI) are of little diagnostic value for concussions per se, because structural imaging results are usually normal in concussions that are uncomplicated by a skull fracture or hematoma. Typically, individuals recover from a concussion within 2 weeks of the injury, but in 10 to 20 percent of cases, the concussive symptoms persist for a number of weeks, months, or even years. In these cases, the individuals may be said to be experiencing post-concussion syndrome.

Neuropsychological testing has a long tradition in measuring cognitive function after TBI and is one of several tools (along with symptom assessment, clinical evaluation, etc.) that may aid in the diagnosis and management of concussions in youth. Studies of the effectiveness of these tests to predict diagnosis and track recovery are mixed and individuals' performances on neuropsychological tests can be influenced by many factors, including effort and the presence of concussion symptoms (e.g., fatigue resulting from sleep disturbance). It appears that high scores on neuropsychological tests, indicating good cognitive function, are predictive of *not* having a concussion. In group studies these tests have been shown to be useful for tracking cognitive recovery for up to 2 weeks post injury, with a majority of concussions considered to be resolved by that time. The results of reliability studies for computerized neuropsychological tests are quite variable, with some studies demonstrating adequate reliability and others indicating less than adequate reliability. There are many possible reasons for this variability, including differences in sample sizes, testing conditions, and variable item pools. Most computerized tests produce multiple forms through a quasi-randomization of items. All commercial test batteries reviewed had some studies indicating acceptable reliability.

Newer imaging techniques—e.g., magnetic resonance spectroscopy, positron emission tomography, single-photon emission computed tomography, functional magnetic resonance imaging, and diffusion tensor imaging—may be useful in the future for assessing sports-related concussions, but at present they have not been validated for clinical use. There is some consensus in the literature that both quantitative electroencephalography and event-related potential procedures can detect differences in performance and neural responses in concussed versus non-concussed student athletes in high school and college even when behavior measures fail. However, these findings are true for a relatively small set of tasks that assess a limited array of cognitive abilities. Use of a broader range of tasks that measure different aspects of cognitive processes is necessary to provide a comprehensive view of behaviors most likely affected and those more likely spared by concussion. There is little research on the use of serum biomarkers in pediatric concussion. Although appropriately sensitive and specific serum biomarkers could be of great diagnostic and prognostic value in sports-related concussion, there currently is no evidence to support their use. There is some evidence, however, to suggest that normal levels of S-100B following head injury may predict individuals who do not have intracranial injury.

Treatments for Sports-Related Concussions

The expert consensus opinion is that an individualized treatment plan including physical and cognitive rest is beneficial for recovery from concussion. There is little empirical evidence for the optimal degree and duration of physical rest needed to promote recovery or the best timing and approach for returning to full physical activity, including the use of graded return-to-play protocols. However, there is evidence that the brain is more susceptible to injury while recovering; thus, common sense dictates reducing the risks of a repeat injury. Similarly, there is little evidence regarding the efficacy of cognitive rest following concussion or to inform the best timing and approach for return to cognitive activity following concussion, including protocols for returning students to school. There are no randomized clinical trials testing the efficacy of psychosocial or psychopharmacological treatments for children and adolescents with post-concussion symptoms and prolonged recovery.

Randomized controlled trials or other appropriately designed studies on the management of concussion in youth are needed in order to develop empirically based clinical guidelines, including studies to determine the efficacy of physical and cognitive rest following a concussion, the optimal period of rest, and the best protocol for returning individuals to full physical activity as well as to inform the development of evidence-based protocols and appropriate accommodations for students returning to school.

To address the many information gaps highlighted in these findings, the committee identified several recommendations for further research. These are provided in Box S-1.

BOX S-1
Committee's Recommendations

Recommendation 1. The Centers for Disease Control and Prevention, taking account of existing surveillance systems and relevant federal data collection efforts, should establish and oversee a national surveillance system to accurately determine the incidence of sports-related concussions, including those in youth ages 5 to 21. The data collected should include, but not be limited to, demographic information (e.g., age, sex, race and ethnicity), preexisting conditions (e.g., attention deficit hyperactivity disorder, learning disabilities), concussion history (number and dates of prior concussions), the use of protective equipment and impact monitoring devices, and the qualifications of personnel making the concussion diagnosis. Data on the cause, nature, and extent of the concussive injury also should be collected, including

- Sport or activity
- Level of competition (e.g., recreational or competitive level)
- Event type (e.g., practice or competition)
- Impact location (e.g., head or body) and nature (e.g., contact with playing surface, another player, equipment)
- Signs and symptoms consistent with a concussion

Recommendation 2. The National Institutes of Health and the Department of Defense should support research to (1) establish objective, sensitive, and specific metrics and markers of concussion diagnosis, prognosis, and recovery in youth and (2) inform the creation of age-specific, evidence-based guidelines for the management of short- and long-term sequelae of concussion in youth.

Recommendation 3. The National Institutes of Health and the Department of Defense should conduct controlled, longitudinal, large-scale studies to assess short- and long-term cognitive, emotional, behavioral, neurobiological, and neuropathological consequences of concussions and repetitive head impacts over the life span. Assessments should also include an examination of the effects of concussions and repetitive head impacts on quality of life and activities of daily living. It is critical that such studies identify predictors and modifiers of outcomes,

---

REFERENCES

Agel, J., and E. J. Harvey. 2010. A 7-year review of men's and women's ice hockey injuries in the NCAA. *Canadian Journal of Surgery* 53(5):319-323.

CDC (Centers for Disease Control and Prevention). 2013. Concussion in Sports. http://www.cdc.gov/concussion/sports/index.html (accessed March 28, 2013).

Datalys Center (Datalys Center for Sports Injury Research and Prevention, Inc.). 2013a. NATA NATION Preliminary Concussion Rates, 2010-2012. Institute of Medicine-National Research Council request. October 3.

including the influence of socioeconomic status, race, ethnicity, sex, and comorbidities. To aid this research, the National Institutes of Health should maintain a national brain tissue and biological sample repository to collect, archive, and distribute material for research on concussions.

Recommendation 4. The National Collegiate Athletic Association, in conjunction with the National Federation of State High School Associations, national governing bodies for youth sports, and youth sport organizations, should undertake a rigorous scientific evaluation of the effectiveness of age-appropriate techniques, rules, and playing and practice standards in reducing sports-related concussions and sequelae. The Department of Defense should conduct equivalent research for sports and physical training, including combatives, at military service academies and for military personnel.

Recommendation 5. The National Institutes of Health and the Department of Defense should fund research on age- and sex-related biomechanical determinants of injury risk for concussion in youth, including how injury thresholds are modified by the number of and time interval between head impacts and concussions. These data are critical for informing the development of rules of play, effective protective equipment and equipment safety standards, impact-monitoring systems, and athletic and military training programs.

Recommendation 6. The National Collegiate Athletic Association and the National Federation of State High School Associations, in conjunction with the Centers for Disease Control and Prevention, the Health Resources and Services Administration, the National Athletic Trainers' Association, and the Department of Education, should develop, implement, and evaluate the effectiveness of large-scale efforts to increase knowledge about concussions and change the culture (social norms, attitudes, and behaviors) surrounding concussions among elementary school through college-age youth and their parents, coaches, sports officials, educators, athletic trainers, and health care professionals. These efforts should take into account demographic variations (e.g., socioeconomic status, race and ethnicity, and age) across population groups. The Department of Defense should conduct equivalent research for military personnel and their families.

Datalys Center. 2013b. NCAA Concussion Rates, 2004-2009 and 2009-2013. Institute of Medicine-National Research Council request. September 23.

DVBIC (Defense and Veterans Brain Injury Center). 2013. DoD worldwide numbers for TBI. http://www.dvbic.org/dod-worldwide-numbers-tbi (accessed June 27, 2013).

Gessel, L. M., S. K. Fields, C. L. Collins, R. W. Dick, and R. D. Comstock. 2007. Concussions among United States high school and collegiate athletes. *Journal of Athletic Training* 42:495-503.

Gilchrist, J., K. E. Thomas, L. Xu, L. C. McGuire, and V. Coronado. 2011. Nonfatal traumatic brain injuries related to sports and recreation activities among persons ≤19 years—United States, 2001-2009. *Morbidity and Mortality Weekly Report* 60(39):1337-1342.

Giza, C. C., J. S. Kutcher, S. Ashwal, J. Barth, T. S. D. Getchius, G. A. Gioia, G. S. Gronseth, K. Guskiewicz, S. Mandel, G. Manley, D. B. McKeag, D. J. Thurman, and R. Zafonte. 2013. *Evidence-Based Guideline Update: Evaluation and Management of Concussion in Sports.* Report of the Guideline Development Subcommittee of the American Academy of Neurology. American Academy of Neurology.

Goldman, S. B. 2013. Army TBI Program Overview. Presentation before the committee, Washington, DC, February 25.

Halstead, M. E., K. D. Walter, and American Academy of Pediatrics, Council on Sports Medicine and Fitness. 2010. Sport-related concussion in children and adolescents. *Pediatrics* 126(3):597-615.

Harmon, K. G., J. A. Drezner, M. Gammons, K. M. Guskiewicz, M. Halstead, S. A. Herring, J. S. Kutcher, A. Pana, M. Putakian, and W. O. Roberts. 2013. American Medical Society of Sports Medicine position statement: Concussion in sport. *British Journal of Sports Medicine* 47(1):15-26.

Hootman, J., R. Dick, and J. Agel. 2007. Epidemiology of collegiate injuries for 15 sports: Summary and recommendations for injury prevention initiatives. *Journal of Athletic Training* 42(2):311-319.

IOM (Institute of Medicine). 2002. *Is Soccer Bad for Children's Heads?: Summary of the IOM Workshop on Neuropsychological Consequences of Head Impact in Youth Soccer.* Washington, DC: National Academy Press.

IOM. 2008. *Gulf War and Health: Volume 7: Long-Term Consequences of Traumatic Brain Injury.* Washington, DC: The National Academies Press.

IOM and NRC (National Research Council). 2000. *From Neurons to Neighborhoods: The Science of Early Childhood Development.* Washington, DC: National Academy Press.

Kelly, T. 2013. Sports and Physical Training-Related Concussion in Military Personnel. Presentation before the committee, Washington, DC, February 25.

Langlois, J., W. Rutland-Brown, and M. Wald. 2006. The epidemiology and impact of traumatic brain injury: A brief overview. *Journal of Head Trauma Rehabilitation* 21(5):375-378.

Lincoln, A., S. Caswell, J. Almquist, R. Dunn, J. Norris, and R. Hinton. 2011. Trends in concussion incidence in high school sports: A prospective 11-year study. *American Journal of Sports Medicine* 39(5):958-963.

Marar, M., N. McIlvain, S. Fields, and R. Comstock. 2012. Epidemiology of concussions among United States high school athletes in 20 sports. *American Journal of Sports Medicine* 40(4):747-755.

McCrory, P., W. H. Meeuwisse, M. Aubry, B. Cantu, J. Dvořák, R. J. Echemendia, L. Engebretsen, K. Johnston, J. S. Kutcher, M. Raftery, A. Sills, B. W. Benson, G. A. Davis, R. G. Ellenbogen, K. Guskiewicz, S. A. Herring, G. L. Iverson, B. D. Jordan, J. Kissick, M. McCrea, A. S. McIntosh, D. Maddocks, M. Makdissi, L. Purcell, M. Putukian, K. Schneider, C. H. Tator, and M. Turner. 2013. Consensus statement on concussion in sport: The 4th International Conference on Concussion in Sport held in Zurich, November 2012. *British Journal of Sports Medicine* 47(5):250-258.

Sapien, J., and D. Zwerdling. 2012. Army study finds troops suffer concussions in training. http://www.propublica.org/article/army-study-finds-troops-suffer-concussions-in-training# comments (accessed October 13, 2013).

Tsao, J. W. 2013. Navy and Marine Corps TBI Efforts. Presentation before the committee, Washington, DC, February 25.

Wilde, E. A., S. R. McCauley, G. Hanten, G, Avci, A. P. Ibarra, and H. S. Levin. 2012. History, diagnostic considerations, and controversies. In *Mild Traumatic Brain Injuries in Children and Adolescents: From Basic Science to Clinical Management*, edited by M. Kirkwood and K. O. Yeates. New York: Guilford Press. Pp. 3-21.

Wolfe, C. L. 2013. West Point health care providers focus on brain injury prevention, diagnosis, treatment. (March 28). http://www.army.mil/article/99664 (accessed July 25, 2013).

1

Introduction

In the past decade, few issues at the intersection of medicine and sports have had as high a profile or have generated as much public interest as sports-related concussions. Historically most concussions were not considered serious, and athletes who sustained them might be said to have been "dinged" or had their "bell rung." The injured player would "shake it off" and return to play. Recent years have seen an increasing awareness and understanding that all concussions involve some level of injury to the brain and that athletes suspected of having a concussion should be removed from play for further evaluation (Aubry et al., 2002; CDC, 2013a; Halstead et al., 2010; Harmon et al., 2013; McCrory et al., 2005, 2009, 2013a).

The acknowledgment of the seriousness of sports-related concussions has initiated a culture change, as evidenced by campaigns to educate athletes, coaches, physicians, and parents of young athletes about concussion recognition and management (e.g., CDC, 2013c; NCAA, 2013; NFHS, 2013; USA Football, 2013a; USA Hockey, 2013); rule changes designed to reduce the risk of head injury (e.g., Pop Warner Little Scholars, 2012, p. 44; USA Hockey, 2011, p. 58); and the enactment of legislation designed to protect young athletes suspected of having a concussion (NCSL, 2013). Despite such efforts, there are indications that the culture shift is not complete. For example, a 2012 survey of high school football players suggests that even when knowledgeable about the symptoms and dangers of concussions, a majority of players thought it was "okay" to play with a concussion and agreed they would "play through any injury to win a game" (Anderson et al., 2013). Some youth baseball rules pertaining to the use of a continuous batting order, in which all available players are in the line-up, penalize teams if a player must leave the game for any reason, including injury (USSSA Baseball, 2013, p. 10, Rule 7.02.D.1[c]). There are also anecdotal reports of players attempting to subvert pre-season baseline neurocognitive tests (Pennington, 2013).

Despite the increased attention to and recent proliferation of research on sports-related concussion, confusion and controversy persist in many areas, from agreement on how to define a concussion and the effects of multiple concussions on the vulnerability of athletes to future injuries, to when it is safe for a player to return to sports and the effectiveness of protective devices and other interventions in reducing the incidence and severity of concussive injuries (Wilde et al., 2012). Parents worry about choosing sports that are safe for their children to play, about selecting the equipment that can best protect their children, and, if a child does receive a concussion, about when is it safe for him or her to return to play or when it might be time to quit a much-loved sport entirely.

It is against this background that the Institute of Medicine (IOM) and National Research Council (NRC) convened the Committee on Sports-Related Concussions in Youth to review the science and prepare a report on sports-related concussions in youth from elementary school through young adulthood, including military personnel and their dependents (see Box 1-1 for the statement of task). The 17-member committee included experts in the areas of basic neuroscience, neuropathology, clinical expertise with head trauma in pediatric populations, sports medicine, emergency medicine, cognitive and educational psychology, psychiatry, bioengineering with an emphasis in pediatric biomechanics, youth sports organization representatives, active duty military training, epidemiology, statistics or statistical analysis and evaluation, and health communication (Appendix B). The committee was charged with reviewing the available literature on concussions, within the context of developmental neurobiology, regarding the causes of concussions, their relationship to impacts to the head or body during sports, the effectiveness of protective devices and equipment in preventing or ameliorating concussions, screening for and diagnosis of concussions, their treatment and management, and their long-term consequences. Specific topics of interest included

- the subacute, acute, and chronic effects of single and repetitive concussive and non-concussive head impacts on the brain;
- risk factors for sports concussion, post-concussion syndrome, and chronic traumatic encephalopathy;
- the spectrum of cognitive, affective, and behavioral alterations that can occur during acute, subacute, and chronic posttraumatic phases;
- physical and biological triggers and thresholds for injury;

- the effectiveness of equipment and sports regulations for the prevention of injury;
- hospital- and non-hospital-based diagnostic tools; and
- the treatment of sports-related concussions.

BOX 1-1
Statement of Task

An ad hoc committee will conduct a study and prepare a report on sports-related concussions in youth, from elementary school through young adulthood, including military personnel and their dependents. The committee will review the available literature on concussions, in the context of developmental neurobiology, in terms of their causes, relationship to hits to the head or body during sports, effectiveness of protective devices and equipment, screening and diagnosis, treatment and management, and long-term consequences. Specific topics of interest include

- the acute, subacute, and chronic effects of single and repetitive concussive and non-concussive head impacts on the brain;
- risk factors for sports concussion, post-concussive syndrome, and chronic traumatic encephalopathy;
- the spectrum of cognitive, affective, and behavioral alterations that can occur during acute, subacute, and chronic posttraumatic phases;
- physical and biological triggers and thresholds for injury;
- the effectiveness of equipment and sports regulations for prevention of injury;
- hospital- and non-hospital-based diagnostic tools; and
- treatments for sports concussion.

Based on currently available evidence, the report will include findings on all the above and provide recommendations to specific agencies and organizations (governmental and nongovernmental) on factors to consider when determining the concussive status of a player. The report will include a section focused on youth sport concussion in military dependents as well as concussion resulting from sports and physical training at Service academies and recruit training for military personnel between the ages of 18 and 21. Recommendations will be geared toward research funding agencies (NIH, CDC, AHRQ, MCHB, DoD), legislatures (Congress, state legislatures), state and school superintendents and athletic directors, athletic personnel (athletic directors, coaches, athletic trainers), parents, and equipment manufacturers. The report will also identify the need for further research to answer questions raised during the study process.

COMMITTEE'S APPROACH TO ITS CHARGE

Terminology and Parameters of Study

Recognizing that concussion is a subgroup of mild traumatic brain injury (mTBI) (see Figure 1-1), the committee chose to use the term "concussion" throughout the report.

However, given the variable use of the terms "concussion" and "mild traumatic brain injury" in the literature, the committee decided to use whichever term was used by the source when referring to specific studies or articles. For a specific definition of concussion, the committee chose to follow the current international consensus definition (McCrory et al., 2013a). Not only does it capture and provide more detail on the common elements of concussion, but the definition was developed through a formal consensus process and has been subject to review and revision on a regular basis (Aubry et al., 2002; McCrory et al., 2005, 2009, 2013a), which has permitted it to evolve along with the science of concussion. It is the committee's expectation that this definition will continue to evolve.

The current international consensus definition of *concussion*, as determined at the Fourth International Conference on Concussion in Sport (McCrory et al., 2013a), is

> Concussion is a brain injury and is defined as a complex pathophysiological process affecting the brain, induced by biomechanical forces. Several common features that incorporate clinical, pathologic and biomechanical injury constructs that may be utilised in defining the nature of a concussive head injury include:
> 1. Concussion may be caused either by a direct blow to the head, face, neck or elsewhere on the body with an "impulsive" force transmitted to the head.
> 2. Concussion typically results in the rapid onset of short-lived impairment of neurologic function that resolves spontaneously. However, in some cases, symptoms and signs may evolve over a number of minutes to hours.
> 3. Concussion may result in neuropathological changes, but the acute clinical symptoms largely reflect a functional disturbance rather than a structural injury and, as such, no abnormality is seen on standard structural neuroimaging studies.
> 4. Concussion results in a graded set of clinical symptoms that may or may not involve loss of consciousness. Resolution of the clinical and cognitive symptoms typically follows a sequential course. However it is important to note that in some cases symptoms may be prolonged.

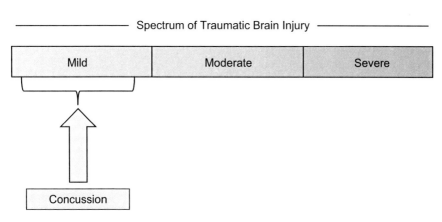

FIGURE 1-1 Relationship of concussions to the spectrum of traumatic brain injury.

In approaching its charge to examine many facets of sports-related concussions in youth, the committee first identified the age range of young people upon which it would focus and what types of activities it would recognize as a being "sports related." On the question of age range, the committee chose to focus on children and youth ages 5 to approximately 21 years (i.e., elementary school through college age). Five years is the approximate age of most children entering elementary school (kindergarten) in the United States (Mulligan et al., 2012). Around that age, children also are becoming more developmentally ready to begin participation in organized sports and recreational activities (Purcell et al., 2005). In selecting the upper boundary for the age range, the committee agreed that, despite the continuation of brain development into the mid-twenties (see Chapter 2), sufficient development occurs by age 21 to use that as a convenient cutoff. Although there is a significant body of literature on sports-related concussion among college athletes, there is little that uniquely captures post-college-age individuals (approximately ages 21 to 23 years) through age 26 years. This age group tends to be included in studies that capture older adults as well. For this reason the committee chose "college age" (approximately 21 years) as the upper age boundary.

On the question of which activities should be regarded as "sports related," the committee recognized that sports can be competitive or recreational, including everything from football and cheerleading to mountain climbing and extreme sports, and it further recognized that concussions can result from other types of physical activity that are not traditionally considered sports, such as playground activities, physical education classes, and ropes and combatives courses during military training. Thus, the committee took a broad view of sports, defining it for the purpose of this report as any sort of vigorous physical activity that does not involve motorized vehicles.

Information Gathering Process

The committee conducted an extensive review of the literature pertaining to sports-related concussions. The committee began with an English-language literature search of online databases, including Academic Search Premier, the Cochrane Database of Systematic Reviews, Embase, Google Scholar, Lexis Law Reviews Database, Medline, PsychINFO, PubMed, Science Direct, Scopus, Web of Science, and WorldCat/First Search. Additional literature and other resources were identified by committee members and project staff using traditional academic research methods and online searches. Attention was given to consensus and position statements issued by relevant experts and professional organizations.

The current evidence base (i.e., research and publications in peer reviewed journals) has notable limitations. As noted already, the poorly defined and inconsistent use of terminology (e.g., "concussion," "mild traumatic brain injury") often makes it difficult to determine the applicability of the literature specifically to concussion. In addition, there is relatively little literature devoted specifically to concussion, compared with the published research available on more severe traumatic brain injury (TBI), especially in the younger age groups (i.e., 5 to 12 years). There are few rigorous evaluations of interventions to reduce the incidence of concussion, there is limited analysis of outcomes associated with the implementation of "concussion" laws, and there are relatively few data on the psychometric properties of sideline screening tools.

The committee focused its review of the literature on research published in peer-reviewed scientific literature and consensus or position statements from groups of experts and professional organizations relevant to the diagnosis and management of sports-related concussion. The committee found considerable variation in the quality of the research studies it reviewed. However, given the current paucity of research in the field, the committee determined that even studies of limited strength could provide some useful information. The committee was careful to include appropriate qualifications when it cited such research. In addition, the committee made every effort to include the most current research. However, strong evidence was sometimes found in older studies, and as some of these studies had not been replicated in recent years, in some cases they were the only available sources of data. In some areas, large-scale studies have not been done, and so the committee looked for whatever data were available from smaller-scale studies. Ultimately, the committee included in this study what it judged to be the best empirical literature available.

Given the limitations of the published literature, the committee used a variety of sources to supplement its review of the literature. The committee met in person five times and held two public workshops to hear from invited experts in areas pertinent to sports-related concussions in youth. Speakers included experts in the diagnosis, management, and rehabilitation of concussed athletes, including their reintegration into academic and athletic settings; genetic and neurogenetic sources of increased risk; the development of biomarkers and imaging technologies for concussion diagnosis and evaluation; protective equipment safety standards and effectiveness; and the role of sports rules and training in the prevention of sports-related concussion. The committee also heard from active duty military experts specializing in concussion policy and care and a representative from service academies specializing in training programs; stakeholder representatives, including athletes, parents, coaches, and officials; and representatives from youth sports organizations, such as the National Collegiate Athletic Association, the National Federation of State High School Associations, and the Amateur Athletic Union. (See Appendix A for open session agendas and speaker lists.)

The committee's work was further informed by the work of bodies such as the international Concussion in Sport Group (McCrory et al., 2013a), the American Academy of Neurology (Giza et al., 2013), the American Academy of Pediatrics (Halstead et al., 2010), and the American Medical Society for Sports Medicine (Harmon et al., 2013), as well as by previous IOM and NRC reports, including *Is Soccer Bad for Children's Heads?: Summary of the IOM Workshop on Neuropsychological Consequences of Head Impact in Youth Soccer* (IOM, 2002); *Cognitive Rehabilitation Therapy for Traumatic Brain Injury: Evaluating the Evidence* (IOM, 2011); *Systems Engineering to Improve Traumatic Brain Injury Care in the Military Health System Workshop Summary* (NAE and IOM, 2009); *Gulf War and Health: Volume 7: Long-Term Consequences of Traumatic Brain Injury* (IOM, 2008); *Early Childhood Development and Learning: New Knowledge for Policy* (IOM and NRC, 2001); *From Neurons to Neighborhoods: The Science of Early Childhood Development* (IOM and NRC, 2000); and *How People Learn: Brain, Mind, Experience, and School* (NRC, 1999).

OVERVIEW OF CORE ISSUES

Variability in Defining Concussion

The lack of reliable biomarkers for concussions and the reliance on a subjective symptom-based definition, combined with variations in terminology (e.g., "concussion" versus "mild traumatic brain injury") and in the definition of those terms, as well as evolving descriptions of the severity of concussion (e.g., grading scales, simple versus complex) pose challenges not only for understanding the epidemiology of sports-related concussion but also for interpreting the information on concussions that is available in the lay and professional literature. Recognition of the need for common definitions and terminology has led to recent efforts to develop consensus definitions and common data elements for TBI research, including adult and pediatric concussion/mTBI research (Aubry et al., 2002; Hicks et al., 2013; McCrory et al., 2005, 2009, 2013a; Menon et al., 2010; NINDS, 2013; Thurmond et al., 2010). The Federal Interagency Traumatic Brain Injury Research (FITBIR) informatics system, developed by the Department of Defense and the National Institutes of Health, is a federal database designed to promote data sharing across the field of TBI research (NIH, 2013). The common data elements for TBI research that have been identified through an ongoing federal interagency initiative (Hicks et al., 2013; Thurmond et al., 2010) form the cornerstone of the FITBIR informatics system data dictionary (NIH, 2013). Participation in such collaborative research efforts may help to advance TBI research through the use of common definitions and standards.

A 2010 position statement issued by a working group of the interagency initiative to develop common data elements for TBI research defines TBI as "an alteration in brain function, or other evidence of brain pathology, caused by an external force" (Menon et al., 2010). This definition of TBI has been adopted by the National Institute of Neurological Disorders and Stroke, the National Institute on Disability and Rehabilitation Research, and other members of the International and Interagency Initiative toward Common Data Elements for Research on Traumatic Brain Injury and Psychological Health as well as by the Brain Injury Association of America (BIAA, 2011; Menon et al., 2010). The term "TBI" does not represent a single, uniform condition, but rather refers to a myriad of brain injuries of different types and severity that may result from varied causes. Even within traditional classifications of TBI as mild, moderate, or severe, there are different types of injury and different degrees of severity. This great variation helps to explain why there are no simple answers to the definition, diagnosis, or treatment and management of TBI.

Although some sources explicitly use the terms "mild traumatic brain injury" and "concussion" synonymously (CDC, 2009; DoD, 2012a), the committee has found it most useful to view concussion as a subset of mTBI (see Figure 1-1; Giza et al., 2013; Harmon et al., 2013; McCrory et al., 2013a,b). Even among concussions, one finds variation in the symptoms experienced by individuals as well as differences in the severity and duration of symptoms. Efforts to standardize a definition of concussion date back to the mid-1960s (Congress of Neurological Surgeons, 1966). More recently, a number of professional groups, including the American Academy of Neurology; governmental bodies, such as the U.S. Centers for Disease Control and Prevention (CDC) and the Department of Defense; and a consensus group organized by international sporting bodies (Concussion in Sport Group) have advanced working definitions of concussion (CDC, 2012; DoD, 2012a; Giza et al., 2013; McCrory et al., 2013a). Although the specifics of the definitions differ, there are common elements. A concussion is understood to be a clinical syndrome involving a disturbance in brain function that is generally time-limited and results from biomechanical forces, such as a bump, blow, or jolt to the head or body (DoD, 2012a; Giza et al., 2013; Harmon et al., 2013; McCrory et al., 2013a,b). In addition, a concussion may, but usually does not, involve loss of consciousness and typically does not result in structural changes observable using standard imaging techniques, such as computed tomography or magnetic resonance imaging. These elements are captured in the consensus definition of concussion adopted by the committee (McCrory et al., 2013a).

Epidemiology

The estimates of sports-related concussions provided by published epidemiologic data are most likely conservative, given that many concussions go unreported (Daneshvar et al., 2011; McCrea et al., 2004). Moreover, the lack of consensus on the definition of "concussion" and the reliance on athletes to self-report their symptoms, combined with various methodological differences, including varying study designs (retrospective versus prospective) and sources of data (emergency departments, athletic trainers, coaches, parents) and differences in what is being measured (concussions, mTBIs, all TBIs), have made estimating injury rates difficult, and the accuracy of much of the existing data is unknown (Daneshvar et al., 2011; McCrea et al., 2004). In the interest of accuracy, the following discussion uses the terms (e.g., TBI, mTBI, concussion) employed by the papers cited. The variations in terminology highlight one of the challenges for understanding the epidemiology of sports-related concussion.

One frequently cited paper estimated that as many as 1.6 million to 3.8 million sports- and recreation-related TBIs may occur annually in the United States, although the authors note that this number might be low because many such injuries may go unrecognized (Langlois et al., 2006). The figure is based on estimates generated from the unintentional injury supplement[1] to the 1991 National Health Interview Survey (NHIS), which estimated that the annual number of sports- and recreation-related TBIs

---

[1]NHIS supplements are designed to capture data beyond those generated by the core questionnaire. Supplements may be used only once or repeated as needed (CDC, 2013d).

involving a loss of consciousness was approximately 300,000 across all age groups (Thurman et al., 1998). Citing studies suggesting that only 8 to 19.2 percent of sports-related concussions involve loss of consciousness (Collins et al., 2003; Schultz et al., 2004), Langlois and colleagues (2006) used these percentages to scale up the 300,000 TBIs involving loss of consciousness to 1.6 million to 3.8 million sports- and recreation-related TBIs annually.

A study using data from 15 National Collegiate Athletic Association (NCAA) sports found that between the 1988-1989 and 2003-2004 academic years, the overall reported concussion rate doubled, from 1.7 to 3.4 per 10,000 athletic exposures[2] (AEs), with an average annual increase of 7.0 percent (Hootman et al., 2007). A study of high school athletes in a large public school system showed an increase in the overall rate of reported concussions from 1.2 to 4.9 per 10,000 AEs between the 1997-1998 and 2007-2008 academic years, with an average annual increase of 16.5 percent (Lincoln et al., 2011). There was a substantial increase in reported concussion rate beginning in 2005, the same year that more training staff were added at each of the high schools in the study (Lincoln et al., 2011). Similarly, the CDC has estimated that between 2001 and 2009 the number of children and adolescents age 19 years and younger in the United States who were treated in emergency departments (EDs) for concussions and other nonfatal, sports- and recreation-related TBIs increased from approximately 150,000 to 250,000 (Gilchrist et al., 2011).[3] The rate of ED visits for such injuries increased 57 percent, from 190 to 298 per 100,000 population during that time period (Gilchrist et al., 2011). During the same time period, the number of ED visits for TBIs that required hospitalization varied, but did not show an increasing trend over time (Gilchrist et al., 2011).[4] A num-

---

[2]Athletic exposures are the number of practices and competitions in which an individual actively participates (i.e., in which he or she is exposed to the possibility of athletic injury).

[3]The *NEISS Coding Manual* contains a specific diagnostic code for "concussion" while coding other closed head injuries (TBIs) (e.g., subdural hematoma) as "internal organ injury" with "head" coded as the body part affected (CPSC, 2013b). The CDC report discussed here includes both types of injury.

[4]Using data from the National Hospital Ambulatory Medical Care Survey, another study examined a 5-year sample (2002-2006) of ED visits for diagnosed concussion in children and adolescents age 19 years and younger (Meehan and Mannix, 2010). The study found that 30 percent of all the diagnosed concussions (approximately 43,200 annually) were sports-related. A higher percentage of concussions in adolescents (11 to 19 years) was attributed to sports than in children under 11 years of age (41 percent versus 8 percent), although percentages do not take rates of participation in sports activities into account. The inclusion criteria for this study were more restrictive than in the CDC report. Only patients with a diagnosis of concussion were included. Patients with other diagnoses, such as skull fractures or unspecified intracranial injury, were included only if they also were diagnosed with concussion. Patients diagnosed with an intracranial hemorrhage were automatically excluded.

ber of factors may have contributed to the increases in reported concussion rates, including increased awareness and recognition of such injuries.

Surveillance Systems

Appropriate epidemiological surveillance can provide valuable data on the incidence, causes, and other information pertinent to the occurrence of sports-related concussions. Such data are important for informing the development of appropriate interventions to reduce the incidence of concussions in youth sports and enabling the assessment of the effectiveness of such interventions. Currently most of the reported epidemiologic data on sports-related concussions in youth come from three surveillance systems (see Table 1-1):

1. National Electronic Injury Surveillance System—All Injury Program (NEISS-AIP)
2. NCAA Injury Surveillance System (NCAA ISS)
3. High School RIO™ (Reporting Information Online)

The CDC data that were previously reported come from the NEISS-AIP, which captures data for individuals treated for injuries in emergency departments (CPSC, 2013c; Gilchrist et al., 2011; Hinton, 2012). NEISS-AIP is the only ongoing surveillance system that captures sports injury data from nonacademic settings and for children younger than high school age. Operated by the U.S. Consumer Product Safety Commission, NEISS-AIP is an expansion of the National Electronic Injury Surveillance System (NEISS), which was originally launched in the early 1970s and captures data from a national probability sample of approximately 100 hospitals with emergency departments in the United States and its territories (CPSC, 2013a,b,c). NEISS data inform national estimates of the number of injuries associated with, although not necessarily caused by, specific consumer products. This distinction is important because a head injury might be attributed to "baseball" even though it occurred during a backyard "sword fight" with baseball bats. In 2000 NEISS-AIP was developed as a subset of NEISS to capture information on all injuries treated in the emergency departments, not only those related to products (CPSC, 2013a). Like NEISS, NEISS-AIP captures data on individuals' age, sex, race, ethnicity, injury diagnosis, and affected body parts as well as the incident locale and product involved (if any), where injured person goes when released from the ED, and also a brief narrative description of how the injury occurred (CDC, 2013b; CPSC, 2013a; Hinton, 2012). Although NEISS-AIP includes data on race and ethnicity, an analysis of the NEISS data found that race and ethnicity were not

TABLE 1-1 Primary Surveillance Systems for Sports-Related Concussion Data

Data System	Design	Population and Years Covered
NEISS-AIP (National Electronic Injury Surveillance System—All Injury Program)	• Sub-sample (n=66) of a national probability sample of 100 hospitals with 24-hour emergency departments (EDs) in the United States and its territories	• Individuals treated for injuries in participating EDs • 2001 to date
NCAA ISS (NCAA Injury Surveillance System)	• Sample of NCAA schools across the three divisions, number varies by year and sport, ranging from an average of 53.5 schools in 2004-2009 to an average of 26.5 in 2009-2013 across the sports reported in Table 1-2	• NCAA athletes • 1982-1983 academic year to date (the number of sports covered has increased from only football to 25—men's and women's sports are counted separately)

Source of Data	Strengths	Limitations
• Medical record abstraction	• All age groups	• Only injuries treated in EDs
	• All sports and recreational activities	• Injuries seen in EDs may be more severe
	• Nationally representative ED data over time (years)	• Only captures primary diagnosis
		• Variability in diagnosis of concussion
		• Variable data on mechanism and circumstances of injury, including injuries involving sporting equipment in non-sports scenarios being categorized as sports-related
		• Number of injuries only; cannot be used to calculate injury rate
• Reports by athletic trainers at participating programs	• Includes participation data; can be used to calculate injury rate	• Only college-age athletes
	• Includes data on mechanism of and circumstances of injury (e.g., practice vs. competition, position, event)	• Limited to 16 competitive sports
		• Does not account for differences in playing time
		• Cannot capture unreported injuries
	• Provides data over time (years)	• Has not always recorded non-time-loss injuries

continued

TABLE 1-1 Continued

Data System	Design	Population and Years Covered
High School RIO™ (Reporting Information Online)	• Sample of U.S. high schools that have athletic trainers, number varies by year and sport, ranging from 95 in 2005-2006 to 208 in 2012-2013	• High school athletes • 2005-2006 academic year to date (the number of sports covered has increased from 9 to 20—boys' and girls' sports are counted separately)

captured in 37 percent of cases in 2007,[5] which has prevented assessments of racial and ethnic differences in injury rates (GAO, 2009).[6]

One positive aspect of NEISS-AIP is that it provides nationally representative ED data over a long period of time. However, a major limitation of using NEISS-AIP to estimate the incidence of sports-related concussion is that it captures data only on individuals treated in EDs, whereas many concussions are treated by athletic trainers, physicians, and other qualified personnel in other venues, and many concussions are not reported at all (Gilchrist et al., 2011; Hinton, 2012). Not only will many sports-related concussions not be captured by NEISS-AIP, but individuals who seek care from EDs may be more severely injured than those who receive care from athletic trainers or personal physicians, which may skew the data. Furthermore, NEISS-AIP captures only the primary diagnosis and body part injured and does not capture cases in which concussion was a secondary diagnosis (Gilchrist et al., 2011). In addition, little is known about the consistency of the diagnoses made by the many physicians treating patients in the various sampled hospitals (Bazarian et al., 2006; Powell et al., 2008). Errors also may be introduced during the hospital-based NEISS-AIP coordinator's identification and abstraction of pertinent medical records for inclusion

---

[5]From 1999 through 2007, an average of 26 percent of cases failed to include data for race and ethnicity.

[6]Racial and ethnic differences in rates of reported injury may reflect a number of factors. These include cultural and psychosocial factors, real or perceived experiences of discrimination in the health care system that can affect how and whether individuals seek care and the quality of the care that they receive, socioeconomic status, education, and access to care. Such differences, if they are found to exist, will suggest areas for future investigation.

Source of Data	Strengths	Limitations
• Reports by athletic trainers at participating programs	• Includes participation data; can be used to calculate injury rate • Includes data on mechanism of and circumstances of injury (e.g., practice vs. competition, position, event) • Provides data over time (years)	• Only high-school-age athletes • Limited to competitive sports at participating high schools • Does not account for differences in playing time • Cannot capture unreported injuries • Has not always recorded non-time-loss injuries

and coding in NEISS-AIP (CPSC, 2013a). Yet another limitation is the variable quality of the data on the mechanism of injury that are captured. As previously noted, an injury may be attributed to a product (e.g., baseball bat, ice skates) even when the injury occurred through some non-sports-related scenario, such as twirling around with a baseball bat or being hit in the head with an ice skate while cleaning out a closet. The narrative section of the report may include information about how the injury actually occurred—for example, during organized or informal athletic activity, during competition or practice, or in some non-sports-related accident—but the quality of the information in the narrative section also varies (Gilchrist et al., 2011; Hinton, 2012). Finally, NEISS-AIP collects information only on the number of injured individuals treated in emergency departments and not on the size of the populations among which the injuries occurred (Gilchrist et al., 2011; Knowles et al., 2010). Consequently, NEISS-AIP data cannot be used to estimate injury rates per 1,000 AEs or relative risks (e.g., for specific sports).

The NCAA ISS, begun in 1982, collects injury and exposure data from a representative sample of institutions across the NCAA's three divisions in a variety of sports (Dick et al., 2007). In 2004, the NCAA injury surveillance program began using an online reporting system, and in 2009, the Datalys Center for Sports Injury Research and Prevention, Inc., assumed management of the program (Datalys Center, 2013b). The number of NCAA institutions participating in the NCSS ISS has varied over time and among sports. Prior to 2009, schools were recruited to report all applicable sports, although not all participating schools offered and hence reported on every sport. Since 2009, schools are recruited on a per sport basis, so data may be reported for only one sport from a given school. From 2004 to 2009, an average of 53.5 schools across the 14 sports listed in Table 1-2 reported data for those sports—ranging from less than 20 schools for men's and women's ice hockey to approximately 90 schools for men's and women's basketball (Datalys Center, 2013b). From 2009 to 2013, the average number of schools reporting across the 14 sports dropped to 26.5—ranging from 10 for field hockey to 41 for women's soccer (Datalys Center, 2013b).

Data are collected by athletic trainers on male and female participants in 25 sports from the first day of official pre-season practice through the final day of any postseason competition (personal communication with Datalys Center for Sports Injury Research and Prevention, Inc., September 23, 2013), although, as stated, not all schools report data for every sport. The athlete-related data captured include year in school, age, height, weight, and sex. Data on race and ethnicity are not collected. The NCAA ISS captures data on participation as well as on injury, and, in contrast to NEISS-AIP, it can be used to calculate injury rates for the sports it tracks.

TABLE 1-2 Reported Concussion Rates by Sport, Sex, and Competition Level (High School and College) (Rates per 10,000 Athletic Exposures)

| Sport | High School | | | |
	Lincoln et al. (1997-2008)	Gessel et al. (2005-2006)	Marar et al. (2008-2010)	Datalys Center[a] (2010-2012)
Football	6.0	4.7	6.4	11.2
Ice Hockey (W)	—	—	—	—
Ice Hockey (M)	—	—	5.4	—
Lacrosse (W)	2.0	—	3.5	5.2
Lacrosse (M)	3.0	—	4.0	6.9
Soccer (W)	3.5	3.6	3.4	6.7
Soccer (M)	1.7	2.2	1.9	4.2
Wrestling	1.7	1.8	2.2	6.2
Field Hockey	1.0	—	2.2	4.2
Basketball (W)	1.6	2.1	2.1	5.6
Basketball (M)	1.0	0.7	1.6	2.8
Softball	1.1	0.7	1.6	1.6
Baseball	0.6	0.5	0.5	1.2
Volleyball	—	0.5	0.6	2.4

[a]Reported rates are based on preliminary data from NATA NATION reported by athletic trainers in participating high schools. Data collection began with 25 schools in 2010-2011 and currently has more than 100 participants in the 2013-2014 academic year.

[b]The data from Hootman and colleagues (2007) represent 16 years (1988-2004), except in the case of women's ice hockey for which data collection began in 2000.

Participation data are recorded in terms of athletic exposures, generally defined as one individual participating in one practice or competition in which he or she is exposed to the possibility of athletic injury, regardless of the time associated with that participation. As constructed, this definition cannot take into account the greater duration of exposure experienced by athletes with significantly more playing time compared with those who have less playing time. Because the NCAA ISS captures information only on injuries receiving medical attention by the team athletics trainers or physicians, it will not include data on concussions in athletes who did not report injury. Another weakness of the system in earlier years is that it recorded only time-loss injuries (i.e., those for which participation was restricted for 1 or more days beyond the day of injury) (Dick et al., 2007), which means it failed to capture data on any athletes with a concussion who return to full physical activity on the same day as the injury. This problem has since been rectified. From 2004 to 2009, data were captured on all concussion and dental injuries regardless of time lost, and since 2009, data are captured on all injuries regardless of time lost (Datalys Center, 2013b). The final limitation to the NCAA data is that, by definition, they are limited to

College				
Hootman et al. (1988-2004)	Gessel et al. (2005-2006)	Agel and Harvey (2000-2007)	Datalys Center[c] (2004-2009)	Datalys Center[c] (2009-2013)
3.7	6.1	—	6.0	6.3
9.1[b]	—	8.2	7.0	5.0
4.1	—	7.2	6.0	8.2
2.5	—	—	6.2	5.5
2.6	—	—	6.0	3.1
4.1	6.3	—	6.7	6.5
2.8	4.9	—	4.2	3.1
2.5	4.2	—	4.9	12.4
1.8	—	—	4.0	14.5[d]
2.2	4.3	—	4.8	6.1
1.6	2.7	—	3.4	3.5
1.4	1.9	—	2.3	3.5
0.7	0.9	—	1.1	0.7[e]
0.9	1.8	—	1.8	3.3

[c]Data for the period 2004-2009 are from the NCAA Injury Surveillance System. The Datalys Center for Sports Injury Research and Prevention, Inc., assumed management of the NCAA injury surveillance program in 2009.

[d]Rate calculated with fewer than 30 raw frequencies.

[e]Average of participating teams over the time period.

SOURCES: Agel and Harvey, 2010; Datalys Center, 2013a,b; Gessel et al., 2007; Hootman et al., 2007; Lincoln et al., 2011; Marar et al., 2012.

college-age athletes and also do not include injuries for athletes participating in intramural, club, or recreational sports.

Modeled on the NCAA ISS and implemented in the 2005-2006 academic year, the High School RIO™, begun under the auspices of the Center for Injury Research and Policy at Nationwide Children's Hospital in Columbus, Ohio, captures injury data annually for male and female athletes from a sample of high schools throughout the country that have athletic trainers (Center for Injury Research and Policy, 2013; Hinton, 2012; PIPER Program, 2013a). The number of schools that participate varies from year to year but has ranged from 95 in 2005-2006 to 208 in the 2012-2013 academic year (PIPER Program, 2013b). The number of sports represented has also increased over time from the 9 original sports to more than 20, although not every school reports data for all sports (Center for Injury Research and Policy, 2013; PIPER Program, 2013b). Data are collected on athletes' year in school, age, sex, height, and weight, but not on their race or ethnicity. Athletic trainers report data weekly on athletic exposures and injuries, including information on the body site, diagnosis, severity, and injury event (e.g., mechanism of injury, activity, position or event, field or court location) (PIPER Program, 2013a). As with the NCAA ISS, the High School RIO captures participation data in terms of athletic exposures, permitting the calculation of injury rates for the sports it tracks, although it too does not take into account differences in playing time among athletes. Like the NCAA ISS, the High School RIO captures information only on concussions reported to or observed by the athletic trainers at the participating high schools, which means it may underestimate the occurrence of concussions. In addition, it too has not always captured data on non-time-loss injuries. Finally, by definition, the High School RIO captures data only on high-school-age youth and is further limited to those participating in the school-sponsored sports followed by the data system. As a result, it cannot provide complete epidemiologic data on sports-related concussion even within the high-school-age population.

The National Athletic Trainers' Association National Athletic Treatment, Injury and Outcomes Network (NATA NATION) project is a 3-year effort sponsored by the NATA Research and Education Foundation and BioCrossroads to examine not only sports-related injuries but also treatments and patient-reported outcomes among high school athletes (Datalys Center, 2013a). Under the auspices of the Datalys Center for Sports Injury Research and Prevention, Inc., the project employs the same data collection technology and methodology used in the NCAA Injury Surveillance System. The NATA NATION project began in 2010-2011 with 25 schools participating and now has more than 100 participants in the 2013-2014 academic year. The number of schools reporting data on any one sport ranges from 25 to 51 for the 14 sports reported in Table 1-2 (Datalys Center, 2013a).

Coordinated efforts to collect sports-injury data for middle-school- and younger-aged youth are limited. A 2011-2012 Middle School RIO study, modeled on the High School RIO and NCAA ISS systems, collected injury data from a national sample of middle school and Pop Warner football players (Middle School RIO™, 2013). In addition, a 2-year study (2012 and 2013 seasons) of 10 youth football leagues of various sizes and demographics across six states is being conducted (USA Football, 2013b). The collection of data is under the auspices of the Datalys Center for Sports Injury Research and Prevention, Inc.

Factors Associated with Increased Incidence Rates of Reported Concussions

Despite the limitations of the surveillance data on sports- and recreation-related concussion, some patterns have emerged. Studies suggest that several factors may be associated with increased rates of reported concussion, such as competition level (youth, high school, college), sports setting (competition, practice), sex (female, male), and sport (e.g., football, soccer) (Covassin et al., 2003; Gessel et al., 2007; Hootman et al., 2007; Lincoln et al., 2011; Marar et al., 2012).

Competition level College athletes had higher overall rates of concussion than did high school students (4.3 versus 2.3 per 10,000 AEs) in nine sports during the 2005-2006 academic year, based on injury data from the NCAA ISS and the High School RIO surveillance systems (Table 1-2; Gessel et al., 2007). The relationship held true across all the sports, for female and male athletes, and for competition and practice, with the exception of practices in baseball, in which the college and high school rates were the same, and practices in softball, in which the high school rate was slightly higher than the college rate (Gessel et al., 2007). More recent data from the NCAA Injury Surveillance Program (2009-2013) and NATA NATION (2010-2012) indicate higher reported concussion rates among high school versus college athletes in football, men's lacrosse, men's soccer, and baseball (Table 1-2; Datalys Center, 2013a,b).

There are few equivalent data available to compare rates of reported concussion among younger athletes with those for high school and college athletes. USA Football (2013b) has commissioned a 2-year study of injury incidence, including concussion, among youth football players. During the 2012 season (the first year of the study), fewer than 4 percent of the 1,913 players ages 7 to 14 sustained a reported concussion from more than 60,000 athletic exposures, including practices and games (USA Football, 2013b), which suggests an overall approximate rate of 11.1 per 10,000 AEs. This is similar to the rate of 11.2 per 10,000 AEs reported for high school students in the preliminary data from the NATA NATION project. A smaller study of youth football players ages 8 to 12 years found an overall reported concussion rate of 17.6 per 10,000 AEs during the 2011 season (Kontos et al., 2013). The study also found that players ages 11 to 12 were approximately 2.5 times more likely to sustain a reported concussion than players ages 8 to 10 years (25.3 versus 9.3 per 10,000 AEs) (Kontos et al., 2013).

Sports setting Several studies have examined the incidence of concussion during practice and competition. In general, reported concussion incidence is consistently higher in competition than in practice for both male and female athletes across all sports and age groups (Gessel et al., 2007; Hootman et al., 2007; Marar et al., 2012).[7] In addition, the two studies of concussion incidence among youth football players also show a higher rate of concussion in competition than in practice (Kontos et al., 2013; USA Football, 2013b). The exception to this trend is in cheerleading, for which a study using High School RIO data for 2005-2006 showed a slightly higher absolute rate of reported concussion during practice than in competition (1.4 versus 1.2 per 10,000 AEs) (Marar et al., 2012).

Sex Studies that compared the rates of reported concussions for male and female athletes in three high school and college sports played by both sexes (soccer, basketball, and softball/baseball) found that females had a higher rate of reported concussions than did their male counterparts (Covassin et al., 2003; Datalys Center, 2013a,b; Dick, 2009; Gessel et al., 2007; Hootman et al., 2007; Lincoln et al., 2011; Marar et al., 2012). Although women's lacrosse generally has demonstrated lower rates of reported concussion than has men's lacrosse, the rules differ sufficiently to preclude direct comparison between the sexes (Datalys Center, 2013a; Hootman et al., 2007; Lincoln et al., 2011; Marar et al., 2012). Recent NCAA data, however, show equivalent or higher rates of reported concussion in women's lacrosse than in men's (Datalys Center, 2013b). Data on collegiate ice hockey also traditionally has shown a higher rate of reported concussion

---

[7]The data reported by Gessel and colleagues (2007) showed a concussion rate for practice that was equal or higher than the rate in competition for high school and college volleyball and high school softball during the 2005-2006 academic year. However, the total number of reported concussions in each group was low (6, 14, and 10, respectively). The 2 years of data reported by Marar and colleagues (2012) follow the trend of concussion rates being higher in competition than in practice for high school volleyball and softball. No additional data were available to evaluate the relative concussion rates for college volleyball.

for females than males (Agel and Harvey, 2010; Hootman et al., 2007),[8] although the 2009-2013 NCAA data indicate a higher rate in men's hockey than in women's (8.2 versus 5.0 per 10,000 AEs) (Datalys Center, 2013b). (See Table 1-2.)

Sport The incidence of reported concussion appears to vary substantially by sport (see Table 1-2). For male athletes in the United States, football, ice hockey, lacrosse, wrestling, and soccer consistently are associated with the highest rates of reported concussions at the high school and college levels (Datalys Center 2013a,b; Gessel et al., 2007; Hootman et al., 2007; Lincoln et al., 2011; Marar et al., 2012). For female athletes, the high school and college sports associated with the highest rates of reported concussions are soccer, lacrosse, and basketball (Datalys Center, 2013a,b; Gessel et al., 2007; Hootman et al., 2007; Lincoln et al., 2011; Marar et al., 2012).[9] In addition, women's ice hockey has one of the highest rates of reported concussions at the college level (Agel and Harvey, 2010; Datalys Center, 2013b; Hootman et al., 2007), but no data are reported on the incidence of reported concussion for female athletes at the high school level.

There are very few studies that have examined sports-related concussions in youth outside of the high school and college settings and very few data on the incidence of reported concussions in different sports for youth younger than high school age (approximately age 14). The ED data captured in the NEISS-AIP database and reported by the CDC (see Table 1-3) and others provide some indication of the distribution by age of sports- and recreation-related activities and that have resulted in an ED visit for concussions or other nonfatal TBIs (Bakhos et al., 2010; Gilchrist et al., 2011), but the absence of participation data (the equivalent of the AEs captured by the NCAA ISS and High School RIO databases) precludes the calculation of injury rates. This is a problem because an activity such as bicycling, the activity most commonly associated with ED visits for nonfatal TBIs among girls ages 10 to 14 years, has a much different participation rate than, for example, horseback riding, which is the fourth most commonly associated activity for the same group (see Table 1-3). Assuming the participation rate for bicycling is much higher than that for horseback riding, the injury rate for bicycling would be lower than for horseback riding even though there were a greater number of injuries. As previously discussed, another

---

[8]Although Hootman and colleagues (2007) reported rates based on 16 years of NCAA ISS data for men's ice hockey and 4 years of data for women's ice hockey, for which data collection only began in the 2000-2001 academic year, Agel and Harvey (2010) used the same 7 years (2000-2007) of data for men's and women's ice hockey.

[9]The rate of reported concussion for field hockey from the NCAA data for 2009-2013 is uncharacteristically high (14.5 per 10,000 AEs), but was calculated from less than 30 raw observations and may not be reliable (Datalys Center, 2013b).

TABLE 1-3 Sports- and Recreation-Related Activities Most Commonly Associated with Emergency Department Visits for Nonfatal TBIs by Age and Sex—NEISS-AIP, United States, 2001-2009

Rank	Male Age Group (years)			Female Age Group (years)		
	5-9 No. (%)[a]	10-14 No. (%)	15-19 No. (%)	5-9 No. (%)	10-14 No. (%)	15-19 No. (%)
1	Bicycling 5,997 (23.6)	Football 8,988 (20.7)	Football 13,667 (30.3)	Playground 3,455 (30.3)	Bicycling 2,051 (12.2)	Soccer 2,678 (16.0)
2	Playground 4,790 (18.9)	Bicycling 8,302 (19.1)	Bicycling 4,377 (9.7)	Bicycling 2,361 (20.7)	Basketball 1,863 (11.1)	Basketball 2,446 (14.6)
3	Baseball 2,227 (8.8)	Basketball 4,009 (9.2)	Basketball 4,049 (9.0)	Baseball 541 (4.7)	Soccer 1,843 (11.0)	Gymnastics[c] 1,513 (9.1)
4	Football 1,657 (6.5)	Baseball 3,061 (7.0)	Soccer 3,013 (6.7)	Scooter riding 525 (4.6)	Horseback riding 1,301 (7.7)	Softball 1,171 (7.0)
5	Basketball 1,133 (4.5)	Skateboarding 2,613 (6.0)	All-terrain vehicle riding[b] 2,546 (5.6)	Swimming 504 (4.4)	Playground 1,041 (6.2)	Horseback riding 1,028 (6.2)

[a]Percent of emergency department visits for nonfatal TBI by age and sex.
[b]Although the committee specifically excluded use of motorized vehicles from its definition of "sport," the information is included here for the sake of completeness.
[c]Includes cheerleading and dance.
SOURCE: Gilchrist et al., 2011.

disadvantage of the NEISS-AIP data is that it is limited to individuals who were treated in EDs, thereby not capturing youth with concussions and other nonfatal TBIs who received medical care in other venues, or who were never treated at all. The data may also represent more severe injuries than those treated in non-emergency settings.

Extreme Sports

So-called extreme sports are rapidly gaining in popularity, especially in the younger population. Examples of extreme sports include competitive skateboarding, mountain biking, and snowboarding jumps and tricks (e.g., half-pipes and terrain parks). Between 1998 and 2008, participation in skateboarding increased by 49 percent and participation in snowboarding increased by 51 percent; mountain biking, the second most popular extreme sport, also saw an increase in participation (Extreme Sport, 2008). Because extreme sports by definition involve a high level of inherent danger, either because of the environment in which they are played or as a result of the sport, they would seem to place participants at high risk for injury, including concussion. However, there are limited epidemiologic data on rates and types of injuries experienced by those participating in extreme sports. A prospective survey of 249 downhill mountain bike riders showed an overall injury rate of 16.8 injuries per 1,000 hours of exposure (Becker et al., 2013). The rate of all reported injuries for expert riders was significantly higher than was the rate of reported injuries for professional riders (17.9 versus 13.4 injuries per 1,000 hours of exposure), and the injury rate reported during competition was significantly higher than the rate for practice (20 versus 13 injuries per 1,000 hours of exposure). Extremities (lower leg and forearm) are the areas of the body most often reported injured. The rate of reported concussions was not provided. Another study reported that serious injuries to the head and neck are more likely to occur when a rider falls over the handlebars than when he or she falls off to the side, which implies that women are at higher risk than men for head and neck injuries because they generally weigh less and are more likely to fall over the handlebars (Kronisch et al., 1996). There is no discussion specifically of concussions, however.

Kyle and colleagues (2002) used NEISS-AIP ED injury data and participation data from the National Sporting Goods Association annual survey to calculate the rate of injuries seen in EDs for several sports. The rate of skateboard injuries seen in the ED (8.9 per 1,000 participants) was lower than that for snowboarding and bicycling (11.2 and 11.5 per 1,000 participants) and much lower than that for football and basketball (20.7 and 21.2 per 1,000 participants).

Military Personnel and Dependents

The committee was specifically asked to examine sports-related concussions among military dependents as well as concussions in military personnel ages 18 to 21 resulting from sports and physical training at military service academies and during recruit training. There are limited data available pertaining to this type of injury among the populations specified. With respect to the dependents of military personnel, there is no evidence about whether the risks for concussion are different for these youth than for youth in general, although there is no reason to think that they would be (Goldman, 2013; Tsao, 2013).

Among the U.S. military personnel worldwide (including the continental United States), approximately 26,000 concussions or mTBIs were diagnosed in 2012, representing about 85 percent of all TBIs in that population (DVBIC, 2013). Although TBI has become the signature injury of the wars in Iraq and Afghanistan, more than 80 percent of TBIs in the military do not occur in the deployed setting (DVBIC, 2013). These TBIs most commonly occur from motor vehicle crashes (privately owned and military vehicles), falls, sports and recreation activities, and military training (DVBIC, 2013).

Service academy students and the majority of military recruits fall within the age range specified by the committee. In fiscal year 2010, approximately 85 percent of active military recruits were between 18 and 24 years of age (DoD, 2012b). Although there is no reason to suspect that military personnel ages 18 to 21 who play intramural or service academy sports have different concussion risks than nonmilitary athletes of the same age participating in the same activities do, military service academies, such as West Point, require physical training activities, such as combatives and ropes courses, and offer other activities, such as boxing, that are not generally available at other collegiate institutions and that pose a high risk of concussion (Kelly, 2013; Wolfe, 2013). In an effort to reduce the number of concussions among cadets, West Point has substituted flag football for intramural football and eliminated intramural rugby altogether (Wolfe, 2013). Outside of the academies, there are anecdotal reports that many military personnel sustain concussions during hand-to-hand (combatives) courses during basic training (Sapien and Zwerdling, 2012), but data on the occurrence of concussions during such training have not been published in the peer-reviewed literature.

Overview of Outcomes and Reintegration

Eighty to 90 percent of individuals who sustain sports-related concussions fully recover within 2 weeks following injury (Covassin et al., 2010;

Eisenberg et al., 2013; Field et al., 2003; Makdissi et al., 2013; McClincy et al., 2006; McCrea et al., 2009, 2013), although high school athletes (14 to 18 years of age) seem to recover more slowly than do college-age athletes and those 11 to 13 years of age (Covassin et al., 2010; Eisenberg et al., 2013; Field et al., 2003). The other 10 to 20 percent have more protracted recovery periods, lasting weeks, months, or longer, as discussed in Chapter 4. Consensus has emerged that individuals suspected of having sustained a concussion should be immediately removed from the activity in which they are engaged and should not return to physical activity until they have been cleared by a health care provider knowledgeable about concussion diagnosis and management (Giza et al., 2013; Halstead et al., 2010; Harmon et al., 2013; McCrory et al., 2013a).

Athletes who return to play before their concussions have fully resolved may place themselves at an increased risk for prolonged recovery (Eisenberg et al., 2013) or more serious consequences if they sustain a second head injury (Cantu, 1998; Cantu and Voy, 1995; Collins et al., 2002; McCrory and Berkovic, 1998; Saunders and Harbaugh, 1984). Although very rare, the potential for catastrophic head injuries, including what has sometimes been called "second impact syndrome," is the primary concern. While catastrophic head injury is uncommon, it may occur more frequently in younger athletes between the ages of 12 to 18 years (Boden et al., 2007, 2013; Cantu, 1998; Cantu and Voy, 1995; McCrory and Berkovic, 1998; Saunders and Harbaugh, 1984; Thomas et al., 2011). Due to development of the brain, adolescence has been suggested to be a time of increased risk of adverse consequences following concussion (Field et al., 2003).

Among youth, the primary focus of reintegration after a concussion often is a return to school, although reintegration also can encompass a return to work or, for members of the armed services, a return to duty. Because concussion symptoms may resolve before full cognitive recovery, students who are recovering from a concussion may require short-term accommodations upon returning to school. As discussed in Chapter 3, a number of states have developed plans or recommended resources for helping students return to academic activity.

Consensus guidelines for the return of athletes to athletic activity recommend a graded return-to-play protocol. Once an individual is symptom-free, the individual moves through a series of increasingly rigorous sport-specific activities, progression through which is governed in part by recurrence of symptoms (Halstead et al., 2010; McCrory et al., 2013a).

From the committee's research, the public testimony it heard, and its collective expertise, the role of "culture" in the recognition and management of concussions in young athletes became apparent. Culture is created by the sum of beliefs and behaviors within a group. It is clear that currently the seriousness of the threat to the health of an athlete suffering a concussion is too often not fully appreciated by athletes, their teammates, and, in some cases, coaches and parents (see, e.g., Anderson et al., 2013; Coyne, 2013; Echlin, 2012; Kroshus et al., 2013; McCrea et al., 2004; Register-Mihalik, et al., 2013a,b; Torres et al., 2013; Wolverton, 2013). In addition, athletes profess that the game and the team are more important than their individual health and often believe that by admitting to having symptoms of a concussion, they will be "letting down" their teammates, coaches, schools, and even parents (Anderson et al., 2013; Kroshus et al., 2013). A culture that encourages "playing through" a potentially concussive injury or returning to play too soon following a concussion can endanger the physical and cognitive well-being of the young athlete. Perhaps because concussions are "invisible" they are easier to ignore than torn ligaments or broken bones are. But each of these types of injury requires the athlete to be removed from play, cared for appropriately in both the acute stage and during the healing process, and judiciously returned to play only when he or she is demonstrably recovered. Increased knowledge about concussions in the absence of changes in attitudes may not be enough to modify reporting behavior among athletes (Anderson et al., 2013; Coyne, 2013; Kroshus et al., 2013; Register-Mihalik et al., 2013a,b; Torres et al., 2013). If the youth sports community can adopt the belief that concussions are serious injuries and institute behaviors and adopt attitudes that emphasize care for players with concussions until they are fully recovered, then the "culture" in which young athletes perform and compete will become much safer.

Similarly, military recruits are immersed in military values and culture, including devotion to duty, commitment, and service before self, and the idea that "there is no greater bond than the one they share with the people 'to their left and their right'" (Halvorson, 2010), which may make them reluctant to self-report symptoms of concussion. The military has acknowledged the need for a culture change, as reflected in such efforts as teaming up with the National Football League to increase awareness about TBI and to effect a culture change in which military personnel and athletes are willing to seek help (and not be stigmatized) if they experience concussive symptoms (AP, 2012; Vergun, 2012).

The Policy Environment

In light of the potential for returning to play too soon having catastrophic results, lawmakers in the United States have passed legislation designed to address the need for concussion education for young athletes and their parents, particularly at the high school level, along with procedures to protect athletes from returning to play before it is deemed appropriate by health care providers. As of October 2013, 49 states and the District of Columbia had enacted concussion laws of some sort; legislation was introduced in Mississippi, but it did not pass (NCSL, 2013; Network for Public Health Law, 2013; Sun, 2013). In May 2009, Washington became the first state to enact legislation designed to protect student athletes suspected of having sustained a concussion. Named after Zackery Lystedt, a 13-year-old football player who was permanently disabled when he returned to a game after having sustained a concussion, Washington's law specifies several principles that have come to be viewed as the three tenets of model concussion legislation:

(1) education of coaches, parents, and athletes about the nature and risk of concussions in sports and a requirement that parents sign a form acknowledging receipt of the information;

(2) immediate removal from play of any youth athlete suspected of having sustained a concussion or head injury; and

(3) a requirement that an athlete who has been removed from play be evaluated by and receive written clearance from a health care professional trained in the evaluation and management of concussion before returning to play.

Although legislation in most of the states that have concussion laws includes some version of the three tenets in the Washington law, there is significant variation among states regarding specific requirements (NCSL, 2013; Network for Public Health Law, 2013).

Since 2009, there have been several federal legislative efforts directed at various aspects of sports-related concussions in youth. Legislation introduced in the House of Representatives—the Concussion Treatment and Care Tools (ConTACT) Act of 2009, later renamed the ConTACT Act of 2010 (H.R. 1347)—called on the Secretary of Health and Human Services to establish guidelines for "the prevention, identification, treatment, and management of concussions" in children 5 to 18 years of age, including return-to-play standards (H.R. 1347). In addition, the bill called for funding for states to collect data on the incidence and prevalence of sports-related concussion among school-aged children, to adopt and implement the aforementioned guidelines, and to implement pre-season baseline and post-injury testing for school-aged children (H.R. 1347). The bill eventually passed the House and was referred to the Senate (S. 2840), where it stalled in committee.

The Protecting Student Athletes from Concussions Act, originally introduced in the House in 2010 (H.R. 6172) and reintroduced in 2011 (H.R. 469), was directed toward state and local educational agencies and was, in part, designed to bring some uniformity to the proliferation of state "Lystedt laws." The bill, which never moved out of committee, would have required as a condition of federal funding the development and implemen-

tation of a concussion safety and management plan that would include a
concussion education component for students, parents, and school personnel; supports for students during recovery from concussion; and best
practices to ensure uniformity in safety standards treatment, and management (H.R. 6172). Other elements of the bill called on school personnel
to remove any student suspected of having sustained a concussion from
the activity in which it occurred and to prohibit participation in athletic
activities until the student was cleared by a health care provider, including
recognition that the provider might specify a gradual, progressive return to
cognitive and physical activity.

The Children's Sports Athletic Equipment Act, jointly introduced in the
House and Senate in 2011 (H.R. 1127; S. 601), was directed to the Consumer Product Safety Commission (CPSC) and addressed issues pertaining
to the development of and compliance with standards for "youth football
helmets, reconditioned helmets, and new helmet concussion resistance."
The 2011 bills died in committee, but similar legislation, the Youth Sports
Concussion Act of 2013, was introduced in the House and Senate in May
2013 (H.R. 2118; S. 1014). The current legislation, which is in committee, is directed to the CPSC and addresses safety standards for protective
equipment to reduce the risk of sports-related injury, to improve the safety
of reconditioned protective equipment, and to modify warning labels on
protective equipment. The legislation also addresses the issue of false or
misleading claims in the marketing of protective equipment.

In February 2013, a resolution was introduced in the House (H.R. 72)
supporting the goals and ideals of the Secondary School Student Athletes'
Bill of Rights (YSSA, 2013), which highlights the importance of proper
safety measures and trained personnel, timely medical assessments, and
appropriate environmental conditions in ensuring the health and well-being
of secondary school student athletes.

State legislative efforts are addressed in more detail in Chapter 6.

REPORT ORGANIZATION

Chapter 2 gives an overview of normal brain development, which provides the basis for understanding the pathophysiology and natural history
of concussion. In addition the chapter discusses the mechanics of concussive injury, physical and biological thresholds for injury, and physical and
behavioral risk and protective factors. Chapter 3 reviews considerations
pertaining to the recognition, diagnosis, and acute management of concussions, including the reintegration of concussed individuals into academic
and athletic activities. Chapter 4 discusses the treatment and management
of individuals with concussion symptoms that persist beyond the typical
1- to 2-week recovery period. The chapter also includes a discussion of

special considerations that arise in the provision of concussion care, such as geographic variation in access to specialized care. Chapter 5 examines the issues surrounding repetitive head impacts that do not produce signs and symptoms of a concussion, as well as multiple concussions. Topics include short- and long-term outcomes, risk factors, neuropathology, and neuroimaging findings. Chapter 6 addresses interventions that may reduce the risk of sports-related concussions and includes discussions of the effectiveness of equipment such as helmets, mouthguards, and other devices; alternative playing surfaces; sport-specific rules and regulations; and legislation directed toward concussion education and athlete protection through policies governing athletes' removal from and return to play following a suspected concussion. Chapter 7 contains the committee's conclusions and recommendations.

FINDINGS

The committee offers the following findings:

- The published literature includes numerous working definitions of concussion and inconsistent use of terminology (e.g., concussion, mTBI [despite the latter including more severe brain injury]), which pose challenges for interpreting and comparing findings across research studies on concussion.
- Concussion rates tend to be higher during competition than in practice (except for cheerleading), higher among female athletes than male athletes in comparable sports, and higher in certain sports.
- The National Collegiate Athletic Association Injury Surveillance System and High School RIO™ (Reporting Information Online) data systems are the only ongoing, comprehensive sources of sports-related injury data, including data on concussions, in youth athletes. Equivalent data are not available for athletes younger than high school age, nor are they available for participants in club sports or for youth engaging in competitive and recreational sports outside of an academic setting. There is no comprehensive system (individually or collectively) for acquiring accurate data on the incidence of sports- and recreation-related concussion across all youth age groups and sports.
- Data captured on sports- and recreation-related concussions do not routinely include race and ethnicity.
- There are no published data on the incidence of reported concussions during basic training for military recruits.

- Despite increased knowledge and a growing recognition in recent years that concussions involve some level of injury to the brain and therefore need to be diagnosed promptly and managed appropriately, there is still a culture among athletes and military personnel that resists the self-reporting of concussions and compliance with appropriate concussion management plans.

REFERENCES

Agel, J., and E. J. Harvey. 2010. A 7-year review of men's and women's ice hockey injuries in the NCAA. *Canadian Journal of Surgery* 53(5):319-323.

Anderson, B. L., W. J. Pomerantz, J. K. Mann, and M. A. Gittelman. 2013. "I Can't Miss the Big Game": High School (HS) Football Players' Knowledge and Attitudes about Concussions. Presented at the Pediatric Academic Societies Annual Meeting, Washington, DC, May 6.

AP (Associated Press). 2012. NFL, Army starts concussion program. http://espn.go.com/nfl/story/_/id/8318684/nfl-teams-us-army-concussion-program (accessed August 5, 2013).

Aubry, M., R. Cantu, J. Dvořák, T. Graf-Baumann, K. Johnston, J. Kelly, M. Lovell, P. McCrory, W. Meeuwisse, and P. Schamasch. 2002. Summary and agreement statement of the first International Conference on Concussion in Sport, Vienna 2001. *British Journal of Sports Medicine* 36(1):6-10.

Bakhos, L. L., G. R. Lockhart, R. Myers, and J. G. Linakis. 2010. Emergency department visits for concussion in young child athletes. *Pediatrics* 126(3):e550-e556.

Bazarian, J. J., P. Veazie, S. Mookerjee, and E. B. Lerner. 2006. Accuracy of mild traumatic brain injury case ascertainment using ICD-9 codes. *Academic Emergency Medicine* 13(1):31-38.

Becker, J., A. Runer, D. Neunhäuserer, N. Frick, H. Resch, and P. Moroder. 2013. A prospective study of downhill mountain biking injuries. *British Journal of Sports Medicine* 47(7):458-462.

BIAA (Brain Injury Association of America). 2011. BIAA adopts new TBI definition (February 6, 2011). http://www.biausa.org/announcements/biaa-adopts-new-tbi-definition (accessed March 28, 2013).

Boden, B. P., R. L. Tacchetti, R. C. Cantu, S. B. Knowles, and F. O. Mueller. 2007. Catastrophic head injuries in high school and college football players. *American Journal of Sports Medicine* 35(7):1075-1081.

Boden, B. P., I. Breit, J. A. Beachler, A. Williams, and F. O. Mueller. 2013. Fatalities in high school and college football players. *American Journal of Sports Medicine* 41(5): 1108-1116.

Cantu, R. C. 1998. Second-impact syndrome. *Clinics in Sports Medicine* 17(1):37-44.

Cantu, R. C., and R. Voy. 1995. Second impact syndrome a risk in any contact sport. *Physician and Sportsmedicine* 23(6):27-34.

CDC (Centers for Disease Control and Prevention). 2009. Heads up: Facts for physicians about mild traumatic brain injury (mTBI). http://www.cdc.gov/concussion/headsup/pdf/facts_for_physicians_booklet-a.pdf (accessed April 3, 2013).

CDC. 2012. Concussion and mild TBI. http://www.cdc.gov/concussion/index.html (accessed March 28, 2013).

CDC. 2013a. Concussion in sports. http://www.cdc.gov/concussion/sports/index.html (accessed March 28, 2013).

CDC. 2013b. Data Sources for WISQARS™ Nonfatal. http://www.cdc.gov/ncipc/wisqars/nonfatal/datasources.htm#5.2 (accessed September 19, 2013).

CDC. 2013c. Heads up: Concussion in youth sports. http://www.cdc.gov/concussion/HeadsUp/youth.html (accessed July 2, 2013).

CDC. 2013d. National Health Interview Survey. http://www.cdc.gov/nchs/nhis/about_nhis.htm (accessed August 29, 2013).

Center for Injury Research and Policy. 2013. High School RIO™. http://www.nationwidechildrens.org/cirp-high-school-rio (accessed May 3, 2013).

Collins, M. W., M. R. Lovell, G. L. Iverson, R. C. Cantu, J. C. Maroon, and M. Field. 2002. Cumulative effects of concussion in high school athletes. *Neurosurgery* 51(5):1175-1181.

Collins, M. W., G. L. Iverson, M. R. Lovell, D. B. McKeag, J. Norwig, and J. Maroon. 2003. On-field predictors of neuropsychological and symptom deficit following sports-related concussion. *Clinical Journal of Sports Medicine* 13(4):222-229.

Congress of Neurological Surgeons. 1966. Committee on head injury nomenclature: Glossary of head injury. *Clinical Neurosurgery* 12:386-394.

Covassin, T., C. Swanik, and M. Sachs. 2003. Sex differences and the incidence of concussions among collegiate athletes. *Journal of Athletic Training* 38(3):238-244.

Covassin, T., R. Elbin, and Y. Nakayama. 2010. Examination of recovery time from sport-related concussion in high school athletes. *Physician and Sportsmedicine* 4(38):1-6.

Coyne, C. 2103. *Experiencing Concussion in Youth Sports: An Athlete's Perspective.* Presentation before the committee, Seattle, WA, April 15.

CPSC (U.S. Consumer Product Safety Commission). 2013a. National Electronic Injury Surveillance System (NEISS). CPSC document #3002. http://www.cpsc.gov/en/Safety-Education/Safety-Guides/General-Information/National-Electronic-Injury-Surveillance-System-NEISS (accessed May 3, 2013).

CPSC. 2013b. *NEISS Coding Manual.* http://www.cpsc.gov/PageFiles/106513/completemanual.pdf (accessed June 4, 2013).

CPSC. 2013c. NEISS injury data: National Electronic Injury Surveillance System (NIESS). http://www.cpsc.gov/Research--Statistics/NEISS-Injury-Data (accessed May 3, 2013).

Daneshvar, D. H., C. J. Nowinski, A. C. McKee, and R. C. Cantu. 2011. The epidemiology of sport-related concussion. *Clinical Journal of Sports Medicine* 30(1):1-17. DOI:10.1016/j.csm.2010.08.006.

Datalys Center (Datalys Center for Sports Injury Research and Prevention, Inc.). 2013a. NATA NATION Preliminary Concussion Rates, 2010-2012. Institute of Medicine-National Research Council request. October 3.

Datalys Center. 2013b. NCAA Concussion Rates, 2004-2009 and 2009-2013. Institute of Medicine-National Research Council request. September 23.

Dick, R. W. 2009. Is there a gender difference in concussion incidence and outcomes? *British Journal of Sports Medicine* 43(Suppl I):i46-i50.

Dick, R., J. Agel, and S. W. Marshall. 2007. National Collegiate Athletic Association Injury Surveillance System commentaries: Introduction and methods. *Journal of Athletic Training* 42(2):173-182.

DoD (Department of Defense). 2012a. Instruction Number 6490.11. DoD Policy Guidance for Management of Mild Traumatic Brain Injury/Concussion in the Deployed Setting (September 18). http://www.usaisr.amedd.army.mil/assets/cpgs/DODI_6490.11_Policy_Guidance_for_Mgmt_of_Mild_Traumatic_Brain_Injury_or_Concussion_in_the_Deployed_Setting.pdf (accessed April 9, 2013).

DoD. 2012b. *Population Representation in the Military Services: Fiscal Year 2010 Summary Report.* http://prhome.defense.gov/rfm/MPP/ACCESSION%20POLICY/PopRep2010/summary/PopRep10summ.pdf (accessed August 29, 2013).

DVBIC (Defense and Veterans Brain Injury Center). 2013. DoD worldwide numbers for TBI. http://www.dvbic.org/dod-worldwide-numbers-tbi (accessed June 27, 2013).

Echlin, P. S. 2012. Editorial: A prospective study of physician-observed concussion during a varsity university ice hockey season. Part 1 of 4. *Neurosurgical Focus* 33(6):E1:1-7.

Eisenberg, M. A., J. Andrea, W. Meehan, and R. Mannix. 2013. Time interval between concussions and symptom duration. Pediatrics. DOI: 10.1542/peds.2013-0432, originally published online June 10, 2013. http://pediatrics.aappublications.org/content/early/2013/06/05/peds.2013-0432 (accessed July 18, 2013).

Extreme Sport. 2008. Extreme sport growing in popularity. http://xtremesport4u.com/extreme-land-sports/extreme-sport-growing-in-popularity (accessed June 7, 2013).

Field, M., M. W. Collins, M. R. Lovell, and J. Maroon. 2003. Does age play a role in recovery from sports-related concussion? A comparison of high school and collegiate athletes. *Journal of Pediatrics* 142(5):546-553.

GAO (U.S. Government Accountability Office). 2009. *Consumer Product Safety Commission: Better Data Collection and Assessment of Consumer Information Efforts Could Help Protect Minority Children.* Report number GAO-09-731. Washington, DC: Government Printing Office.

Gessel, L. M., S. K. Fields, C. L. Collins, R. W. Dick, and R. D. Comstock. 2007. Concussions among United States high school and collegiate athletes. *Journal of Athletic Training* 42:495-503.

Gilchrist, J., K. E. Thomas, L. Xu, L. C. McGuire, and V. Coronado. 2011. Nonfatal traumatic brain injuries related to sports and recreation activities among persons ≤19 years—United States, 2001–2009. *Morbidity and Mortality Weekly Report* 60(39):1337-1342.

Giza, C. C., J. S. Kutcher, S. Ashwal, J. Barth, T. S. D. Getchius, G. A. Gioia, G. S. Gronseth, K. Guskiewicz, S. Mandel, G. Manley, D. B. McKeag, D. J. Thurman, and R. Zafonte. 2013. *Evidence-Based Guideline Update: Evaluation and Management of Concussion in Sports.* Report of the Guideline Development Subcommittee of the American Academy of Neurology. American Academy of Neurology.

Goldman, S. B. 2013. Army TBI Program Overview. Presentation before the committee, Washington, DC, February 25.

Halstead, M. E., K. D. Walter, and American Academy of Pediatrics, Council on Sports Medicine and Fitness. 2010. Sport-related concussion in children and adolescents. *Pediatrics* 126(3):597-615.

Halvorson, A. 2010. *Understanding the Military: The Institution, the Culture, and the People.* http://partnersforrecovery.samhsa.gov/docs/military_white_paper_final.pdf (accessed August 29, 2013).

Harmon, K. G., J. A. Drezner, M. Gammons, K. M. Guskiewicz, M. Halstead, S. A. Herring, J. S. Kutcher, A. Pana, M. Putakian, and W. O. Roberts. 2013. American Medical Society of Sports Medicine position statement: Concussion in sport. *British Journal of Sports Medicine* 47(1):15-26.

Hicks, R., J. Giacino, C. Harrison-Felix, G. Manley, A. Valadka, and E. A. Wilde. 2013. Progress in developing common data elements for traumatic brain injury research: Version two—the end of the beginning. *Journal of Neurotrauma.* September 9, doi:10.1089/neu.2013.2938.

Hinton, R. Y. 2012. Sports injury surveillance systems. *Sports Medicine Update* January/February:2-7.

Hootman, J., R. Dick, and J. Agel. 2007. Epidemiology of collegiate injuries for 15 sports: Summary and recommendations for injury prevention initiatives. *Journal of Athletic Training* 42(2):311-319.

IOM (Institute of Medicine). 2002. *Is Soccer Bad for Children's Heads?: Summary of the IOM Workshop on Neuropsychological Consequences of Head Impact in Youth Soccer.* Washington, DC: National Academy Press.

IOM. 2008. *Gulf War and Health: Volume 7: Long-Term Consequences of Traumatic Brain Injury.* Washington, DC: The National Academies Press.

IOM. 2011. *Cognitive Rehabilitation Therapy for Traumatic Brain Injury: Evaluating the Evidence.* Washington, DC: The National Academies Press.

IOM and NRC (National Research Council). 2000. *From Neurons to Neighborhoods: The Science of Early Childhood Development.* Washington, DC: National Academy Press.

IOM and NRC. 2001. *Early Childhood Development and Learning: New Knowledge for Policy.* Washington, DC: National Academy Press.

Kelly, T. 2013. *Sports and Physical Training-Related Concussion in Military Personnel.* Presentation before the committee, Washington, DC, February 25.

Knowles, S. B., K. L. Kucera, and S. W. Marshall. 2010. The injury proportion ratio: What's it all about? *Journal of Athletic Training* 45(5):475-477.

Kontos, A. P., R. J. Elbin, V. C. Fazzio-Sumrock, S. Burkhart, H. Swindell, J. Maroon, and M. W. Collins. 2013. Incidence of sports-related concussion among youth football players aged 8-12 years. *Journal of Pediatrics* 163(3):717-720.

Kronisch, R. L., R. P. Pfeiffer, and T. K. Chow. 1996. Acute injuries in cross country and downhill road cycle racing. *Medicine and Science in Sports and Exercise* 28(11):1351-1355.

Kroshus, E., D. H. Daneshvar, C. M. Baugh, C. J. Nowinski, and R. C. Cantu. 2013. NCAA concussion education in ice hockey: An ineffective mandate. *British Journal of Sports Medicine*, in press. doi: 10.1136/bjsports-2013-092498.

Kyle, S. B., M. L. Nance, G. W. Rutherford, Jr., and F. K. Winston. 2002. Skateboard-associated injuries: Participation-based estimates and injury characteristics. *Journal of Trauma-Injury Infection and Critical Care* 53(4):686-690.

Langlois, J., W. Rutland-Brown, and M. Wald. 2006. The epidemiology and impact of traumatic brain injury: A brief overview. *Journal of Head Trauma Rehabilitation* 21(5):375-378.

Lincoln, A., S. Caswell, J. Almquist, R. Dunn, J. Norris, and R. Hinton. 2011. Trends in concussion incidence in high school sports: A prospective 11-year study. *American Journal of Sports Medicine* 39(5):958-963.

Makdissi, M., R. C. Cantu, K. M. Johnston, P. McCrory, and W. H. Meeuwisse. 2013. The difficult concussion patient: What is the best approach to investigation and management of persistent (>10 days) postconcussive symptoms? *British Journal of Sports Medicine* 47(5):308-313.

Marar, M., N. McIlvain, S. Fields, and R. Comstock. 2012. Epidemiology of concussions among United States high school athletes in 20 sports. *American Journal of Sports Medicine* 40(4):747-755.

McClincy, M. P., M. R. Lovell, J. Pardini, M. W. Collins, and M. K. Spore. 2006. Recovery from sports concussion in high school and collegiate athletes. *Brain Injury* 20(1):33-39.

McCrea, M., T. Hammeke, G. Olsen, P. Leo, and K. M. Guskiewicz. 2004. Unreported concussion in high school football players: Implications for prevention. *Clinical Journal of Sports Medicine* 14(1):13-17.

McCrea, M., K. Guskiewicz, C. Randolph, W. B. Barr, T. A. Hammeke, S. W. Marshall, and J. P. Kelly. 2009. Effects of a symptom-free waiting period on clinical outcome and risk of reinjury after sport-related concussion. *Neurosurgery* 65(5):876-882; discussion 876-882.

McCrea, M., K. Guskiewicz, C. Randolph, W. B. Barr, T. A. Hammeke, S. W. Marshall, M. R. Powell, K. Woo Ahn, Y. Wang, and J. P. Kelly. 2013. Incidence, clinical course, and predictors of prolonged recovery time following sport-related concussion in high school and college athletes. *Journal of the Inernational Neuropsychological Society* 19(1):22-33.

McCrory, P. R., and S. F. Berkovic. 1998. Second impact syndrome. *Neurology* 50(3):677-683.

McCrory, P., K. Johnston, W. Meeuwisse, M. Aubry, R. Cantu, J. Dvořák, T. Graf-Baumann, J. Kelly, M. Lovell, and P. Schamasch. 2005. Summary and agreement statement of the 2nd International Conference on Concussion in Sport, Prague 2004. *British Journal of Sports Medicine* 39(Suppl I):i78-i86.

McCrory, P., W. Meeuwisse, K. Johnston, J. Dvořák, M. Aubry, M. Molloy, and R. Cantu. 2009. Consensus statement on concussion in sport: The 3rd International Conference on Concussion in Sport held in Zurich, November 2008. *British Journal of Sports Medicine* 43(Suppl 1):i76-i84.

McCrory, P., W. H. Meeuwisse, M. Aubry, B. Cantu, J. Dvořák, R. J. Echemendia, L. Engebretsen, K. Johnston, J. S. Kutcher, M. Raftery, A. Sills, B. W. Benson, G. A. Davis, R. G. Ellenbogen, K. Guskiewicz, S. A. Herring, G. L. Iverson, B. D. Jordan, J. Kissick, M. McCrea, A. S. McIntosh, D. Maddocks, M. Makdissi, L. Purcell, M. Putukian, K. Schneider, C. H. Tator, and M. Turner. 2013a. Consensus statement on concussion in sport: The 4th International Conference on Concussion in Sport held in Zurich, November 2012. *British Journal of Sports Medicine* 47(5):250-258.

McCrory, P., W. H. Meeuwisse, R. J. Echemendia, G. L. Iverson, J. Dvořák, and J. S. Kutcher. 2013b. What is the lowest threshold to make a diagnosis of concussion? *British Journal of Sports Medicine* 47(5):268-271.

Meehan, W. P., III, and R. Mannix. 2010. Pediatric concussions in United States emergency departments in the years 2002 to 2006. *Journal of Pediatrics* 157(6):889-893.

Menon, D. K., K. Schwab, D. W. Wright, and A. I. Maas, on behalf of The Demographics and Clinical Assessment Working Group of the International and Interagency Initiative toward Common Data Elements for Research on Traumatic Brain Injury and Psychological Health. 2010. Position statement: Definition of traumatic brain injury. *Archives of Physical Medicine and Rehabilitation* 91(11):1637-1640.

Middle School RIO™. 2013. http://www.nationwidechildrens.org/cirp-middle-school-rio (accessed June 28, 2013).

Mulligan, G. M., S. Hastedt, and J. C. McCarroll. 2012. *First-Time Kindergartners in 2010-11: First Findings From the Kindergarten Rounds of the Early Childhood Longitudinal Study, Kindergarten Class of 2010-11 (ECLS-K:2011).* NCES 2012-049.

NAE (National Academy of Engineering) and IOM. 2009. *Systems Engineering to Improve Traumatic Brain Injury Care in the Military Health System Workshop Summary.* Washington, DC: The National Academies Press.

NCAA (National Collegiate Athletic Association, Sports Sciences Institute). 2013. Concussion resources. http://www.ncaa.org/wps/wcm/connect/public/NCAA/SSI/Resources/concussion+resources/Partnership+strives+to+reduce+concussions+in+youth+football (accessed September 18, 2013).

NCSL (National Conference of State Legislatures). 2013. Traumatic brain injury legislation. http://www.ncsl.org/issues-research/health/traumatic-brain-injury-legislation.aspx (accessed October 4, 2013).

Network for Public Health Law. 2013. Summary matrix of state laws addressing concussions in youth sports (December 31, 2012). http://www.networkforphl.org/_asset/7xwh09/StateLawsTableConcussions_2-19-13.pdf (accessed October 4, 2013).

NFHS (National Federation of State High School Associations). 2013. Concussion in sports: What you need to know. http://www.nfhslearn.com/electiveDetail.aspx?courseID=38000 (accessed September 18, 2013).

NIH (National Institutes of Health). 2013. FITBIR informatics system. https://fitbir.nih.gov (accessed September 12, 2013).

NINDS (National Institute of Neurological Disorders and Stroke). 2013. NINDS common data elements: Traumatic brain injury, data standards. http://www.commondataelements. ninds.nih.gov/tbi.aspx#tab=Data_Standards (accessed September 12, 2013).

NRC. 1999. *How People Learn: Brain, Mind, Experience, and School*. Washington, DC: National Academy Press.

Pennington, B. 2013. Flubbing a baseline test on purpose is often futile. *New York Times* (May 6):D7. http://www.nytimes.com/2013/05/06/sports/sandbagging-first-concussion-test-probably-wont-help-later.html?_r=0 (accessed July 17, 2013).

PIPER Program (Pediatric Injury Prevention, Education and Research Program). 2013a. High School RIO™: Reporting Information Online. http://www.ucdenver.edu/academics/ colleges/PublicHealth/research/ResearchProjects/piper/projects/RIO/Pages/default.aspx (accessed October 4, 2013).

PIPER Program. 2013b. High School RIO™ study reports. http://www.ucdenver.edu/ academics/colleges/PublicHealth/research/ResearchProjects/piper/projects/RIO/Pages/ Study-Reports.aspx (accessed October 4, 2013).

Pop Warner Little Scholars. 2012. *2012 Pop Warner Rule Book*. Langhorne, PA: Pop Warner Little Scholars, Inc.

Powell, J. M., J. V. Ferraro, S. S. Dikmen, N. R. Temkin, and K. R. Bell. 2008. Accuracy of mild traumatic brain injury diagnosis. *Archives of Physical Medicine and Rehabilitation* 89(8):1550-1555.

Purcell, L., C. LeBlanc, M. McTimoney, J. Philpott, and M. Zetaruk. 2005. Sport readiness in children and youth. *Paediatrics and Child Health* 10(6):343-344.

Register-Mihalik, J. K., K. M. Guskiewicz, T. C. Valovich McLeod, L. A. Linnan, F. O. Mueller, and S. W. Marshall. 2013a. Knowledge, attitude, and concussion-reporting behaviors among high school athletes: A preliminary study. *Journal of Athletic Training* 48(5):645-653.

Register-Mihalik, J. K., L. A. Linnan, S. W. Marshall, T. C. Valovich McLeod, F. O. Mueller, and K. M. Guskiewicz. 2013b. Using theory to understand high school aged athletes' intentions to report sport-related concussion: Implications for concussion education initiatives. *Brain Injury* 27(7-8):878-886.

Sapien, J., and D. Zwerdling. 2012. Army study finds troops suffer concussions in training. http://www.propublica.org/article/army-study-finds-troops-suffer-concussions-in-training#comments (accessed June 7, 2013).

Saunders, R. L., and R. E. Harbaugh. 1984. Second impact in catastrophic contact-sports head trauma. *JAMA* 252(4):538-539.

Schultz, M. R., S. W. Marshall, F. O. Mueller, J. Yang, N. L. Weaver, W. D. Kalsbeek, and J. M. Bowling. 2004. Incidence and risk factors for concussion in high school athletes, North Carolina, 1996–1999. *American Journal of Epidemiology* 160(10):937-944.

Sun, J. F. 2013. See where your state stands on concussion law. http://usafootball.com/news/ featured-articles/see-where-your-state-stands-concussion-law (accessed October 4, 2013).

Thomas, M., T. S. Haas, J. J. Doerer, J. S. Hodges, B. O. Aicher, R. F. Garberich, F. O. Mueller, R. C. Cantu, and B. J. Maron. 2011. Epidemiology of sudden death in young, competitive athletes due to blunt trauma. *Pediatrics* 128(1):e1-e8.

Thurman, D. J., C. M. Branche, and J. E. Sniezek. 1998. The epidemiology of sports-related traumatic brain injuries in the United States: Recent developments. *Journal of Head Trauma Rehabilitation* 13(2):1-8.

Thurmond, V. A., R. Hicks, T. Gleason, A. C. Miller, N. Szuflita, J. Orman, and K. Schwab. 2010. Advancing integrated research in psychological health and traumatic brain injury: Common data elements. *Archives of Physical Medicine and Rehabilitation* 91(11): 1633-1636.

Torres, D. M., K. M. Galetta, H. W. Phillips, E. M. S. Dziemianowicz, J. A. Wilson, E. S. Dorman, E. Laudano, S. L. Galetta, and L. J. Balcer. 2013. Sports-related concussion: Anonymous survey of a collegiate cohort. *Neurology Clinical Practice* 3(4):279-287.

Tsao, J. W. 2013. *Navy and Marine Corps TBI Efforts.* Presentation before the committee, Washington, DC, February 25.

USA Football. 2013a. Concussion awareness. http://usafootball.com/health-safety/concussion-awareness (accessed September 18, 2013).

USA Football. 2013b. USA Football releases preliminary data in study examining youth football player health and safety. News Release, May 20. http://usafootball.com/health-safety/usa-football-releases-preliminary-date-study-examining-youth-football-player-health-an (accessed July 25, 2013).

USA Hockey. 2011. *2011-2013 Official Rules of Ice Hockey.* Colorado Springs, CO: USA Hockey, Inc.

USA Hockey. 2013. Concussion information. http://www.usahockey.com/page/show/908034-concussion-information (accessed September 18, 2013).

USSSA Baseball (U.S. Specialty Sports Association Baseball). 2013. *Official Baseball National By-Laws & Rules.* Kissimmee, FL: U.S. Specialty Sports Association.

Vergun, D. 2012. NFL, Army both work to combat traumatic brain injury. http://www.army.mil/article/86544 (accessed August 5, 2013).

Wilde, E. A., S. R. McCauley, G. Hanten, G. Avci, A. P. Ibarra, and H. S. Levin. 2012. History, diagnostic considerations, and controversies. In *Mild Traumatic Brain Injuries in Children and Adolescents: From Basic Science to Clinical Management,* edited by M. Kirkwood and K. O. Yeates. New York: Guilford Press. Pp. 3-21.

Wolfe, C. L. 2013. West Point health care providers focus on brain injury prevention, diagnosis, treatment. (March 28). http://www.army.mil/article/99664 (accessed July 25, 2013).

Wolverton, B. 2013. Coach makes the call. *Chronicle of Higher Education* (September 2). http://chronicle.com/article/Trainers-Butt-Heads-With/141333?cid=megamenu (accessed September 15, 2013).

YSSA (Youth Sports Safety Alliance). 2013. *Secondary School Student Athletes' Bill of Rights.* http://www.youthsportssafetyalliance.org/docs/Athletes-Bill-of-Rights.pdf (accessed August 5, 2013).

2

Neuroscience, Biomechanics, and Risks of Concussion in the Developing Brain

Over the past 30 years, a number of experimental models of traumatic brain injury (TBI) have been developed to study various aspects of TBI in humans. This area of research originally focused on adult animal models of moderate to severe brain injuries, and these models have significantly contributed to our understanding of the biomechanics and neurochemical changes that occur after TBI. More recently, research efforts have focused on animal models of mild TBI (mTBI) and concussions, but only a few studies have addressed age and sex differences in injuries of this severity. TBI of any severity in the developing brain is complicated by ongoing cerebral maturation. The goal of this chapter is to (1) summarize the normal changes that occur with brain maturation; (2) explain the biomechanics involved in generating brain injuries of a range of severities; (3) summarize what is known about the neurochemical and metabolic changes that occur after concussions; and (4) describe risk factors for concussions in youth. In the section on the biomechanics of concussion, the committee responds to the portion of its charge concerning physical and biological thresholds for concussive injury.

NORMAL BRAIN DEVELOPMENT

The human brain is a complex system of connections that continues to be refined and reshaped throughout an individual's lifespan. During development, rapid changes in synapses, myelination, and metabolism occur, with the brain achieving adult-like connections by the mid-20s (see Figure 2-1). The changes in both the structural architecture and the func-

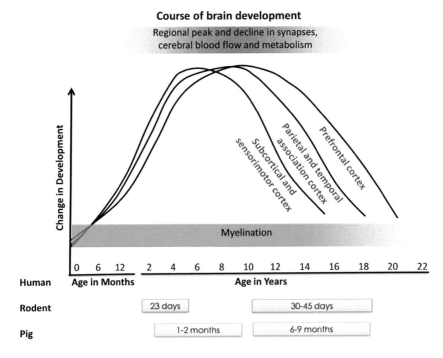

FIGURE 2-1 Profiles of parameters of human brain development and the estimated age ranges for research animal models. This figure illustrates the timing of changes in the number of brain synapses, cerebral blood flow, and metabolism (blue) and in brain myelination (green). The colored bars below the figure reflect the approximated human age equivalent of the rat (blue) and pig (green) based on species specific developmental profiles.
SOURCE: Adapted from Casey et al., 2005.

tional organization of the brain reflect a dynamic interplay of progressive and regressive events that occur simultaneously as the developing individual interacts with the environment. Although total brain size is about 90 percent of adult size by age 6 years, the brain continues to undergo dynamic changes throughout adolescence and into young adulthood (Yakovlev and Lecours, 1967). Current neuroimaging methods do not have the resolution to delineate the processes that underlie the observed developmental changes beyond observations of the brain's gray and white matter subcomponents. The techniques do, however, allow for assessment of functional sequelae of concussions and, together with animal models, suggest that the developing brain responds differently to concussion than does the mature brain (Choe et al., 2012; Shrey et al., 2011).

Synaptic Density

Brain cells communicate with each other through synapses, which are dynamic points of contact between cells where chemicals called neurotransmitters are transferred. During brain development there are dramatic changes in the number of synapses in the brain, with different regions of the brain developing at different rates and times (Bourgeois et al., 1994; Huttenlocher and Dabholkar, 1997). There is a dramatic increase in the number of synapses during the first few years of life. This production of synapses is followed by a prolonged period of synaptic pruning that, based on an individual's experiences, eliminates weaker synaptic contacts while retaining and strengthening the stronger connections. This pruning process occurs earlier in the auditory and visual cortex (by approximately 12 years of age), than in areas of the prefrontal cortex, which plays a role in executive functions such as problem solving and decision making (by approximately 18 years of age) (Bourgeois et al., 1994; Huttenlocher and Dabholkar, 1997).

Gray and White Matter

Gray and white matter are two major components of the central nervous system (CNS), which includes the brain and the spinal cord. Gray matter is associated with processing and cognition, while white matter is involved in coordinating communication between different brain regions. Longitudinal studies using magnetic resonance imaging (MRI) to map the developmental time-course of structural changes in the normal brain indicate that increases in white matter are linear throughout childhood and adolescence and continue well into young adulthood. In contrast, the growth in gray matter volume shows an inverted U-shaped course, first increasing during the first few years of life and then decreasing during adolescence (Giedd, 2004; Giedd et al., 1999, 2012; Gogtay et al., 2004; Sowell et al., 2004). These changes do not occur uniformly throughout an individual's development. The primary sensorimotor regions mature during early adolescence, while parietal and prefrontal regions, which are important for attention and working memory, have a more protracted development, lasting into young adulthood (Gogtay et al., 2004; Sowell et al., 2004). In general, regions of cortical gray matter (parietal, frontal, and temporal) develop earlier in females than in males during adolescence (Giedd et al., 2012). Concussions and other head injuries can result in changes to the integrity of gray and white matter.

Cerebral Blood Flow and Glucose Metabolism

In parallel with the structural changes that occur with brain development, there are changes in cerebral glucose metabolism and cerebral blood flow (CBF), which refers to the blood supply to the brain. Normal CBF at birth is lower than the adult rate of 50ml/min/100g (Chiron et al., 1992). Blood flow rates increase rapidly during the first year of life and are 50 to 80 percent higher than flow rates in adults by the time a child is 5 to 6 years of age. CBF rates then decrease gradually during childhood and adolescence, reaching adult values when an individual is between 15 and 19 years of age. CBF varies with age and sex (Tontisirin et al., 2007; Udomphorn et al., 2008; Vavilala et al., 2005), with adolescents and adult females showing greater middle cerebral artery flow rates than male adults (Bakker et al., 2004; Vavilala et al., 2002a).

Given that cerebral substrate supply and utilization are linked, it is not surprising that the developmental profile of cerebral glucose uptake mirrors that of CBF in both animals and humans (Nehlig et al., 1989). Positron emission tomography (PET) has been used to image the regional changes in glucose uptake of the normal developing brain. This research shows that the overall cerebral metabolic rate of glucose consumption (CMRglc) at birth are 30 percent lower than they are for adults and that glucose uptake increases sharply after birth to peak at approximately 4 years of age (Chugani, 1998). CMRglc plateaus at 50-60 µmol/min/100g between 4 and 10 years, followed by a decline in glucose uptake until the uptake reaches adult rates by the age of 16 to 18 years.

Changes in CBF, cerebral metabolic rates for oxygen, and CMRglc mirror one another as they peak during early childhood and gradually decrease to adult levels (Udomphorn et al., 2008). CBF is coupled to glucose metabolism, partial pressure of carbon dioxide, partial pressure of oxygen, and blood viscosity (Len and Neary, 2011). Several studies have demonstrated that females from 4 to 8 years of age and between 10 and 16 years of age show greater middle cerebral artery and basilar artery blood flow velocities relative to males of the same age (Tontisirin et al., 2007; Vavilala et al., 2005). Compared with adults, youth ages 12 to 17 years show lower autoregulation of blood flow and higher blood flow velocities (Vavilala et al., 2002b). While evidence in the literature sufficiently demonstrates the existence of age and sex differences in the maturation of these couplings, it is also clear that much more research needs to be done to understand the extent and significance of these differences in regard to how they affect cerebral response to concussions and other brain injuries.

Behavioral Changes

Sleep patterns change dramatically during brain maturation. The average sleep duration for infants is 12.7 hours and for toddlers is 11.9 hours (Galland et al., 2012). Sleep duration is influenced by the start of school attendance, which begins around 5 or 6 years of age. The average sleep duration gradually decreases from approximately 10.5 hours during elementary school (5- to 10-year-olds) to about 9.3 hours during middle school (11- to 13-year-olds) (Iglowstein et al., 2003). During adolescence, biological sleep patterns shift toward later times for both sleeping and waking (Malone, 2011). Although the optimal sleep duration for adolescents is about 9 hours each night (Carskadon et al., 2004), the average high schooler (14- to 18-year-olds) gets between 6 and 8 hours of sleep each night, largely due to early school start times and wake-inducing activities (e.g., social and academic activities) that interfere with sleep. This reduction in sleep coincides with the period of adolescent cortical synaptic pruning. The possibility of interactive factors at work, with changes in sleep altering cognitive, linguistic, and emotional behaviors, should be considered when identifying sleep and cognitive impairments in youths following a concussion.

Adolescence is also a period of brain development that is marked by an increase in risk behaviors and addiction. The prefrontal cortex is important in executive decision making, the regulation of emotions, and the assessment of risk and reward (Bechara et al., 2000; Kelley et al., 2004; Romer, 2010; Spear, 2010). Protracted development of the prefrontal cortex may contribute to an increase in risk-taking behaviors in adolescence (Bava and Tapert, 2010; Casey and Jones, 2010; Dayan et al., 2010; Pharo et al., 2011). Such behaviors may include those that result in increased risk of injury. Compared with previous generations, today's youth, due to an earlier average age of puberty (Biro et al., 2010), may have a greater mismatch between the propensity to engage in risk taking (which arises with the onset of puberty) and behavioral inhibition (which is associated with development of the prefrontal cortex).

BIOMECHANICS OF CONCUSSION

The biomechanics of TBI (including concussions) is defined broadly as the interrelationships among the forces experienced during impact, head and neck movements, stiffness of the tissue that composes the head/neck complex, deformation of structures at the macroscopic and microscopic level, and the biological responses to the various loading conditions imposed on the head. The biological responses may be structural (torn vessels and axons) or functional (changes in blood flow or neurological status), and they may be immediate or delayed.

Understanding the biomechanics of sports-related concussions in youth requires knowledge about what head and neck movements and applied forces occur in an array of sporting environments, how the developing head and neck mechanical and biological properties change with age and gender, how mechanical responses change during development, and how tissue deformations or changes in physiology (e.g., CBF, metabolism) produced by these motions and forces may directly or indirectly cause a concussion. This information plays a pivotal role in understanding risk factors and designing practices and equipment to reduce the incidence of concussions in sports. The studies employed for biomechanics investigations typically include direct measurements of loading conditions and responses in humans, animals, and anthropomorphic surrogates (i.e., crash test dummies); visualization of tissue responses to prescribed loads in order to characterize the responses of complex geometries or composite structures; mechanical property testing of individual components in order to identify changes with age; computational models to predict how tissues will deform during impact or rapid head rotations; and identification of the time-course of cell or tissue responses to specified deformations in order to define thresholds associated with various types of injuries. Note that blast injuries are typically associated with exposure to extremely rapid pressure waves that cause rapid expansion and contraction of brain tissue as they pass through the brain; the biomechanics and characteristics of these types of brain injuries are distinct from most brain injuries that occur in sporting environments (Holbourn, 1945; Ommaya et al., 1971), and they will not be discussed further in this section. Non-blast-related impacts to the head that occur in the military setting may be governed by similar mechanics as those on the athletic field, however, and the concepts discussed in the following section are applicable.

Understanding the relationships between biomechanics and concussions in the developing brain is an essential step in creating protective devices to reduce the incidence of sports-related concussion and in developing rule changes aimed at reducing individuals' exposure to hazardous conditions. This section summarizes the range of experimental platforms used to study brain injury, what has been learned from these studies about how brain injuries occur, and the many gaps in our understanding of how concussions occur in a youth sports environment.

Overview of Common Experimental Platforms for Understanding the Biomechanics of Traumatic Brain Injury

Investigators can use human data obtained in the field during sporting events to help understand what scenarios cause concussion. Typically, a sensor affixed to a helmet or a mouthpiece is used to measure the magnitude, direction, and type (i.e., linear, rotational, centroidal, or non-centroidal) of head motion (see, for example, Camarillo et al., 2013; Crisco et al., 2010; Daniel et al., 2012; Rowson and Duma, 2013; Rowson et al., 2012). These sensors do not usually measure head impact forces directly (for an exception, see Ouckama and Pearsall, 2011), but rather they measure the head's movement (acceleration or velocity) in response to an impact. The mechanical data recorded by the sensors are correlated with clinical assessments of injuries sustained on the sport field. However, such human data are influenced by equipment design limitations. For example, some devices are unable to measure actual head movements because of slipping between head and sensor, some cannot measure linear motions independently from angular motions or only report motion in a single plane of motion or a composite, and some sensors have errors or measurement variability that exceed reasonable standards. The human data may also be limited by inaccuracies in self-reports of concussions and difficulties in adequately adjusting for varying histories of previous impact exposures. Furthermore, the lack of control over the direction, extent, and number of head movements each subject experiences impedes the ability to determine whether the person-to-person variability in outcome measures is attributable to differences in impact forces or head motions or to differences in sex, age, and previous history of head injuries. As the current obstacles related to biomechanical measurements are addressed and objective clinical measures of concussion are improved, human data collected from on-field settings will play an increasingly valuable role in understanding what biomechanical conditions or predisposing factors contribute to concussions.

In 2012 the U.S. Army began using sensors to collect data on the effects of blasts on the body, including the mechanisms that lead to concussions and other traumatic brain injury in soldiers. Results are not yet published (Hoffman, 2012).

To obtain kinematic information in more controlled settings, human-like anthropomorphic surrogates (i.e., crash test dummies) and laboratory-based studies are used to reenact film and witness accounts of sports-related events in order to estimate the forces of impact and head movements (kinematics). Surrogates and humans are also used to document the kinematics associated with non-injurious activities (Feng et al., 2010; Funk et al., 2011; Lloyd et al., 2011), which are important for identifying both tolerable and injurious kinematic conditions. It is important to note that surrogates measure only kinematic responses and that at this time, in the absence of accepted tolerance values, surrogates cannot be used to predict or measure concussions or tissue distortions. Instead, results obtained using surrogates must be correlated with animal studies, autopsy reports, and patient records to infer biological responses to kinematic loading conditions or with computational models to infer tissue deformations resulting from a head rotation or impact. A final issue is that there are few surrogates for youth and no surrogate has been validated as representative of human responses in sports settings, where kinematic conditions are often considerably lower than in car crashes.

Computational models are used to estimate the tissue distortions and stresses that may result from the kinematics of a rapid head motion or head impact, but they are valuable for understanding mechanics only when they use life-like tissue stiffnesses. Brain and skull tissue stiffnesses are available for young children (infants and toddlers) and adults (Coats and Margulies, 2006; Elkin et al., 2010; Kaster et al., 2011; Prange and Margulies, 2002; Prevost et al., 2011), but there are few data for older youth. As is the case with surrogates, computational models cannot be used to directly measure concussion or axonal injury, skull fracture, or vessel rupture; instead, predicted deformations or stresses from the model must be compared to published tissue-specific thresholds in order to infer injury. An important point is that early data have demonstrated that the brain tissue distortions and stresses in the skull that are associated, respectively, with axonal injury and skull fracture are smaller in young children than in adults (Coats and Margulies, 2006; Ibrahim et al., 2010; Raghupathi and Margulies, 2002; Robbins and Wood, 1969), but there are no concussion tissue threshold data for older youth.

It is important to note that, typically, biomechanical thresholds of injury correspond to the risk of acute injury. Rarely is biomechanics used to develop injury thresholds for long-term consequences, repeated exposures, or predisposing biological conditions. The physiological response to an initial injury may continue for days or weeks (see discussion on the neurochemistry of concussion later in this chapter), potentially creating a prolonged period when the brain may respond differently to a second event (discussed in Chapter 5). It is unknown whether deformation injury thresholds for previously injured tissue, which may be hypoxic or metabolically compromised, are lower than for normally functioning tissue. Research at the intersection of biomechanics and physiology is required before investigators can predict whether a subsequent head rotation or impact after a concussion may be more damaging than a single event.

Another common application of computational models is to simulate the head response to an impact and, if human data for that event are known, to use the model's estimates of tissue distortions to infer tissue deformations that may be associated with brain injury (Kimpara and Iwamoto, 2012; Kleiven, 2007; Takhounts et al., 2008). This indirect prediction of brain injury is hampered by the drawbacks described above and, given that brain injury is now understood to be heterogeneous, by the challenge of defining the critical deformations associated with various types and severity of the specific brain injury of interest (Saatman et al., 2008). Previous biomechanics studies have linked tissue deformations to a spectrum of brain injuries and have demonstrated that deformation thresholds are age- and injury-specific and that the magnitude and rate of the distortion required to rupture a blood vessel are different from those required to injure an axon or cause a concussion (Coats et al., 2012; Monson et al., 2003; Smith et al., 1999; Zhu et al., 2006). It is widely accepted that smaller deformations may be associated with brief functional changes (deficits in synaptic transmission, signaling pathways, and membrane permeability; see Meaney and Smith, 2011) and that larger deformations may cause permanent structural changes (Cater et al., 2006; Elkin and Morrison, 2007). Thus, tissue distortions and the rates of tissue deformation associated with concussion (with no lingering neural or vascular structural changes visible in radiological imaging or pathology) are probably lower than those for more severe brain injuries (Gennarelli et al., 2003), so it is inappropriate to rely on a single threshold for all head injuries. Moreover, it is unknown whether a concussion is produced when a critical proportion of the entire brain experiences deformation above a threshold level or whether only certain brain locations must be exposed to deformation (King et al., 2003; Ommaya and Gennarelli, 1974). Furthermore, the research community has not reached a consensus regarding whether the most appropriate injury thresholds should be defined as an average value, a threshold associated with zero injury risk, or one associated with some modest acceptable chance of injury. For comparison, in automotive safety, vehicles and restraint systems are designed so that body regions experience mechanical loads below a threshold value associated with a chance of moderate to serious injury of anywhere from 15 to 50 percent (Kleinberger et al., 1998). Each of these gaps in knowledge about concussion thresholds limits the ability of computational models to predict whether a concussion would occur from a specific head rotation or impact. However, when appropriate and acceptable tissue thresholds specific to concussions in youth are determined in the future, computational models of the human head will be powerful platforms to identify dominant and secondary factors that contribute to the biomechanics of concussion, to integrate future data regarding synergistic effects of biology and biomechanics, and to develop rational guidelines for protective equipment.

Presently, because human data and computational models are limited, researchers use alternative idealized experimental preparations such as animals, tissues, and isolated cells to create controllable settings with similar predisposing conditions among subjects and reproducible mechanical loads. Animal models are useful for measuring physiological responses (e.g., reflexes, blood flow, tissue oxygen content, metabolic derangements); injuries to the vessels, axons, and neural cell bodies; and changes in motor, memory, learning, and behavioral aptitudes at prescribed time-points after injury.

Although they are the best substitute for humans, there are four challenges in using animal models to understand sports-related concussion youth. First, human concussion includes changes in mental status without a loss of consciousness, and no metrics have been developed to assess these subtle alterations in animals immediately after injury. Thus, the definition of brain injury in an animal model includes loss of consciousness, often accompanied with demonstrable changes in axon structure or function, appearance of hemorrhages, or longer-term alterations in neurological function. Because concussions may not be associated with axonal injury, hemorrhage, and loss of consciousness, animal models, even those of mTBI, most commonly involve more severe brain injuries than concussion. Second, informative injury models need to mimic the injuries seen in sporting environments (Wall and Shani, 2008), yet most brain injury models create focal hemorrhagic cortical lesions caused by direct impact to the skull or exposed brain (Xiong et al., 2013), while the human concussed brain is more commonly associated with distributed white matter alterations (Benson et al., 2007; Kraus et al., 2007). Third, most models use adult animals, and, given the developmental differences described earlier in this chapter, extensions to youth should be made with caution. Fourth, animal models most commonly involve mice and rats but have also included ovine, porcine, and nonhuman primate models (Browne et al., 2011; Durham et al., 2000; Finnie et al., 2012; Gennarelli et al., 1981, 1982; Viano et al., 2012). Recent reports indicate that rodents have limited fidelity to human genomic and proteomic responses, injury time-courses, and gray and white brain matter distribution (Duhaime et al., 2006; Seok et al., 2013), which implies that there are challenges in applying what is learned about injury in the developing rodent brain to the human child. Despite these four substantial challenges, animal models are a valuable tool for understanding how head impacts and sudden head movements translate to brain deformations and how brain deformations result in a spectrum of brain injuries, from mild to severe.

What Has Been Learned About How Traumatic Brain Injuries Occur

Using the tools described above, researchers have determined that with or without a helmet, when the head contacts a stationary or moving object there is a rapid change in velocity and a possible deformation of the skull. Skull deformation may produce a local contusion or hemorrhage if the deformations of the tissues exceed their injury thresholds. When the properties of the contact surfaces are softer or allow sliding or deformation, the rate of velocity change (acceleration or deceleration, depending on whether the velocity is increasing or decreasing) is lower. Similarly, if there is no head contact but only body contact (e.g., in a tackle), the deceleration of the moving head is usually lower than when the head is contacted directly.

After the initial rapid change in velocity caused by impact to the head or body, the subsequent motion of the head is influenced by the location of that initial point of contact and the interaction between the head, neck, and body. There are three possible kinematic responses to head contact. First, if the contact is directed through the center of mass of the brain (i.e., is centroidal), there may be linear motion and no rotation of the head (e.g., a weight dropping down onto the top of the head or a blow to the back of the head that moves the ears and nose forward without neck flexion or extension). Animal studies have shown that these purely linear motions produce little brain motion or distortion and no concussion (Hardy et al., 2001; Ommaya and Gennarelli, 1974; Ommaya et al., 1971). However, most often the contact force is not directed centroidally through the brain, a situation that is referred to as a *non-centroidal impact*. After a non-centroidal contact, the head may rotate without a linear motion (e.g., shaking the head "no"). This purely rotational motion produces a distortion of the brain's neural and vascular structures within the skull because the brain is softer than the skull and loosely coupled to the skull. More commonly, though, a head impact produces a change in head velocity that is associated with both linear acceleration and rotation of the head. This combined rotational and linear motion may occur because the contact is glancing (further away from the rotation center) or the body continues to move after the head is restrained by the contact surface or the head bounces or rebounds after contact. For these combined rotation/linear head responses, computational simulations have illuminated the relationship between the location of the head impact, the kinematic responses of the head (linear and rotational accelerations), and the predicted brain tissue deformations (Aare et al., 2004; Kleiven, 2007; Post et al., 2011). Specifically, for those unusual instances when the head impact is through the center of mass of the head, linear acceleration correlates with the rotational acceleration response and the average deformation response in the brain. In these situations, linear acceleration is a reasonable surrogate for the brain tissue distortion response. By contrast, in the more common non-centroidal head impacts, linear and rotational accelerations are not correlated significantly, and the rotational acceleration component of the head response correlates most strongly with the average and peak brain deformations. Thus, for the most common head contact events, the linear acceleration component does not describe all of the brain's deformation response, and therefore when used alone, is not a robust predictor of injury risk.

Internal structures of the head, such as the falx cerebri and tentorium, influence how the brain moves within the skull and may cause local brain regions with very high deformations only in certain directions of head rotation, so that sagittal and coronal rotations may produce more severe injuries in primates at lower accelerations and velocities (Gennarelli et al., 1982). In addition, animal and human studies have shown a general trend that higher rotational velocities and accelerations—rather than linear accelerations—can cause larger diffuse brain deformations and worse diffuse brain injuries (Gennarelli et al., 2003, Kimpara and Iwamoto, 2012; Ommaya et al., 1971) and that head injuries depend on the direction of head motion as well as on the magnitude of rotational kinematics (Eucker et al., 2011, Gennarelli et al., 1981).

Previous research attempted to tease out if it is the change in rotational velocity ("delta v"), or the rate of change in rotational velocity (rotational acceleration or deceleration), or the acceleration duration that best predicts injury. Kimpara and Iwamoto (2012) demonstrated that head impact scenarios have shorter durations and higher accelerations than non-head contact events. Ommaya and colleagues showed that unconsciousness occurred more readily in adult nonhuman primates when rapid head rotations were achieved via direct blows to the head than when they were achieved via a non-head contact whiplash motion (Ommaya et al., 1973); other research showed that unconsciousness occurred less frequently for a given change in velocity when a cervical collar was used to decrease rotation of the head (Ommaya, 1985). Similarly, animal models that allow more head rotation after impact or enhanced head or brain movement produce more severe brain injuries (Foda and Marmarou, 1994; Marmarou et al., 1994). It is difficult to determine whether change in rotational velocity and acceleration contribute independently to concussion because no studies have used high and low rotational accelerations for the same change in rotational velocity to determine the relative importance of these kinematic variables on injury risk.

Animal studies have indicated that it is important to limit the duration of exposure to acceleration, as research has shown that concussions occur when the duration of rotational acceleration is increased (Ommaya et al., 1966). Furthermore, animal studies have demonstrated that the location of brain deformation may affect the resulting injury, suggesting that even a concussion-specific brain deformation threshold may vary with region (Cater et al., 2006; Elkin and Morrison, 2007; Vink et al., 2001; Yoshino et al., 1991).

In summary, further research is needed to define the direction-specific and brain-region-specific thresholds for linear and rotational accelerations associated with concussions in youth. These thresholds may differ between youth and adults and may vary across the pediatric age spectrum. Finally, as mentioned above, the deformations associated with functional and structural impairment may differ, and tools need to be developed to accurately assess functional derangement. The physio-mechanical link between multiple impacts must be defined. Until these foundational biomechanics are defined, it will be premature to make predictions of concussions based upon computational model simulations and head kinematic measurements in humans and surrogates.

NEUROCHEMISTRY OF CONCUSSION

Damage to brain tissue resulting from movement of the brain within the skull, as may occur with a head impact, initiates a cascade of molecular events that disrupt normal brain cell function. In this section the molecular processes that have been shown to characterize brain injuries are discussed in the context of age and sex. It should be noted that much of what is currently known about these processes is drawn from research involving animals and subjects sustaining moderate to severe brain injuries. Box 2-1 describes some of the experimental models that were used in the research described in this section to study the physiological response to brain injury in animal models.

Ionic Flux and Neurotransmitter Release

TBI induces immediate changes in brain neurochemistry (see Figure 2-2, Steps 1-3). Normally, significant cellular energy is used to keep ions distributed across the plasma membranes in such a way so as to maintain a membrane potential between −40 and −80 millivolts (mVs). Studies primarily involving rodents show that an indiscriminate efflux of potassium and glutamate (Katayama et al., 1990) and an influx of calcium follow immediately after a concussive fluid percussion brain injury (Enerson and Drewes, 2003; Osteen et al., 2001). The magnitude of the potassium rise in the extracellular space increases with injury severity (Katayama et al., 1990), with as much as a fivefold increase observed at 1.5 minutes post injury. These rapid increases resolve after approximately 2.5 minutes in mild injuries and within 6 minutes after more severe injuries. Increases in extracellular glutamate concentrations showed a similar time-course following TBI in the adult rat. The release of excitatory amino acids following severe brain injury in humans has been observed with microdialysis probes (Bullock et al., 1995, 1998; Persson and Hillered, 1992; Vespa et al., 1998). Research involving humans also provides evidence for neurotransmitter release after concussive injuries. In a study involving 12 concussed athletes (mean age 22.5 years) and 12 non-concussed athletes, Henry and colleagues used (1)H magnetic resonance spectroscopy ((1)H-MR) to noninvasively study acute metabolic changes post injury. The concussed athletes showed more symptoms and a significant decrease in N-acetylaspartylglutamic acid (NAA) in the primary motor cortex between 1 and 6 days post injury as compared with the non-concussed controls (Henry et al., 2010). The findings of decreased glutamate are in contrast to the changes seen in studies

---

BOX 2-1
Overview of Commonly Used Experimental
Models of Traumatic Brain Injury

The **fluid percussion device** is commonly used to produce general brain movement injuries. Saline is injected rapidly into the epidural space of the brain of an experimental animal through a craniotomy upon release of a pendulum that generates a fluid wave pulse in a saline-filled cylinder (Lindgren and Rinder, 1965; Stålhammar, 1990). Various injury severities can be generated with this model, and the location of the impact site has been shown to determine histopathology (Vink et al., 2001). Lateral mild injuries produce general brain tissue deformation that produces metabolic derangements with no overt cell loss (Fineman et al., 1993; Prins et al., 1996). In contrast, mid-lateral injuries do generate a developing contusion core (Vink et al., 2001). This model has been used in numerous age groups to generate diffuse brain injuries with measurable cognitive deficits, and mild fluid percussion injuries mimic numerous aspects of concussive injuries (Prins and Hovda, 1998, 2001; Prins et al., 1996).

The **weight drop injury model** involves the release of a known weight onto either the unrestrained exposed skull to produce diffuse injury (Marmarou model) or directly onto the brain through a craniotomy to produce a focal contusion (Feeney model) (see Feeney et al., 1981). In both cases injury severity can be adjusted by the amount of weight and the height from which the weight is released. The Marmarou weight drop injury has been applied to the developing brain, both are well characterized in the adult brain, and milder injuries can replicate aspects of concussive injuries (Kane et al., 2012; Milman et al., 2005).

The **controlled cortical impact** (CCI) model uses a pneumatic piston that is driven a known depth and velocity into the exposed brain to produce an evolving contusion (Lighthall, 1988), or it can be applied to the closed skull to produce "concussive" types of injuries (Huh et al., 2007; Laurer et al., 2001; Prins et al., 2010). As with the other models, the depth of penetration and velocity can be varied to produce different injury severities in different age groups.

Fluid percussion, weight drop, and CCI injuries have been applied to various animal species, including mice, rats, cats, and piglets. Rotational injuries have been applied to rats (Davidsson and Risling, 2011; Li et al., 2010) as well as to piglets and primates (Browne et al., 2011; Ståhlhammer, 1986; Sullivan et al., 2013).

---

involving animals and more severe TBI, but the time-course of changes was not examined in this study. Scans collected between 1 and 6 days post injury were averaged and may not reflect the same time-course of changes observed in other studies. The animal studies were conducted immediately after impact, and the clinical studies were conducted 1 to 6 days post injury. There is currently little research that examines the time-course of these changes over longer periods and at different injury severities.

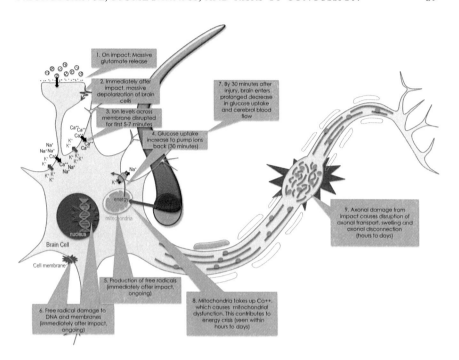

FIGURE 2-2 Neurochemical cascade observed after moderate traumatic brain injuries. Many of these events are believed to be involved to a lesser extent following mild and concussive brain injuries. Step 1 shows the indiscriminate release of glutamate and other neurotransmitters immediately after impact. These neurotransmitters bind to the post-synaptic membrane, causing rapid large-scale depolarization of brain cells (Step 2). The depolarization opens ionic channels, allowing many ions to flow down their concentration gradients and disrupting cell membrane potential (Step 3). Na+/K+ pumps work harder to reestablish the normal ionic gradient, but this requires cellular energy in the form of adenosine triphosphate, or ATP (Step 4). Glucose uptake into the brain transiently increases shortly after injury (Step 4), but within 30 minutes enters a prolonged stage of decreased glucose uptake (Step 7). During these early metabolic changes there are also increases in free radical production by the mitochondria (Step 5), which are increasingly compromised by their attempt to buffer intracellular calcium (Step 8). The free radicals contribute to protein, DNA, and lipid damage (Step 6). Additionally, the mechanical disruption of the impact can cause damage to microtubules, leading to axonal swelling, disruption of axonal transport, and eventual disconnection (Step 9).

Collectively, the animal studies of moderate brain injuries suggest that such injuries cause a release of signaling molecules which results in a disruption of the ionic balance across the cell membrane immediately after the injury event. Unless these ions are pumped back to the correct side of the cell membranes, the brain cells will not be able to be activated again. While it is thought that these events occur to a lesser degree or for a shorter duration following milder or concussive injuries, human studies examining acute neurochemical changes following concussive injuries in youth as well as adults or that address sex differences in response are lacking.

Metabolic Cascade After Traumatic Brain Injury: Glucose and Cerebral Blood Flow

The energy required to resolve the disruption of the neurochemical environment seen after injury triggers an immediate increase in brain glucose uptake or CMRglc. The immediate release of glutamate after impact plays a significant role in this transient increase in glucose uptake (Kawamata et al., 1992). In an adult rat, CMRglc rates increase 30 to 46 percent immediately after moderate fluid percussion impact and remain elevated for 30 minutes (Yoshino et al., 1991) (see Figure 2-2, Step 4). The early increase in cerebral glucose uptake following brain injury is thought to reflect the increased energy demands associated with reestablishing ionic homeostasis and maintaining neuronal membrane potential (Hovda et al., 1994; Sutton et al., 1994; Yoshino et al., 1991). While [^{18}F]-fluorodeoxyglucose positron emission tomography (FDG-PET) studies have shown increased glucose uptake following severe TBI in humans (Bergsneider et al., 1997), no studies have examined this immediate increase in glucose uptake after mild or concussive brain injuries.

TBI-induced increases in cerebral glucose uptake are followed by a reduction of adenosine triphosphate (ATP) levels and prolonged CMRglc depression (see Figure 2-2, Step 7). This post-injury decrease in CMRglc has been established as a hallmark response after TBI. It is a response that is observed in animals following experimental fluid percussion that results in concussive injuries and cortical contusion (Andersen and Marmarou, 1992; Buczek et al., 2002; Chen et al., 2004; Kawamata et al., 1992; Richards et al., 2001; Yoshino et al., 1991, 1992) and that is also observed in humans who have sustained severe TBI (Bergsneider et al., 1997; O'Connell et al., 2005). On the other hand, there is no evidence of these changes from studies involving humans who have sustained concussions.

Relationship Between Injury Severity and CMRglc Depression

Research involving adult rats has found glucose metabolic depression to remain for 5, 10, or 14 days after experimental mild, moderate, or severe fluid percussion injury, respectively (Hovda et al., 1994). Focal injuries from controlled cortical impact (CCI) appear to produce a more profound and longer-lasting depression than the more diffuse fluid percussion injury does (Prins and Hovda, 2009; Sutton et al., 1994). TBIs that do not cause overt cell death or gross pathology can still produce metabolic dysfunction. Studies involving humans show that mTBI, which may involve axonal damage or dysfunction as detected by diffusion tensor imaging, is associated with measurable decreases in CMRglc (Gross et al., 1996; Humayun et al., 1989). The decreases in CMRglc in mTBI patients are correlated with persistent post-concussive symptoms (Gross et al., 1996; Umile et al., 2002). PET studies in 14 human TBI patients (mean age 36 years) with a mean Glasgow coma score scale of 6.5 (mild-severe) showed CMRglc depression between 5 and 28 days for all levels of injury severity (Bergsneider et al., 2001). This duration of CMRglc depression has been estimated to be five to six times longer in humans than in rats. Initial injury severity in adult human TBI patients does not appear to correlate with the magnitude or time-course of cortical metabolic recovery (Bergsneider et al., 2001). However, the CMRglc rates for thalamus, brain stem, and cerebellum correlate significantly with the level of consciousness at the time of PET imaging in adult TBI patients (Hattori et al., 2003). This pattern may suggest that concussions would result in a shorter duration of decreased metabolic depression than would moderate and severe brain injuries.

Relationship Between Age, Sex, and CMRglc Depression

Animal research suggests that the magnitude and duration of CMRglc depression following a brain injury increases with age. For example, 17-day-old rats (analogous to human newborns) that were injured via fluid percussion showed glucose metabolic recovery to age-matched shams within 3 days (Thomas et al., 2000), whereas adult (70-day-old) rats took 10 days for recovery. After CCI injury, 35-day-old rats (human adolescent) showed recovery of metabolic rates of subcortical structures within 3 days, as compared with 7 days in 90-day-old rats and also exhibited better metabolic recovery in the cortex by day 7 (Prins and Hovda, 2009). It is important to note that these are metabolic recoveries observed in animal models and that pediatric CMRglc after various severities of TBI has not been measured. While these studies all modeled injuries that are more severe than concussions, there was one experimental study that measured CMRglc after concussive-like injuries in the adolescent rat; in this case CMRglc depression was observed at 24 hours after a closed-head concussive injury, and recovery was observed in all structures by 5 days (Prins et al., 2013).

There have been no studies in humans on age and sex differences in the metabolic alterations that occur after a concussion. Some research has used PET imaging of TBI in youth populations as a way of measuring metabolic activity, but these studies did not evaluate whether there were differences in the findings by age (Gross et al., 1996; Roberts et al., 1995; Worley et al., 1995). In one study, abnormal CMRglc rates were positively correlated with the number of clinical symptoms reported and with neuropsychological test results following mTBI in patients 12 to 59 years old at 3.5 years post injury (Gross et al., 1996). Worley and colleagues (1995) demonstrated that abnormalities on PET images obtained within 12 weeks following severe TBI were associated with poorer clinical outcomes in children 4 months to 19 years of age. The limited data from research involving human subjects suggests that younger and female youth may take longer to become symptom-free following a concussion and that younger youth may take longer than older youth to return to baseline on neurocognitive measures (Berz et al., 2013; Zuckerman et al., 2012). Future clinical studies comparing the time-course between children and adults after similar types of injuries may give insight into whether the experimental evidence translates to the human condition.

Changes in Cerebral Blood Flow After TBI

There have been hundreds of studies on changes in CBF after TBI, but relatively few of them have focused on CBF changes in pediatric populations, and even fewer have addressed changes following a concussion or mTBI. Only a couple of studies have evaluated sex differences in changes in CBF following TBI. As with CMRglc responses, CBF decreases immediately following both moderate to severe TBIs and mTBIs, and it can remain depressed for extended durations (Bonne et al., 2003; Giza and Hovda, 2001; Golding et al., 1999; Grindel, 2003; McQuire et al., 1998; Werner and Engelhard, 2007). Younger TBI patients can show a different response to injury than do older individuals, with acute hyperemia followed by decreases in CBF (Mandera et al., 2002). This pattern has also been observed in experimental studies with 3.5- to 4.5-week-old rats (human adolescent), which demonstrated age differences in CBF response to weight drop injury, with young adult animals showing a greater reduction in blood flow at the injury site 2 hours post injury (Grundl et al., 1994). Subsequent study found that both 3- to 4-week-old and 2- to 3-month-old (young adult) rats show hyperemia between 24 and 48 hours post injury (Biagas et al., 1996). Dramatic decreases in CBF were also measured within 1 hour after rapid head rotations that caused diffuse white matter injury in 3- to 5-day-old infant piglets and 4-week-old toddler piglets (Eucker et al., 2011; Friess et al., 2011; Zhou et al., 2009), with significant reductions even 24 hours after diffuse brain injury (Kilbaugh et al., 2011). Decreases were also detected in 1- and 4-month-olds at 3 hours after CCI injury (Durham et al., 2000). Differing ages, injury severity, and injury type may also result in different CBF responses. Fluid percussion injury in 1- to 3-day-old piglets showed greater reductions in CBF than did the same injury in juvenile (3- to 4-week-old) pigs (Armstead, 1999). The different CBF age responses among piglets of different ages versus among rats of different ages may be related to differences in the types and severities of the injuries as well as differences in the time that the CBF was measured. There are fewer studies examining the effects of mild or concussive injuries on CBF in the younger brain. A recent study of 12 concussed children ages 11 to 15 showed that CBF, as measured by phase-contrast magnetic resonance angiography, was decreased relative to controls immediately after injury and that this decrease persisted beyond 30 days after injury even after symptoms resolved (Maugans et al., 2012).

In addition to causing changes in CBF, TBI can also affect cerebral autoregulation. Autoregulation is the ability of the brain to maintain a constant CBF in response to changes in blood pressure between 50 and 150 mmHg. TBI can directly affect the brain's ability to maintain appropriate blood flow. Age and severity-dependent impairment in autoregulation has been observed. Mild brain injury has been shown to impair autoregulation and vascular reactivity in children (Becelewski and Pierzchala, 2003; Choe et al., 2012; Junger et al., 1997; Vavilala et al., 2004). Clinical studies examining changes in autoregulation after pediatric TBI have shown that the prevalence of impaired autoregulation increases with injury severity (Vavilala et al., 2004). Sex differences in CBF or autoregulation following TBI of any injury severity have not been addressed in the literature. Given that children and adolescents have higher normal blood flow rates, age-dependent definitions for "hyperemia" and "hypoperfusion" have been established for patient management (Vavilala et al., 2004). The risks for secondary ischemia versus elevations in intracranial pressure must be established by age and sex following all injury severities.

In summary, changes in brain glucose metabolism and blood flow after brain injury have been shown to be important biomarkers of TBI pathophysiology in all age groups and injury severities. However, there is a lack of data on changes in blood flow and glucose metabolism following mTBI and concussions in both males and females and at different ages during childhood and adolescence.

Oxidative Damage

In addition to TBI-induced metabolic crisis, there are also various pathways that result in oxidative damage that are activated acutely after TBI. It is unclear whether oxidative damage occurs after concussion, but given the potentially additive nature of multiple concussions it is important to discuss this common finding in animal models. Free radicals are molecules with unpaired electrons that will react with surrounding compounds to gain electrons. TBI-induced increases in reactive oxygen species (ROS) and reactive nitrogen species can generate hydroxyl radicals ($\bullet$OH) and peroxynitrite (ONOO-). While normal mitochondrial metabolism produces ROS, they are managed by cellular antioxidant systems. Studies have shown that trauma to the brain and CNS can result in greater production of ROS, resulting in oxidative damage to proteins, lipids, and DNA (Hall and Braughler, 1993; Kerr et al., 1996; O'Connell and Littleton-Kearney, 2013) (see Figure 2-2, Steps 5 and 6).

It is difficult to quantify the level of the short-lived free radicals precisely, but the level has been shown to be elevated shortly after experimental brain injury. Hydroxyl radical ($\bullet$OH) production has been observed to increase 60 percent within the first minute, peak within 30 minutes, and then subsequently decrease after a weight drop resulting in a concussive-like injury in adult mice (Althaus et al., 1993; Hall et al., 1993). CCI injury in adult rats produced a 250 percent increase in $\bullet$OH production, which was sustained for 90 minutes (Marklund et al., 2001; Sen et al., 1993). Focal CCI injury produced a rapid increase in nitrate levels, with the peak at 5 minutes and a return to baseline by 6 hours post injury (Rao et al., 1998). Longer-lasting changes in cortical levels of the inducible isoform of nitric oxide synthase (iNOS) were observed by immunostaining 3 to 7 days following adult concussive fluid percussion injury (Wada et al., 1998). Fluid percussion injury induces iNOS expression after 24 to 28 hours in immature vascular smooth muscle cells and neutrophils (Clark et al., 1996). Until recently, it was not possible to measure free radicals in human TBI patients. Biomarkers for oxidative damage in human severe head injuries have been explored in adults and children through microdialysis sampling (Bayir et al., 2009; Clausen et al., 2012; Cristofori et al., 2005), which remains too invasive for concussion patients. Free radical production has not been quantified after concussive injuries in any age group.

Laboratory measurement of free radicals is difficult because their persistence in the body is generally short-lived. Thus, researchers have focused on the measurement of damage produced by free radicals by quantifying the lipid peroxidation, protein nitration, and DNA oxidation that occurs after moderate to severe TBI. In rodent models, increases in lipid peroxidation were observed 1 to 24 hours after weight drop injury (severity not always noted) (Hall et al., 2004; Hsiang et al., 1997; Léwen and Hillered, 1998; Marmarou et al., 1994; Tyurin et al., 2000; Vagnozzi et al., 1999), after CCI (Singh et al., 2006), and after moderate fluid percussion injury (Praticò et al., 2002). Similarly, protein oxidation or nitration products were significantly elevated 30 minutes after CCI injury in adult mice and returned to baseline within 12 hours (Singh et al., 2006). DNA damage as measured by poly-ADP ribose polymerase (PARP) activity has also been shown to be elevated between 1 and 21 days after CCI injury in adult rodents (Satchell et al., 2003). Although there are a limited number of studies directly measuring PARP, research shows the inhibition of PARP to improve lesion volume after moderate fluid percussion injury (LaPlaca et al., 2001) and shows preserved cellular NAD^+ concentrations with improved functional performance in the Morris water maze[1] (Satchell et al., 2003) in rodents.

While significant strides have been made toward understanding the effects of free radicals after more severe TBI, far fewer studies have addressed oxidative stress after mild or concussive injuries. Mild TBI produced decreases in cytochrome oxidase activity in the cortex and hippocampus 1 to 10 days after fluid percussion injury in adult rats (Hovda et al., 1991). A threefold increase in protein carbonyls was seen immediately after mild weight drop injury, the protein carbonyls peaked at 3 hours, and they remained elevated at 12 hours (Petronilho et al., 2010). In this study the magnitude and duration of protein oxidative damage was inversely related to the severity of the injury following weight drop injury in adult rats. Another injury severity study with weight drop showed that mild injury did not produce histopathology, astrogliosis, or evidence of acute oxidative stress (Schwarzbold et al., 2010). In this study the degree of pathology and oxidative damage increased with injury severity.

While experimental studies have been used to address oxidative injury in various injury models and for various severities in adult animals, there are very few studies quantifying age- or sex-related differences in oxidative response after brain injury, including concussions. Currently there is only one study that examined the consequences of oxidative injury in the developing brain, and this was done in animals. Tsuru-Aoyagi and colleagues (2009) showed that 21-day-old mice have increases in protein nitration after CCI injury prior to contusion development. Other studies have addressed age-related differences in the antioxidant defense systems after injury. Despite increased thiobarbituric acid reactive substances after CCI, no acute compensatory increase in superoxide dismutase or glutathione

---

[1]The Morris water maze is a procedure used to measure spatial learning and memory in rodents. Rodents are placed into a pool of water from which they may escape onto a platform. Comparison of the performance of normal and injured animals on this test is a way of examining the effects of a brain injury (Morris, 1984).

peroxidase is observed in 7-day-old (Ozdemir et al., 2005) or 21-day-old (Fan et al., 2003) mice. This lack of increase in antioxidant response in the younger brain may increase vulnerability to oxidative damage after injury.

Both clinical and experimental evidence demonstrates that moderate and severe TBI increases oxidative injuries to proteins, membranes, and DNA in both the younger and the adult brain. However, there are currently no studies addressing oxidative injury specifically in concussive injuries with regard to sex or age.

Axonal Injury

In experimental models, axonal damage has been found to be present acutely after TBI of all severities, with the regional distribution and the number of damaged axons increasing with injury severity. Originally, this microscopic pathology was thought to be caused by a mechanical shearing of the axons during impact that resulted in the formation of an axoplasm swelling and axonal disconnection (Strich, 1956; Strich and Oxon, 1961). However, experimental studies have revealed that TBI of any severity can induce disruptions in axonal transport that cause swellings during the first 6 to 24 hours (Povlishock and Christman, 1995; Povlishock et al., 1983) (see Figure 2-2, Step 9). Calcium entry through the compromised plasma membrane has been shown to activate proteases (calpain, calcineurin), resulting in neurofilament degradation, disruption of axonal transport, and functional failure (Schlaepfer, 1974, 1987). Both mechanical disruption of cytoskeletal elements and neurochemical changes contribute to acute and long-term secondary axotomy.

Evidence of axonal damage has been well documented in various experimental adult models and at varying severities of TBI. The disruption of axonal transport of amyloid precursor protein (APP) after TBI led to the use of APP as a marker of axonal injury. Positive APP labeling has been shown in adult animal models after mild fluid percussion injury (Hoshino et al., 2003; Hylin et al., 2013; Shultz et al., 2011), after weight drop (Creed et al., 2011), after CCI injury (Chen et al., 2004; Dunn-Meynell and Levin, 1997; Itoh et al., 2009), and after rotational injury (Browne et al., 2011).

In contrast to the numerous studies on axonal injury in the adult brain, most of which have involved animals, few studies have been conducted in the developing brain, and only a couple of studies have examined mild injuries. Models of greater injury severities in P11-P21 age ranges show axonal bulbs and varicosities with APP staining between 6 hours and 1 week (Adelson et al., 2001; Huh et al., 2006, 2007, 2008; Tong et al., 2002). Studies of mTBI also show positive APP staining. Mild CCI in the P7 mouse produced significant APP labeling in the cingulum/external capsule between 30 minutes and 24 hours post injury, with decreased labeling at 48 hours (Dikranian et al., 2008). While the "mild" impact depth used in these experiments did not produce cortical cavitation, it did produce increases in caspase 3 in the posterior cingulate cortex and anterior thalamus between 16 and 48 hours. Because age was not incorporated into the study design, it remains unclear if these findings suggest a specific vulnerability of the "infant" brain to injury. Studies examining rotational injuries in the neonatal pig have also shown axonal injuries. However, studies examining rotational injuries in the neonatal and toddler pig have shown that a single rapid rotational injury without impact in the 3- to 5-day-old piglet produced more axonal swellings and disconnections at 6 hours post injury than in the adult pig (Raghupathi and Margulies, 2002), and the damage was similar to that seen in the toddler pig (Ibrahim et al., 2010), despite the infant pig's mechanically protective much smaller brain, indicating a vulnerability in the very young brain. Even single mild concussive injury in the infant piglet (Kilbaugh et al., 2011) and adult 35-day-old rat showed significant axonal injury 24 hours after injury (Prins et al., 2010).

In summary, experimental studies have demonstrated damage to neuronal "cables" or axons in mild injuries in both adult and infant age groups. There is not yet enough known to compare regional and time-course differences in axonal pathology across the pediatric age range. There are currently no studies addressing whether sex differences in axonal pathology exist in concussions.

Plasticity and Synaptic Changes

TBI leads to changes in the connectivity of the brain and alterations in the intimate communication between synapses. Experimental models with adult moderate fluid percussion injury have revealed that synaptophysin (a protein within the synapse) labeling increased in the cortex and white matter in a manner that was dependent on the severity of the injury. Western blot analysis also showed that the accumulation of synaptophysin was long lasting (30 days), suggesting that the transportation of synaptic vesicles may be disrupted (Shojo and Kibayashi, 2006). In this same model, decreases in dendritic spine densities were observed 24 hours after injury, but increases above controls were observed 7 days later (Campbell et al., 2012b). These acute synaptic changes are thought to reflect synaptic instability and degeneration (Campbell et al., 2012a) and may have significant implications for the initiation of rehabilitation. Griesbach and colleagues (2004) showed that exercise initiated immediately after a mild fluid percussion injury decreases synaptic plasticity molecules (including phosphorylated CREB [cAMP response element-binding protein], synapsin I, and mitogen activated protein kinase) and worsens spatial learning and memory tasks in the adult rat. By contrast, when exercise was initiated 2 weeks after mild fluid percussion injury, the expression of plasticity proteins (BDNF [brain-derived neurotrophic factor], phosphorylated CREB, synapsin I) increased (Griesbach et al., 2007).

Environmental experiences can induce significant alterations in the brain during normal cerebral maturation. These types of "learning" or "good plasticity" have been shown to produce long-lasting connectivity changes in the brain following environmental enrichment (Greenough et al., 1973). Age differences in this type of plasticity response have been observed following TBI induced by fluid percussion. The brains of young rats raised in an enriched environment (EE) (consisting of toys, tunnels, and ladders placed in a two-level cage) show increased dendritic branching, increased cortical thickness, and improved cognitive performance (Ip et al., 2002). However, when 17- to 21-day-old rats were placed in an EE immediately after mild to moderate injury, their brains failed to show the EE-related plasticity and improved cognitive performance (Fineman et al., 2000; Ip et al., 2002). Recovery of this plasticity response was observed when immature rats were placed in EE 2 weeks after mild fluid percussion injury (Giza et al., 2005). Examination of the molecular signals involved in brain enrichment revealed changes in the N-methyl-D-aspartate (NMDA) receptor after injury. The NR2A subunit of the NMDA receptor increases during normal brain development and also in response to stimulation. Following this concussive-like brain injury, the decrease in NR2A expression in the younger brain is thought to contribute to the failure to show EE plasticity acutely (Giza et al., 2006). Collectively these research findings provide evidence that mTBI results in early synaptic changes that can affect experience-dependent plasticity in the developing brain. More research is needed to further understand the effects of concussive injury on neuroplasticity at different ages and in males and females.

Hormonal and Pituitary Changes

The pituitary gland is responsible for hormonal production essential for normal reproductive, cognitive, social, and emotional maturation. Among adults with mild, moderate, and severe TBI, between 28 and 69 percent showed pituitary dysfunction between 3 months and 23 years post injury (Agha et al., 2004; Bondanelli et al., 2004; Kelly et al., 2000; Lieberman et al., 2001). Case studies of children with moderate to severe brain injuries and clinical studies of such children have reported acute and persistent pituitary dysfunction (Acerini and Tasker, 2007; Ives et al., 2007; Niederland et al., 2007; Norwood et al., 2010). Among pediatric patients with mild to moderate TBI, 42 percent were found to have significantly lower than normal growth hormone levels, with the effect seen predominantly in boys. While deficiency in growth hormone is common after TBI, children can also experience deficiency in adrenocorticotropic hormone,[2] diabetes insipidus, hypothyroidism, and increases in prolactin (Rose and Auble, 2012). Cortisol deficiencies have also been observed in children several months post injury (Niederland et al., 2007). The injury severities in this study ranged from concussions to severe injuries, and the authors report that pituitary dysfunction was not severity-dependent, although these data were not shown. There is evidence for pituitary dysfunction after mild to severe TBI in children (Casano-Sancho et al., 2013; Einaudi and Bondone, 2007; Khadr et al., 2010; Niederland et al., 2007) that may result in acute and long-term disruption of normal growth, but changes that occur specifically after concussions have not been examined. There are currently no experimental models quantifying hormonal deficiencies after concussions by age or sex. Undetected hormonal changes may have effects on memory, attention, executive function, mood, fatigue, and sleep and may thereby increase the duration of recovery.

Window of Vulnerability

The time period during which the brain remains vulnerable to another injury is the time that athletes should remain out of play. Although there are currently consensus-derived return-to-play guidelines for professional and pediatric sports, there are no biological markers of this window of vulnerability. A measurable biological marker would allow physicians to assess the extent of recovery from a concussion.

Although there are no studies addressing biomarkers for increased risk of subsequent concussions, there is evidence to support the idea that cerebral vulnerability increases immediately following a concussion. An experimental study by Meehan and colleagues (2012) showed that as the interval between injuries decreased, the duration of cognitive impairments increased. Adult mice were given five repeat weight drop injuries at 1-, 7-, or 30-day intervals and then assessed in the Morris water maze (MWM) at 1 month and 1 year post last injury. Animals that received daily or weekly injuries showed significant cognitive impairments that remained at 1 year post injury. Animals injured at 1-month intervals showed no significant MWM impairments. The injury model produced no significant edema, hippocampal cell loss, change in cerebral volume, or axonal injury relative to shams, thus indicating the mild nature of the injury. The cumulative effect of cognitive dysfunction when injuries occur at shorter intervals suggests that the impact interval reflects the duration of cerebral vulnerability.

These experimental findings were subsequently tested in human pa-

---

[2]Adrenocorticotropic hormone is released from the pituitary gland in the brain. It helps to modulate the secretion of cortisol and other hormones in the body.

tients using (1)H-MR spectroscopy. The clinical study, which involved 13 concussed athletes, found that NAA/Cr ratios had decreased by 18.5 percent at 3 days post injury and that they had returned to control levels by 30 days. Three of these patients who resumed normal activities shortly thereafter sustained a second concussion, which resulted in more prolonged deficits in NAA/Cr ratios with delayed recovery at 45 days (Vagnozzi et al., 2008). The length of time it takes to recover from the metabolic alterations following a concussion appears to correspond to the duration of adult cerebral vulnerability. Similar metabolic and structural changes have been documented in small groups of concussed athletes who showed no significant changes in neuropsychological test scores (see Henry et al., 2010, 2011).

RISK FACTORS FOR CONCUSSION IN THE DEVELOPING BRAIN

The concussion literature has identified several factors that appear to modify an individual's risk of sustaining a concussion. In this section, the risk factors for concussion as they pertain to the developing brain, including sex, age, genetics, and history of prior concussions, are addressed. A discussion of factors that influence concussion outcomes and recovery appears in Chapter 4.

Sex

As discussed in Chapter 1, data from sports played by both males and females show higher reported rates of concussions for females. Cross-sex comparisons of the mechanics of concussion have included heading in soccer, which is one of the few sports in which the rules, protective equipment, and playing style are similar for the two sexes. Tierney and colleagues (2005, 2008) found that female soccer players exhibited greater head-neck segment peak acceleration and angular displacement than males did when exposed to a similar force. Reduced neck musculature and larger ball-to-head size ratios in females relative to males may explain this difference, but the literature is not clear on the influence of cervical muscle strength on kinematic measures such as head acceleration (Garces et al., 2002; Mansell et al., 2005; Queen et al., 2003; Schneider and Zernicke, 1988; Tierney et al., 2008). The data from the soccer studies were collected under controlled loading conditions such that the force applied to male and female participants was equivalent. In order to translate these laboratory-based data to the playing field, one must take into account that males and females may experience different loading conditions while playing sports. For example, two studies in which head acceleration data were collected under normal play conditions in ice hockey and boxing demonstrated that males experienced greater accelerations on average than did females (Brainard et al.,

2012; Stojsih et al., 2010). Furthermore, from a mechanics perspective, although player-to-player contact appears to be a primary mechanism for sustaining a concussion overall, player contact is responsible for a major proportion of concussions in male athletes (65 to 81 percent), while contact with the playing surface or the ball is a more common cause of concussions in female athletes (Dick, 2009). However, no details exist concerning whether impacts with the playing surface impart more energy to the female head than do impacts with other players. Further research on the biomechanics of concussions in male and female athletes is warranted, especially in sports in which males and females have similar rules, equipment, and environment. It is important that comparisons across the sexes be made in circumstances with similar loading environments. Finally, some of the difference in concussion rates between males and females may be explained by a lower rate of reporting of concussion symptoms by male athletes (Daneshvar et al., 2011; Granite and Carroll, 2002; Harmon et al., 2013), although there is no definitive evidence that this is the case.

Age

There is currently a lack of data to determine whether there are variations in concussion rates across the pediatric age spectrum. Most studies comparing concussion incidence in high school and collegiate athletes have focused on football, with less attention being given to other sports, including those played by females (Gessel et al., 2007). Few studies of sports-related concussions have focused on pre-high-school-age youth. Immaturity of the developing CNS, a larger head-to-body ratio, thinner cranial bones, reduced development of neck and shoulder musculature, a larger subarachnoid space in which the brain can move, and differences in cerebral blood volume have been proposed as possible sources of increased susceptibility to concussions for youth relative to adults (Karlin, 2011; Meehan et al., 2011). In addition, it has been speculated that the gains in weight and mass that occur during the adolescent growth spurt may increase force and momentum during collisions without corollary increases in neck strength (Buzzini and Guskiewicz, 2006; Karlin, 2011). Incomplete myelination of the brain tissue may put the developing brain at greater risk for shear injury (Cook et al., 2006; Kieslich et al., 2002; Ommaya et al., 2002). Relative to adults, children demonstrate more widespread and prolonged cerebral swelling and increased metabolic sensitivities following a head injury, and these physiological changes may result in more apparent (i.e., more severe and persistent) symptoms (Biagas et al., 1996; Field et al., 2003; Giza and Hovda, 2001; Karlin et al., 2011; Reddy et al., 2008).

Genetics

There has been little research done on how genetic factors influence susceptibility to concussion. In a retrospective survey of collegiate male football players (n=163) and female soccer players (n=33), those with three alleles (E2, E4, and promoter) of the apolipoprotein E (APOE) gene (four participants) were nearly 10 times more likely to self-report that they had experienced a concussion in the past than were individuals who did not carry these alleles. Furthermore, athletes possessing the promoter allele (nine participants) were 8.4 times more likely to report a history of multiple concussions (Tierney et al., 2010). An earlier retrospective study of intercollegiate football and soccer players (n=195) showed that those with the APOE promoter genotype were nearly three times as likely to have a history of concussion, after adjusting for age, sport, school, and years in their primary sport (Terrell et al., 2008). On the other hand, a few prospective studies of high school and collegiate athletes found no significant differences in the frequency of concussions between individuals with or without the APOE or tau genotype, although these studies were limited by relatively small sample sizes (Kristman et al., 2008; Terrell et al., 2012, 2013). Genetic studies beyond APOE are lacking. Prospective research with larger samples sizes that control for athletic exposure, prior concussion history, and other predisposing factors may help to clarify the role that genetics play in risk for and recovery from concussions in youth populations (Harmon et al., 2013).

History of Prior Concussion

A history of previous concussions is a relatively well-established predictor of increased risk for future concussions. (See Chapter 5 for a more complete discussion of multiple concussions.) Studies of high school and college athletes suggest that, compared with those who have never had a concussion, individuals with a history of prior concussion are 2 to 5.8 times more likely to sustain a (subsequent) concussion (Collins et al., 2002; Guskiewicz et al., 2000, 2003; Harmon et al., 2013; Hollis et al., 2009; Schulz et al., 2004; Zemper, 2003). It is not known the extent to which the increased risk is due to changes in the brain after an initial concussion that may make it more vulnerable to future impacts as opposed to factors (e.g., playing style, position, musculature) that might make an individual more susceptible to concussion in general. A prospective study of 2,905 college football players found a dose-response relationship between number of self-reported previous concussions and incident concussions after controlling for division of play, playing position, years of participation in organized football, academic year in school, and body mass index (Guskiewicz et al., 2003). Brain injury models indicate that brain function may be altered for several days to weeks after brain injury, including concussion. Additional research is needed to elucidate how physiological factors, including enduring changes in the brain that may occur after an individual appears to have clinically recovered from a concussion, may influence future concussion risk.

FINDINGS

The committee offers the following findings on the neuroscience, biomechanics, and risks of concussion in the developing brain:

- There are normal changes in brain structure, blood flow, and metabolism that occur with brain development that may influence susceptibility to and prognosis following concussions in youth.
- Research primarily involving animals and individuals with more severe head injury has provided a limited framework for understanding the neuroscience of concussion. This research indicates that there are a series of molecular and functional changes that take place in the brain following head injury, some of which may serve as important biomarkers for the pathophysiology of concussion. However, little research has been conducted specifically on changes in the brain following concussions in youth or has attempted to evaluate the differences in such changes between female and male youth. Research using newer noninvasive imaging techniques in the first hours and days following injury may help to improve understanding of the neurobiology of concussion.
- Existing studies of head injury biomechanics have limited applicability to youth and thus are inadequate to define the direction- and age-related thresholds for linear and rotational acceleration specifically associated with concussions in youth.
- Available data indicate that female youth athletes and youth with a history of prior concussion have higher rates of reported sports-related concussions. The extent to which these findings are due to physiological, biomechanical, and other factors (e.g., possible differences between males and females in the reporting of concussion symptoms or player aggressiveness) is not yet well understood.
- While it has been suggested that physiological and biomechanical risks for concussion may differ between younger children and older youth and adults, there is currently a lack of epidemiologic data from a variety of sports to calculate and compare rates of sports-related concussions across the age spectrum.
- The findings of studies examining associations between genetic variation and risk for concussion have been mixed and are limited by small sample sizes.

REFERENCES

Aare, M., S. Kleiven, and P. Halldin. 2004. Injury tolerances for oblique impact helmet testing. *International Journal of Crashworthiness* 9(1):15-23.

Acerini, C. L., and R. C. Tasker. 2007. Traumatic brain injury induced hypothalamic-pituitary dysfunction: A paediatric perspective. *Pituitary* 10(4):373-380.

Adelson, P. D., L. W. Jenkins, R. L. Hamilton, P. Robichaud, M. P. Tran, and P. M. Kochanek. 2001. Histopathologic response of the immature rat to diffuse traumatic brain injury. *Journal of Neurotrauma* 18(10):967-976.

Agha, A., B. Rogers, M. Sherlock, P. O'Kelly, W. Tormey, J. Phillips, and C. J. Thompson. 2004. Anterior pituitary dysfunction in survivors of traumatic brain injury. *Journal of Clinical Endocrinology and Metabolism* 89(1):4929-4936.

Althaus, J. S., P. K. Andrus, C. M. Williams, P. F. Vonvoigtlander, A. R. Cazers, and E. D. Hall. 1993. The use of salicylate hydroxylation to detect hydroxyl radical generation in ischemic and traumatic brain injury. Reversal by tirilazad mesylate (U-74006F). *Molecular and Chemical Neuropathology* 20(2):147-162.

Andersen, B. J., and A. Marmarou. 1992. Post-traumatic selective stimulation of glycolysis. *Brain Research* 585(1-2):184-189.

Armstead, W. M. 1999. Role of endothelin-1 in age dependent cerebrovascular hypotensive responses after brain injury. *American Journal of Physiology* 274(5 Pt 2): H1884-H1894.

Bakker, S. L., F. E. de Leeuw, T. den Heijer, P. J. Koudstaal, A. Hofman, and M. M. Breteler. 2004. Cerebral haemodynamics in the elderly: The Rotterdam study. *Neuroepidemiology* 23(4):178-184.

Bava, S., and S. F. Tapert. 2010. Adolescent brain development and the risk for alcohol and other drug problems. *Neuropsychology Review* 20(4):398-413.

Bayir, H., P. D. Adelson, S. R. Wisniewski, P. M. Shore, Y. C. Lai, S. D. Brown, K. L. Janeski-Feldman, V. E. Kagan, and P. M. Kochanek. 2009. Therapeutic hypothermia preserves antioxidant defenses after severe traumatic brain injury in infants and children. *Critical Care Medicine* 37(2):689-695.

Becelewski, J., and K. Pierzchala. 2003. Cerebrovascular reactivity in patients with mild head injury. *Polish Journal of Neurology and Neurosurgery* 37(2):339-350.

Bechara, A., H. Damasio, and A. R. Damasio. 2000. Emotion, decision making and the orbitofrontal cortex. *Cerebral Cortex* 10(3):295-307.

Benson, R. R., S. A. Meda, S. Vasudevan, Z. Kou, K. A. Govindarajan, R. A. Hanks, S. R. Millis, M. Makki, Z. Latif, W. Coolin, J. Meythaler, and E. M. Haacke. 2007. Global white matter analysis of diffusion tensor images is predictive of injury severity in traumatic brain injury. *Journal of Neurotrauma* 24(3):446-459.

Bergsneider, M., D. A. Hovda, E. Shalmon, D. F. Kelly, P. M. Vespa, N. A. Martin, M. E. Phelps, D. L. McArthur, M. J. Caron, J. F. Kraus, and D. P. Becker. 1997. Cerebral hyperglycolysis following severe traumatic brain injury in humans: A positron emission tomography study. *Journal of Neurosurgery* 86(2):241-251.

Bergsneider, M., D. A. Hovda, D. L. McArthur, M. Etchepare, S. C. Huang, N. Sehati, P. Satz, M. E. Phelps, and D. P. Becker. 2001. Metabolic recovery following human traumatic brain injury based on FDG-PET: Time course and relationship to neurological disability. *Journal of Head Trauma Rehabilitation* 16(2):135-148.

Berz, K., J. Divine, K. B. Foss, R. Heyl, K. R. Ford, and G. D. Myer. 2013. Sex-specific differences in the severity of symptoms and recovery rate following sports-related concussions in young athletes. *Physician and Sports Medicine* 41(2):64-69.

Biagas, K. V., P. D. Grundl, P. M. Kochanek, J. K. Schiding, and E. M. Nemoto. 1996. Post-traumatic hyperemia in immature, mature, and aged rats: Autoradiographic determination of cerebral blood flow. *Journal of Neurotrauma* 13(4):189-200.

Biro, F. M., M. P. Galvez, L. C. Greenspan, P. A. Succop, N. Vangeepuram, S. M. Piney, S. Teitelbaum, G. C. Windham, L. H. Kushi, and M. S. Wolff. 2010. Pubertal assessment method and baseline characteristics in a mixed longitudinal study of girls. *Pediatrics* 126(3):e583-e590.

Bondanelli, M., M. L. De, M. R. Ambrosio, M. Monesi, D. Valle, M. C. Zatelli, A. Fusco, A. Bianchi, M. Farneti, and E. C. degli Uberti. 2004. Occurrence of pituitary dysfunction following traumatic brain injury. *Journal of Neurotrauma* 21(6):685-696.

Bonne, O., A. Gilboa, Y. Louzoun, O. Kempf-Sherf, M. Katz, Y. Fishman, Y. Z. Ben-Nahum, Y. Krausz, M. Bocher, H. Lester, R. Chisin, and B. Lerer. 2003. Cerebral blood flow in chronic symptomatic mild traumatic brain injury. *Psychiatry Research* 124(3):141-152.

Bourgeois, J. P., P. S. Goldman-Rakic, and P. Rakic. 1994. Synaptogenesis in the prefrontal cortex of rhesus monkeys. *Cerebral Cortex* 4(1):78-96.

Brainard, L. L., J. G. Beckwith, J. J. Chu, J. J. Crisco, T. W. McAllister, A. C. Duhaime, A. C. Maerlender, and R. M. Greenwald. 2012. Gender differences in head impacts sustained by collegiate ice hockey players. *Medicine and Science in Sports and Exercise* 44(2):297-304.

Browne, K. D., X. H. Chen, D. F. Meaney, and D. H. Smith. 2011. Mild traumatic brain injury and diffuse axonal injury in swine. *Journal of Neurotrauma* 28(9):1747-1755.

Buczek, M., J. Alvarez, Y. Zhou, W. D. Lust, W. R. Selman, and R. A. Ratcheson. 2002. Delayed changes in regional brain energy metabolism following cerebral concussion in rats. *Metabolic Brain Disease* 17(3):153-167.

Bullock, R., A. Zauner, J. Woodward, and H. F. Young. 1995. Massive persistent release of excitatory amino acids following human occlusive stroke. *Stroke* 26(11):2187-2189.

Bullock, R., A. Zauner, J. Woodward, J. Myseros, S. C. Choi, J. D. Ward, A. Marmarou, and H. F. Young. 1998. Factors affecting excitatory amino acid release following severe human head injury. *Journal of Neurosurgery* 89(4):507-518.

Buzzini, S. R., and K. M. Guskiewicz. 2006. Sport-related concussion in the young athlete. *Current Opinion in Pediatrics* 18(4):376-382.

Camarillo, D. B., P. B. Shull, J. Mattson, R. Shultz, and D. Garza. 2013. An instrumented mouthguard for measuring linear and angular head impact kinematics in American football. *Annals of Biomedical Engineering* 41(9):1939-1949.

Campbell, J. N., B. Low, J. E. Kurz, S. S. Patel, M. T. Young, and S. B. Churn. 2012a. Mechanisms of dendritic spine remodeling in a rat model of traumatic brain injury. *Journal of Neurotrauma* 29(2):218-234.

Campbell, J. N., D. Register, and S. B. Churn. 2012b. Traumatic brain injury causes an FK506-sensitive loss and an overgrowth of dendritic spines in rat forebrain. *Journal of Neurotrauma* 29(2):201-217.

Carskadon, M. S., C. Acebo, and O. G. Jenni. 2004. Regulation of adolescent sleep: Implications for behavior. *Annals of the New York Academy of Sciences* 1021:276-291.

Casano-Sancho, P., L. Suarez, L. Ibanez, G. Garcia-Fructuoso, J. Medina, and A. Febrer. 2013. Pituitary dysfunction after traumatic brain injury in children: Is there a need for ongoing endocrine assessment? *Clinical Endocrinology* 79(6):853-858.

Casey, B. J., and R. M. Jones. 2010. Neurobiology of the adolescent brain and behavior: Implications for substance use disorders. *Journal of the American Academy of Child and Adolescent Psychiatry* 49(12):1189-1285.

Casey, B. J., N. Tottenham, C. Liston, and S. Durston. 2005. Imaging the developing brain: What have we learned about cognitive development? *Trends in Cognitive Sciences* 9(3):104-110.

Cater, H. L., L. E. Sundstrom, and B. Morrison. 2006. Temporal development of hippocampal cell death is dependent on tissue strain but not strain rate. *Journal of Biomechanics* 39(15):2810-2818.

Chen, J. R., Y. J. Wang, and G. F. Tseng. 2004. The effects of decompression and exogenous NGF on compressed cerebral cortex. *Journal of Neurotrauma* 21(11):1640-1651.

Chiron, C., C. Raynaud, B. Maziere, M. Zilbovicius, L. Laflamme, M. C. Masure, O. Dulac, and M. Bourguignon. 1992. Changes in regional cerebral blood flow during activation during brain maturation in children and adolescents. *Journal of Nuclear Medicine* 33(5):696-703.

Choe, M. C., T. Babikian. J. DiFiori, D. A. Hovda, and C. C. Giza. 2012. A pediatric perspective on concussion pathophysiology. *Current Opinion in Pediatrics* 24(6):689-695.

Chugani, H. T. 1998. A critical period of brain development: Studies of cerebral glucose utilization with PET. *Preventive Medicine* 27(2):184-188.

Clark, R. S., P. M. Kochanek, W. D. Obrist, H. R. Wong, R. R. Billiar, S. R. Wisniewski, and D.W. Marion. 1996. Cerebrospinal fluid and plasma nitrite and nitrate concentrations after head injury in humans. *Critical Care Medicine* 24(7):1243-1251.

Clausen, F., N. Marklund, A. Lewén, P. Enblad, S. Basu, and L. Hillered. 2012. Interstitial F(2)-isoprostane 8-iso-PGF(2α) as a biomarker of oxidative stress after severe human traumatic brain injury. *Journal of Neurotrauma* 29(5):766-775.

Coats, B., and S. S. Margulies. 2006. Material properties of human infant skull and suture at high rates. *Journal of Neurotrauma* 23(8):1222-1232.

Coats, B., S. A. Eucker, S. Sullivan, and S. S. Margulies. 2012. Finite element model predictions of intracranial hemorrhage from non-impact, rapid head rotations in the piglet. *International Journal of Developmental Neuroscience* 30(3):191-200.

Collins, M. W., M. R. Lovell, G. L. Iverson, R. Cantu, J. Maroon, and M. Field. 2002. Cumulative effects of concussion in high school athletes. *Neurosurgery* 51(5):1175-1179.

Cook, R. S., L. Schweer, K. F. Shebesta, K. Hartjes, and R. A. Falcone. 2006. Mild traumatic brain injury in children: Just another bump on the head? *Journal of Trauma Nursing* 13(2):58-65.

Creed, J. A., A. M. DiLeonardi, D. P. Fox, A. R. Tessler, and R. Raghupathi. 2011. Concussive brain trauma in the mouse results in acute cognitive deficits and sustained impairment of axonal function. *Journal of Neurotrauma* 28(4):547-563.

Crisco, J. J., R. Fiore, J. G. Beckwith, J. J. Chu, P. G. Brolinson, S. Duma, T. W. McAllister, A. C. Duhaime, and R. M. Greenwald. 2010. Frequency and location of head impact exposures in individual collegiate football players. *Journal of Athletic Training* 45(6):549-559.

Cristofori, L., B. Tavazzi, R. Gambin, R. Vagnozzi, S. Signoretti, A. M. Amorini, G. Fazzina, and G. Lazzarino. 2005. Biochemical analysis of the cerebrospinal fluid: Evidence for catastrophic energy failure and oxidative damage preceding brain death in severe head injury: A case report. *Clinical Biochemistry* 38(1):97-100.

Daneshvar, D. H., C. J. Nowinski, A. C. McKee, and R. C. Cantu. 2011. The epidemiology of sport-related concussion. *Clinical Journal of Sports Medicine* 30(1):1-17.

Daniel, R. W., S. Rowson, and S. M. Duma. 2012. Head impact exposure in youth football. *Annals of Biomedical Engineering* 40(4):976-981.

Davidsson, J., and M. Risling. 2011. A new model to produce sagittal plane rotational induced diffuse axonal injuries. *Frontiers in Neurology* 2:41.

Dayan, J., A. Bernard, B. Olliac, A. S. Mailhes, and S. Kermarrec. 2010. Adolescent brain development, risk-taking and vulnerability to addiction. *Journal of Physiology, Paris* 104(5):279-286.

Dick, R. W. 2009. Is there a gender difference in concussion incidence and outcomes? *British Journal of Sports Medicine* 43(Suppl 1):I46-I50.

Dikranian, K., R. Cohen, C. Mac Donald, Y. Pan, D. Brakefield, P. Bayly, and A. Parsadanian. 2008. Mild traumatic brain injury to the infant mouse causes robust white matter axonal degeneration which precedes apoptotic death of cortical and thalamic neurons. *Experimental Neurology* 211(2):551-560.

Duhaime, A. C., A. J. Saykin, B. C. McDonald, C. P. Dodge, C. J. Eskey, T. M. Darcey, L. L. Grate, and P. Tomashosky. 2006. Functional magnetic resonance imaging of the primary somatosensory cortex in piglets. *Journal of Neurosurgery* 104(4 Suppl):259-264.

Dunn-Meynell, A. A., and B. E. Levin. 1997. Histological markers of neuronal, axonal and astrocytic changes after lateral rigid impact traumatic brain injury. *Brain Research* 761(1):25-41.

Durham, S. R., R. Raghupathi, M. A. Helfaer, S. Marwaha, and A. C. Duhaime. 2000. Age-related differences in acute physiologic response to focal traumatic brain injury in piglets. *Pediatric Neurosurgery* 33(2):76-82.

Einaudi, S., and C. Bondone. 2007. The effects of head trauma on hypothalamic-pituitary function in children and adolescents. *Current Opinion in Pediatrics* 19(4):465-470.

Elkin, B. S., and B. Morrison. 2007. Region-specific tolerance criteria for the living brain. *Stapp Car Crash Journal* 51:127-138.

Elkin, B. S., A. Ilankovan, and B. Morrison. 2010. Age-dependent regional mechanical properties of the rat hippocampus and cortex. *Journal of Biomechanical Engineering* 132(1): 011010.

Enerson, B. E., and L. R. Drewes. 2003. Molecular features, regulation and function of monocarboxylate transporters: Implications for drug delivery. *Journal of Pharmaceutical Science* 92(8):1531-1544.

Eucker, S. A., C. Smith, J. Ralston, S. H. Friess, and S. S. Margulies. 2011. Physiological and histopathological responses following closed rotational head injury depend on direction of head motion. *Experimental Neurology* 227(1):559-564.

Fan, P., T. Yamauchi, L. J. Noble, and D. M. Ferriero. 2003. Age-dependent differences in glutathione peroxidase activity after traumatic brain injury. *Journal of Neurotrauma* 20(5):437-445.

Feeney, D. M., M. G. Boyeson, R. T. Linn, H. M. Murray, and W. G. Dail. 1981. Response to cortical injury: I. Methodology and local effects of contusions in the rat. *Brain Research* 211(1):67-77.

Feng, Y., T. M. Abney, R. J. Okamoto, R. B. Pless, G. M. Genin, and P. V. Bayly. 2010. Relative brain displacement and deformation during constrained mild frontal head impact. *Journal of the Royal Society* 7(53):1677-1688.

Field, M., M. W. Collins, M. R. Lovell, and J. Maroon. 2003. Does age play a role in recovery from sports-related concussion? A comparison of high school and collegiate athletes. *Journal of Pediatrics* 142(5):546-553.

Fineman, I., D. A. Hovda, M. Smith, A. Yoshino, and D. P. Becker. 1993. Concussive brain injury is associated with a prolonged accumulation of calcium: A 45CA autoradiographic study. *Brain Research* 624(1-2):94-102.

Fineman, I., C. C. Giza, B. V. Nahed, S. M. Lee, and D. A. Hovda. 2000. Inhibition of neocortical plasticity during development by a moderate concussive brain injury. *Journal of Neurotrauma* 17(9):739-749.

Finnie, J. W., P. C. Blumbergs, J. Manavis, R. J. Turner, S. Helps, R. Vink, R. W. Byard, G. Chidlow, B. Sandoz, J. Dutschke, and R. W. Anderson. 2012. Neuropathological changes in a lamb model of non-accidental head injury (the shaken baby syndrome). *Journal of Clinical Neuroscience* 19(8):1159-1164.

Foda, M. A., and A. Marmarou. 1994. A new model of diffuse brain injury in rats. Part II: Morphological characterization. *Journal of Neurosurgery* 80(2):301-313.

Friess, S. H., J. Ralston, S. A. Eucker, M. A. Helfaer, C. Smith, and S. S. Margulies. 2011. Neurocritical care monitoring correlates with neuropathology in a swine model of pediatric traumatic brain injury. *Neurosurgery* 69(5):1139-1147.

Funk, J. R., J. M. Cormier, C. E. Bain, H. Guzman, E. Bonugli, and S. J. Manoogian. 2011. Head and neck loading in everyday and vigorous activities. *Annals of Biomedical Engineering* 39(2):766-776.

Galland, B. C., B. J. Taylor, D. E. Elder, and P. Herbison. 2012. Normal sleep patterns in infants and children: A systematic review of observational studies. *Sleep Medicine Reviews* 16(3):213-222.

Garces, G. L., D. Medina, L. Milutinovic, P. Garavote, and E. Guerado. 2002. Normative database of isometric cervical strength in a healthy population. *Medicine and Science in Sports and Exercise* 34(3):464-470.

Gennarelli, T. A., J. H. Adams, and D. I. Graham. 1981. Acceleration induced head injury in the monkey. I. The model, its mechanical and physiological correlates. *Acta Neuropathologica Supplementum* 7:23-25.

Gennarelli, T. A., L. E. Thibault, J. H. Adams, D. I. Graham, C. J. Thompson, and R. P. Marcincin. 1982. Diffuse axonal injury and traumatic coma in the primate. *Annals of Neurology* 12(6):564-574.

Gennarelli, T. A., F. A. Pintar, and N. Yoganandan. 2003. Biomechanical tolerances for diffuse brain injury and a hypothesis for genotypic variability in response to trauma. *Annual Proceedings from the Association of Advancement in Automotive Medicine* 47:624-628.

Gessel, L. M., S. K. Fields, C. L. Collins, R. W. Dick, and R. D. Comstock. 2007. Concussions among United States high school and collegiate athletes. *Journal of Athletic Training* 42(4):495-503.

Giedd, J. N. 2004. Structural magnetic resonance imaging of the adolescent brain. *Annals of the New York Academy of Sciences* 1021:77-85.

Giedd, J. N., J. Blumenthal, N. O. Jeffries, F. X. Castellanos, H. Liu, A. Zijdenbos, T. Paus, A. C. Evans, and J. L. Rapoport. 1999. Brain development during childhood and adolescence: A longitudinal MRI study. *Nature Neuroscience* 2(10):861-863.

Giedd, J. N., A. Raznahan, K. L. Mills, and R. K. Lenroot. 2012. Review: Magnetic resonance imaging of male/female differences in human adolescent brain anatomy. *Biological Sex Differences* 3(1):19.

Giza, C. C., and D. A. Hovda. 2001. The neurometabolic cascade of concussion. *Journal of Athletic Training* 36(3):228-235.

Giza, C. C., G. S. Griesbach, and D. A. Hovda. 2005. Experience-dependent behavioral plasticity is disturbed following traumatic injury to the immature brain. *Behavioural Brain Research* 157(1):11-22.

Giza, C. C., N. S. Maria, and D. A. Hovda. 2006. N-methyl-D-aspartate receptor subunit changes after traumatic injury to the developing brain. *Journal of Neurotrauma* 23(6):950-961.

Gogtay, N., J. N. Giedd, L. Lusk, K. M. Hayashi, D. Greenstein, A. C. Vaituzis, T. F. Nugent, D. H. Herman, L. S. Clasen, A. W. Toga, J. L. Rapoport, and P. M. Thompson. 2004. Dynamic mapping of human cortical development during childhood through early adulthood. *Proceedings of the National Academy of Sciences of the United States of America* 101(21):8174-8179.

Golding, E. M., C. S. Robertson, and R. M. Bryan. 1999. The consequences of traumatic brain injury on cerebral blood flow and autoregulation: A review. *Clinical and Experimental Hypertension* 21(4):299-332.

Granite, V., and J. Carroll. 2002. Psychological response to athletic injury: Sex differences. *Journal of Sport Behavior* 25(3):243-259.

Greenough, W. T., F. R. Volkmar, and J. M. Juraska. 1973. Effects of rearing complexity on dendritic branching in frontolateral and temporal cortex of the rat. *Experimental Neurology* 41(2):371-378.

Griesbach, G. S., D. A. Hovda, R. Molteni, A. Wu, and F. Gomez-Pinilla. 2004. Voluntary exercise following traumatic brain injury: Brain-derived neurotrophic factor upregulation and recovery of function. *Neuroscience* 125(1):129-139.

Griesbach, G. S., F. Gómez-Pinilla, and D. A. Hovda. 2007. Time window for voluntary exercise-induced increases in hippocampal neuroplasticity molecules after traumatic brain injury is severity dependent. *Neurotrauma* 24(7):1161-1171.

Grindel, S. H. 2003. Epidemiology and pathophysiology of minor traumatic brain injury. *Current Sports Medicine Reports* 2(1):18-23.

Gross, H., A. Kling, G. Henry, C. Herndon, and H. Lavretsky. 1996. Local cerebral glucose metabolism in patients with long-term behavioral and cognitive deficits following mild traumatic brain injury. *Journal of Neuropsychiatry and Clinical Neurosciences* 8(3):324-334.

Grundl, P. D., K. V. Biagas, P. M. Kochanek, J. K. Schiding, M. A. Barmada, and E. M. Nemoto. 1994. Early cerebrovascular response to head injury in immature and mature rats. *Journal of Neurotrauma* 11(2):135-148.

Guskiewicz, K. M., N. L. Weaver, D. A. Padua, and W. E. Garrett. 2000. Epidemiology of concussion in collegiate and high school football players. *American Journal of Sports Medicine* 28(5):643-650.

Guskiewicz, K. M., M. McCrea, S. W. Marshall, R. C. Cantu, C. Randolph, J. A. Onate, and J. P. Kelly. 2003. Cumulative effects associated with recurrent concussion in collegiate football players: The NCAA Concussion Study. *JAMA* 290(19):2549-2555.

Hall, E. D., and J. M. Braughler. 1993. Free radicals in CNS injury. *Research Publications—Association for Research on Nervous in Mental Disease* 71:81-105.

Hall, E. D., P. K. Andrus, and P. A. Yonkers. 1993. Brain hydroxyl radical generation in acute experimental head injury. *Journal of Neurochemistry* 60(2):588-594.

Hall, E. D., M. R. Detloff, K. Johnson, and N. C. Kupina. 2004. Peroxynitrite-mediated protein nitration and lipid peroxidation in a mouse model of traumatic brain injury. *Journal of Neurotrauma* 21(1):9-20.

Hardy, W. N., C. D. Foster, M. J. Mason, K. H. Yang, A. I. King, and S. Tashman. 2001. Investigation of head injury mechanisms using neutral density technology and high-speed biplanar X-ray. *Stapp Car Crash Journal* 45:337-368.

Harmon, K., J. Drezner, M. Gammons, K. M. Guskiewicz, M. Halstead, S. A. Herring, J. S. Kutcher, A. Pana, M. Putukian, and W. O. Roberts. 2013. American Medical Society for Sports Medicine position statement: Concussion in sport. *British Journal of Sports Medicine* 47(1):15-26.

Hattori, N., S. C. Huang, H. M. Wu, E. Yeh, T. C. Glenn, P. M. Vespa, D. McArthur, M. E. Phelps, D. A. Hovda, and M. Bergsneider. 2003. Correlation of regional metabolic rates of glucose with Glasgow coma scale after traumatic brain injury. *Journal of Nuclear Medicine* 44(11):1709-1716.

Henry, L. C., S. Tremblay, Y. Boulanger, D. Ellemberg, and M. Lassonde. 2010. Neurometabolic changes in the acute phase after sports concussions correlate with symptom severity. *Journal of Neurotrauma* 27(1):65-76.

Henry, L. C., J. Tremblay, S. Tremblay, A. Lee, C. Brun, N. Lepore, H. Theoret, D. Ellemberg, and M. Lassonde. 2011. Acute and chronic changes in diffusivity measures after sports concussion. *Journal of Neurotrauma* 28(20):2049-2059.

Hoffman, M. 2012. Army ships next-gen blast sensors. http://www.military.com/daily-news/2012/07/27/army-ships-out-next-gen-blast-sensors.html (accessed October 3, 2013).

Holbourn, A. H. S. 1945. The mechanics of brain injuries. *British Medical Bulletin* 3(6): 147-149.

Hollis, S. J., M. R. Stevenson, A. S. McIntosh, E. A. Shores, M. W. Collins, and C. B. Taylor. 2009. Incidence, risk, and protective factors of mild traumatic brain injury in a cohort of Australian nonprofessional male rugby players. *American Journal of Sports Medicine* 37(12):2328-2333.

Hoshino, S., S. Kobayashi, T. Furukawa, T. Asakura, and A. Teramoto. 2003. Multiple immunostaining methods to detect traumatic axonal injury in the rat fluid-percussion brain injury model. *Neurologia Medico-Chirurgica (Tokyo)* 43(4):165-173.

Hovda, D. A., A. Yoshino, T. Kawamata, Y. Katayama, and D. P. Becker. 1991. Diffuse prolonged depression of cerebral oxidative metabolism following concussive brain injury in the rat: A cytochrome oxidase histochemistry study. *Brain Research* 567(1):1-10.

Hovda, D. A., K. Fu, H. Badie, A. Samii, P. Pinanong, and D. P. Becker. 1994. Administration of an omega-conopeptide one hour following traumatic brain injury reduces 45calcium accumulation. *Acta Neurochirurgica* 60 (Suppl):521-523.

Hsiang, J. N., J. Y. Wang, S. M. Ip, H. K. Ng, A. Stadlin, A. L. Yu, and W. S. Poon. 1997. The time course and regional variations of lipid peroxidation after diffuse brain injury in rats. *Acta Neurochirurgica (Wien)* 139(5):464-468.

Huh, J. W., M. A. Franklin, A. G. Widing, and R. Raghupathi. 2006. Regionally distinct patterns of calpain activation and traumatic axonal injury following contusive brain injury in immature rats. *Developmental Neuroscience* 28(4-5):466-476.

Huh, J. W., A. G. Widing, and R. Raghupathi. 2007. Basic science–Repetitive mild noncontusive brain trauma in immature rats exacerbates traumatic axonal injury and axonal calpain activation: A preliminary report. *Journal of Neurotrauma* 24(1):15-27.

Huh, J. W., A. G. Widing, and R. Raghupathi. 2008. Midline brain injury in the immaturer at induces sustained cognitive deficits, bihemispheric axonal injury and neurodegeneration. *Experimental Neurology* 213(1):84-92.

Humayun, M. S., S. K. Presty, N. D. Lafrance, H. H. Holcomb, H. Loats, D. M. Long, H. N. Wagner, and B. Gordon. 1989. Local cerebral glucose abnormalities in mild closed head injured patients with cognitive impairments. *Nuclear Medicine Communications* 10(5):335-344.

Huttenlocher, P. R., and A. S. Dabholkar. 1997. Regional differences in synaptogenesis in human cerebral cortex. *Journal of Comparative Neurology* 387(2):167-178.

Hylin, M. J., S. A. Orsi, J. Zhao, K. Bockhorst, A. Perez, A. N. Moore, and P. K. Dash. 2013. Behavioral and histopathological alterations resulting from mild fluid percussion injury. *Journal of Neurotrauma* 30(9):702-715.

Ibrahim, N. G., J. Ralston, C. Smith, and S. S. Margulies. 2010. Physiological and pathological responses to head rotations in toddler piglets. *Journal of Neurotrauma* 27(6):1021-1035.

Iglowstein, I., O. G. Jenni, L. Molinari, and R. H. Largo. 2003. Sleep duration from infancy to adolescence: Reference values and generational trends. *Pediatrics* 111(2):302-307.

Ip, E. Y., C. C. Giza, G. S. Griesbach, and D. A. Hovda. 2002. Effects of enriched environment and fluid percussion injury on dendritic arborization within the cerebral cortex of the developing rat. *Journal of Neurotrauma* 19(5):573-585.

Itoh, T., T. Satou, S. Nishida, M. Tsubaki, S. Hashimoto, and H. Ito. 2009. Expression of amyloid precursor protein after rat traumatic brain injury. *Neurological Research* 31(1):103-109.

Ives, J. C., M. Alderman, and S. E. Stred. 2007. Hypopituitarism after multiple concussions: A retrospective case study in an adolescent male. *Journal of Athletic Training* 42(3):431-439.

Junger, E. C., D. W. Newell, G. A. Grant, A. M. Avellino, S. Ghatham, C. M. Dauville, A. M. Lam, R. Aaslid, and H. R. Winn. 1997. Cerebral autoregulation following minor head injury. *Journal of Neurosurgery* 86(3):425-532.

Kane, M. J., M. Angoa-Perez, D. I. Briggs, D. C. Viano, C. W. Kreipke, and D. M. Kuhn. 2012. A mouse model of human repetitive mild traumatic brain injury. *Journal of Neuroscience Methods* 203(1):41-49.

Karlin, A. M. 2011. Concussion in the pediatric and adolescent population: Different population, different concerns. *Physical Medicine and Rehabilitation* 3(Suppl):S369-S379.

Kaster, T., I. Sack, and A. Samani. 2011. Measurement of the hyperelastic properties of ex vivo brain tissue slices. *Journal of Biomechanics* 44(6):1158-1163.

Katayama, Y., D. P. Becker, T. Tamura, and D. A. Hovda. 1990. Massive increases in extracellular potassium and the indiscriminate release of glutamate following concussive brain injury. *Journal of Neurosurgery* 73(6):889-900.

Kawamata, T., Y. Katayama, D. A. Hovda, A. Yohino, and D. P. Becker. 1992. Administration of excitatory amino acid antagonists via microdialysis attenuates the increase in glucose utilization seen following concussive brain injury. *Journal of Cerebral Blood Flow and Metabolism* 12(1):12-24.

Kelley, A. E., T. Schochet, and C. F. Landry. 2004. Risk taking and novelty seeking in adolescence: Introduction to part 1. *Annals of the New York Academy of Sciences* 1021:27-32.

Kelly, D. F., I. T. Gonzalo, P. Cohan, N. Berman, R. Swerdloff, and C. Wang. 2000. Hypopituitarism following traumatic brain injury and aneurysmal subarachnoid hemorrhage: A preliminary report. *Journal of Neurosurgery* 93(5):743-752.

Kerr, M. E., C. M. Bender, and E. J. Monti. 1996. An introduction to oxygen free radicals. *Heart and Lung: The Journal of Critical Care* 25(3):200-208.

Khadr, S. N., P. M. Crofton, P. A. Jones, B. Wardhaugh, J. Roach, A. J. Drake, R. A. Minns, and C. J. Kelnar. 2010. Evaluation of pituitary function after traumatic brain injury in children. *Clinical Endocrinology* 73(5):637-643.

Kieslich, M., A. Fielder, C. Heller, W. Kreuz, and G. Jacobi. 2002. Minor head injury as cause and co-factor in the aetiology of stroke in children: A report of eight cases. *Journal of Neurology, Neurosurgery, and Psychiatry* 7(1)3:13-16.

Kilbaugh, T. J., S. Bhandare, D. H. Lorom, M. Saraswati, C. L. Robertson, and S. S. Margulies. 2011. Cyclosporin A preserves mitochondrial function after traumatic brain injury in the immature rat and piglet. *Journal of Neurotrauma* 29(5):763-774.

Kimpara, H., and M. Iwamoto. 2012. Mild traumatic brain injury predictors based on angular accelerations during impacts. *Annals of Biomedical Engineering* 40(1):114-126.

King, A. I., K. H. Yang, L. Zhang, W. Hardy, and D. C. Viano. 2003. Is head injury caused by linear or angular acceleration? Proceedings of the 2003 International Research Conference on the Biomechanics of Impact. http://www.smf.org/docs/articles/hic/King_IRCOBI_2003.pdf (accessed July 1, 2013).

Kleinberger, M., E. Sun, R. H. Eppinger, S. Kuppa, and R. Saul. 1998. Development of improved injury criteria for the assessment of automotive restraint systems. National Highway Traffic Safety Administration, NHTSA Docket No. NHTSA-98-4405. September.

Kleiven, S. 2007. Predictors for traumatic brain injuries evaluated through accident reconstructions. *Stapp Car Crash Journal* 51:81-114.

Kraus, M. F., T. Susmaras, B. P. Caughlin, C. J. Walker, J. A. Sweeney, and D. M. Little. 2007. White matter integrity and cognition in chronic traumatic brain injury: A diffusion tensor imaging study. *Brain* 130(Part 10):2508-2519.

Kristman, V. L., C. H. Tator, N. Kreiger, D. Richards, L. Mainwaring, S. Jaglal, G. Tomlinson, and P. Comper. 2008. Does the apolipoprotein epsilon 4 allele predispose varsity athletes to concussion? A prospective cohort study. *Clinical Journal of Sport Medicine* 18(4):322-328.

LaPlaca, M. C., J. Zhang, R. Raghupathi, J. H. Li, F. Smith, F. M. Bareyre, S. H. Snyder, D. I. Graham, and T. K. McIntosh. 2001. Pharmacologic inhibition of poly (ADP-ribose) polymerase is neuroprotective following traumatic brain injury in rats. *Journal of Neurotrauma* 18(4):369-376.

Laurer, H., F. M. Bareyre, V. M. Lee, J. Q. Trojanowski, L. Longhi, R. Hoover, K. E. Saatman, R. Raghupathi, S. Hoshino, M. S. Grady, and T. K. McIntosh. 2001. Mild head injury increases the brain's vulnerability to a second traumatic impact. *Journal of Neurosurgery* 95(5):859-870.

Len, T. K., and J. P. Neary. 2011. Cerebrovascular pathophysiology following mild traumatic brain injury. *Clinical Physiology and Functional Imaging* 31(2):85-93.

Lewén, A., and L. Hillered. 1998. Involvement of reactive oxygen species in membrane phospholipid breakdown and energy perturbation after traumatic brain injury in the rat. *Journal of Neurotrauma* 15(7):521-530.

Li, X. Y., J. Li, D. F. Feng, and L. Gu. 2010. Diffuse axonal injury induced by simultaneous moderate linear and angular head accelerations in rats. *Neuroscience* 169(1):357-369.

Lieberman, S. A., A. L. Oberoi, C. R. Gilkison, B. E. Masel, and R. J. Urban. 2001. Prevalence of neuroendocrine dysfunction in patients recovering from traumatic brain injury. *Journal of Clinical Endocrinology and Metabolism* 86(6):2752-2756.

Lighthall, J. W. 1988. Controlled cortical impact: A new experimental brain injury model. *Journal of Neurotrauma* 5(1):1-15.

Lindgren, S., and L. Rinder. 1965. Experimental studies of head injury. I. Some factors influencing results of model experiments. *Biophysik* 2(5):320-329.

Lloyd, R., B. Parr, S. Davies, and C. Cooke. 2011. A kinetic comparison of back-loading and head-loading in Xhosa women. *Ergonomics* 54(4):380-391.

Malone, S. K. 2011. Early to bed, early to rise?: An exploration of adolescent sleep hygiene practices. *Journal of School Nursing* 27(5):348-354.

Mandera, M., D. Larysz, and M. Wojtacha. 2002. Changes in cerebral hemodynamics assessed by transcranial Doppler ultrasonography in children after head injury. *Child's Nervous System* 18(3-4):124-128.

Mansell, J., R. T. Tierney, M. R. Sitler, K. A. Swanik, and D. Stearne. 2005. Resistance training and head-neck segment dynamic stabilization in male and female collegiate soccer players. *Journal of Athletic Training* 40(4):310-319.

Marklund, N., T. Lewander, F. Clausen, and L. Hillered. 2001. Monitoring of reactive oxygen species production after traumatic brain injury in rats with microdialysis and the 4-hydroxybenzoic acid trapping method. *Journal of Neurotrauma* 18(11):1217-1227.

Marmarou, A., M. A. Foda, W. van den Brink, J. Campbell, H. Kita, and K. Demetriadou. 1994. A new model of diffuse brain injury in rats. Part I: Pathophysiology and biomechanics. *Journal of Neurosurgery* 80(2):291-300.

Maugans, T. A., C. Farley, M. Altaye, J. Leach, and K. M. Cecil. 2012. Pediatric sports-related concussion produces cerebral blood flow alterations. *Pediatrics* 129(1):28-37.

McQuire, J. C., J. C. Sutcliffe, and T. J. Coats. 1998. Early changes in middle cerebral artery blood flow velocity after head injury. *Journal of Neurosurgery* 89(4):526-532.

Meaney, D. F., and D. H. Smith. 2011. Biomechanics of concussion. *Clinics in Sports Medicine* 30(1):19-31.

Meehan, W. P., A. M. Taylor, and M. Proctor. 2011. The pediatric athlete: Younger athletes with sport-related concussion. *Clinics in Sports Medicine* 30(1):133-144.

Meehan, W. P., J. Zhang, R. Mannix, and M. J. Whalen. 2012. Increasing recovery time between injuries improves cognitive outcome after repetitive mild concussive brain injuries in mice. *Neurosurgery* 71(4):885-891.

Milman, A., A. Rosenberg, R. Weizman, and C. G. Pick. 2005. Mild traumatic brain injury induces persistent cognitive deficits and behavioral disturbances in mice. *Journal of Neurotrauma* 22(9):1003-1010.

Monson, K. L., W. Goldsmith, N. M. Barbaro, and G. T. Manley. 2003. Axial mechanical properties of fresh human cerebral blood vessels. *Journal of Biomechanical Engineering* 125 (2):288-294.

Morris, R. 1984. Developments of a water maze procedure for studying spatial learning in the rat. *Journal of Neuroscience Methods* 11(1):47-60.

Nehlig, A., A. Pereira de Vasconcelos, and S. Boyet. 1989. Postnatal changes in local cerebral blood flow measured by the quantitative autoradiographic [14C]iodoantipyrine technique in freely moving rats. *Journal of Cerebral Blood Flow and Metabolism* 9(5):579-588.

Niederland, T., H. Makovi, V. Gál, B. Andréka, C. S. Ábrahám, and J. Kovács. 2007. Abnormalities of pituitary function after traumatic brain injury in children. *Journal of Neurotrauma* 24(1):119-127.

Norwood, K. W., M. D. Deboer, M. J. Gurka, M. N. Kuperminc, A. D. Rogol, J. A. Blackman, J. B. Wamstad, M. L. Buck, and P. D. Patrick. 2010. Traumatic brain injury in children and adolescents: Surveillance for pituitary dysfunction. *Clinical Pediatrics (Phila)* 49(11):1044-1049.

O'Connell, K. M., and M. T. Littleton-Kearney. 2013. The role of free radicals in traumatic brain injury. *Biological Research for Nursing* 15(3):253-263.

O'Connell, M. T., A. Seal, J. Nortje, P. G. Al-Rawi, J. P. Coles, T. D. Fryer, D. K. Menon, J. D. Pickard, and P. J. Hutchinson. 2005. Glucose metabolism in traumatic brain injury: A combined microdialysis and [18F]-2-fluoro-2-deoxy-d-glucose-positron emission tomography (FDG-PET) study. *Acta Neurochirurgica Supplement* 95:165-168.

Ommaya, A. K. 1985. Biomechanics of head injury: Experimental aspects. In *Biomechanics of Trauma*, edited by A. M. Nahum and J. W. Melvin. Prentice-Hall, Pp. 245-269.

Ommaya, A. K., and T. A. Gennarelli. 1974. Cerebral concussion and traumatic unconsciousness. Correlation of experimental and clinical observations of blunt head injuries. *Brain* 97(4):633-654.

Ommaya, A. K., A. E. Hirsch, and J. L. Martinez. 1966. The role of whiplash in cerebral concussion. 10th Stapp Car Crash Conference, SAE, 10:314-324.

Ommaya, A. K., R. L. Grubb, and R. A. Naumann. 1971. Coup and contre-coup injury: Observations on the mechanics of visible brain injuries in the rhesus monkey. *Journal of Neurosurgery* 35(5):503-516.

Ommaya, A. K., P. Corrao, and F. S. Letcher. 1973. Head injury in the chimpanzee. Part 1: Biodynamics of traumatic unconsciousness. *Journal of Neurosurgery* 39(2):152-166.

Ommaya, A. K., W. Goldsmith, and L. Thibault. 2002. Biomechanics and neuropathology of adult and paediatric head injury. *British Journal of Neurosurgery* 16(3):220-242.

Osteen, C. L., A. H. Moore, M. L. Prins, and D. A. Hovda. 2001. Age-dependency of 45calcium accumulation following lateral fluid percussion: Acute and delayed patterns. *Journal of Neurotrauma* 18(2):141-162.

Ouckama, R., and D. J. Pearsall. 2011. Evaluation of a flexible force sensor for measurement of helmet foam impact performance. *Journal of Biomechanics* 44(5):904-909.

Ozdemir, D., N. Uysal, S. Gonenc, O. Acikgoz, A. Sonmez, A. Topcu, N. Ozdemir, M. Duman, I. Semin, and H. Ozkan. 2005. Effect of melatonin on brain oxidative damage induced by traumatic brain injury in immature rats. *Physiological Research* 54(6):631-637.

Persson, L., and L. Hillered. 1992. Chemical monitoring of neurosurgical intensive care patients using intracerebral microdialysis. *Journal of Neurosurgery* 76(1):72-80.

Petronilho, F., G. Feier, B. de Souza, C. Guglielmi, L. S. Constantino, R. Walz, J. Quevedo, and R. Dal-Pizzol. 2010. Oxidative stress in brain according to traumatic brain injury intensity. *Journal of Surgical Research* 164(2):316-320.

Pharo, H., C. Sim, M. Graham, J. Gross, and H. Hayne. 2011. Risky business: Executive function, personality, and reckless behavior during adolescence and emerging adulthood. *Behavioral Neuroscience* 125(6):970-978.

Post, A., E. S. Walsh, T. B. Hoshizaki, and M. Gilchrist. 2011. Analysis of loading curve characteristics on the production of brain deformation metrics. International Union of Theoretical and Applied Mechanics Symposium on Impact Biomechanics in Sport, Dublin, Ireland. http://www.ucd.ie/t4cms/proceedings_IUTAM.pdf (accessed July 1, 2013).

Povlishock, J. T., and C. W. Christman. 1995. The pathobiology of traumatically induced axonal injury in animals and humans: A review of current thoughts. *Journal of Neurotrauma* 12(4):555-564.

Povlishock, J. T., D. P. Becker, C. L. Cheng, and G. W. Vaughan. 1983. Axonal change in minor head injury. *Journal of Neuropathology and Experimental Neurology* 42(3):225-242.

Prange, M. T., and S. S. Margulies. 2002. Regional, directional, and age-dependent properties of the brain undergoing large deformation. *Journal of Biomechanical Engineering* 124(2):244-252.

Praticò, D., P. Reiss, L. X. Tang, S. Sung, J. Rokach, and T. K. McIntosh. 2002. Local and systemic increase in lipid peroxidation after moderate experimental traumatic brain injury. *Journal of Neurochemistry* 80(5):894-898.

Prevost, T. P., G. Jin, M. A. de Moya, H. B. Alam, S. Suresh, and S. Socrate. 2011. Dynamic mechanical response of brain tissue indentation in vivo, in situ, and in vitro. *Acta Biomaterialia* 7(12):4090-4101.

Prins, M. L., and D. A. Hovda. 1998. Traumatic brain injury in the developing rat: Effects of maturation on Morris water maze acquisition. *Journal of Neurotrauma* 15(10):799-811.

Prins, M. L., and D. A. Hovda. 2001. Mapping cerebral glucose metabolism during spatial learning: Interactions of development and traumatic brain injury. *Journal of Neurotrauma* 18(1):31-46.

Prins, M. L., and D. A. Hovda. 2009. The effects of age and ketogenic diet on local cerebral metabolic rates of glucose after controlled cortical impact injury in rats. *Journal of Neurotrauma* 26(7):1083-1093.

Prins, M. L., S. M. Lee, C. L. Y. Cheng, D. P. Becker, and D. A. Hovda. 1996. Fluid percussion brain injury in the developing and adult rat: A comparative study of mortality, morphology, intracranial pressure and mean arterial blood pressure. *Developmental Brain Research* 95(2):272-282.

Prins, M. L., A. Hales, M. Reger, C. C. Giza, and D. A. Hovda. 2010. Repeat traumatic brain injury in the juvenile rat is associated with increased axonal injury and cognitive impairments. *Developmental Neuroscience* 32(5-6):510-518.

Prins, M. L., D. Alexander, C. C. Giza, and D. A. Hovda. 2013. Repeated mild traumatic brain injury: Mechanisms of cerebral vulnerability. *Journal of Neurotrauma* 30(1):30-38.

Queen, R. M., P. Weinhold, D. T. Kirkendall, and B. Yu. 2003. Theoretical study of the effect of ball properties on impact force in soccer heading. *Medicine and Science in Sports Exercise* 35(12):2069-2076.

Raghupathi, R., and S. S. Margulies. 2002. Traumatic axonal injury after closed head injury in the neonatal pig. *Journal of Neurotrauma* 19(7):843-853.

Rao, A. M., A. Dogan, J. F. Hatcher, and R. J. Dempsey. 1998. Fluorometric assay of nitrite and nitrate in brain tissue after traumatic brain injury and cerebral ischemia. *Brain Research* 793(1-2):265-270.

Reddy, C. C., M. W. Collins, and G. A. Gioia. 2008. Adolescent sports concussion. *Physical Medicine and Rehabilitation Clinics of North America* 19(2):247-269.

Richards, H. K., S. Simac, S. Piechnik, and J. D. Pickard. 2001. Uncoupling of cerebral blood flow and metabolism after cerebral contusion in the rat. *Journal of Cerebral Blood Flow and Metabolism* 21(7):779-781.

Robbins, D. H., and J. L. Wood. 1969. Determination of the mechanical properties of bones of the skull. *Experimental Mechanics* 9(5):236-240.

Roberts, M. A., F. F. Manshadi, D. L. Bushnell, and M. E. Hines. 1995. Neurobehavioural dysfunction following mild traumatic brain injury in childhood: A case report with positive findings on positron emission tomography (PET). *Brain Injury* 9(5):427-436.

Romer, D. 2010. Adolescent risk taking, impulsivity, and brain development: Implications for prevention. *Developmental Psychobiology* 52(3):263-276.

Rose, S. R., and B. A. Auble. 2012. Endocrine changes after pediatric traumatic brain injury. *Pituitary* 15(3):267-275.

Rowson, S., and S. M. Duma. 2013. Brain injury prediction: Assessing the combined probability of concussion using linear and rotational head acceleration. *Annals of Biomedical Engineering* 41(5):873-882.

Rowson, S., S. M. Duma, J. G. Beckwith, J. J. Chu, R. M. Greenwald, J. J. Crisco, P. G. Brolinson, A. C. Duhaime, T. W. McAllister, and A. C. Maerlender. 2012. Rotational head kinematics in football impacts: An injury risk function for concussion. *Annals of Biomedical Engineering* 40(1):1-13.

Saatman, K. E., A. C. Duhaime, R. Bullock, A. I. Maas, A. Valadka, and G. T. Manley. 2008. Classification of traumatic brain injury for targeted therapies. *Journal of Neurotrauma* 25(7):719-738.

Satchell, M. A., X. Zhang, P. M. Kochanek, C. E. Dixon, L. W. Jenkins, J. Melick, C. Szabo, and R. S. Clark. 2003. A dual role for poly-ADP-ribosylation in spatial memory acquisition after traumatic brain injury in mice involving NAD+depletion and ribosylation of 14-3-3gamma. *Journal of Neurochemistry* 85(3):697-708.

Schlaepfer, W. W. 1974. Calcium-induced degeneration of axoplasm in isolated segments of rat peripheral nerve. *Brain Research* 69(2):203-215.

Schlaepfer, W. W. 1987. Neurofilaments: Structure, metabolism and implications in disease. *Journal of Neuropathology and Experimental Neurology* 46(2):117-129.

Schneider, K., and R. F. Zernicke. 1988. Computer simulation of head impact: Estimation of head-injury risk during soccer heading. *International Journal of Sport Biomechanics* 4(4):358-371.

Schulz, M. R., S. W. Marshall, F. O. Mueller, J. Yang, N. L. Weaver, W. D. Kalsbeek, and J. M. Bowling. 2004. Incidence and risk factors for concussion in high school athletes, North Carolina, 1996–1999. *American Journal of Epidemiology* 160(10):937-944.

Schwarzbold, M. L., D. Rial, T. De Bem, D. G. Machado, M. P. Cunha, A. dos Santos, D. P. dos Santos, C. P. Figueiredo, M. Farina, E. M. Goldfeder, A. L. Rodrigues, R. D. Prediger, and R. Walz. 2010. Effects of traumatic brain injury of different severities on emotional, cognitive, and oxidative stress-related parameters in mice. *Journal of Neurotrauma* 27(10):1883-1893.

Sen, S., H. Goldman, M. Morehead, S. Murphy, and J. W. Phillis. 1993. Oxypurinol inhibits free radical release from the cerebral cortex of closed head injured rats. *Neuroscience Letters* 162(1-2):117-120.

Seok, J., H. S. Warren, A. G. Cuenca, M. N. Mindrinos, H. V. Baker, W. Xu, D. R. Richards, G. P. McDonald-Smith, H. Gao, L. Hennessy, C. C. Finnerty, C. M. Lopez, S. Honari, E. E. Moore, J. P. Minei, J. Cuschieri, P. E. Bankey, J. L. Johnson, J. Sperry, A. B. Nathens, T. B. Billiar, M. A. West, M. G. Jeschke, M. B. Klein, R. L. Gamell, N. S. Gibran, B. H. Brownstein, C. Miller-Graziano, S. E. Calvano, P. H. Mason, J. P. Cobb, L. G. Rahme, S. F. Lowry, R. V. Maier, L. L. Moldawer, D. N. Herndon, R. W. Davis, W. Xiao, R. G. Tompkins, and the Inflammation and Host Response to Injury, Large Scale Collaborative Research Program. 2013. Genomic responses in mouse models poorly mimic human inflammatory diseases. *Proceedings of the National Academy of Sciences of the United States of America* 110(9):3507-3512.

Shojo, H., and K. Kibayashi. 2006. Changes in localization of synaptophysin following fluid percussion injury in the rat brain. *Brain Research* 1078(1):198-211.

Shrey, D. W., G. S. Griesbach, and C.C. Giza. 2011. The pathophysiology of concussions in youth. *Physical Medicine and Rehabilitationl Clinics of North America* 22(4):577-602.

Shultz, S. R., F. Bao, V. Omana, C. Chiu, A. Brown, and D. P. Cain. 2011. Repeated mild lateral fluid percussion brain injury in the rat causes cumulative long-term behavioral impairments, neuroinflammation, and cortical loss in an animal model of repeated concussion. *Journal of Neurotrauma* 29(2):281-294.

Singh, I. N., P. G. Sullivan, Y. Deng, L. H. Mbye, and E. D. Hall. 2006. Time course of posttraumatic mitochondrial oxidative damage and dysfunction in a mouse model of focal traumatic brain injury: Implications for neuroprotective therapy. *Journal of Cerebral Blood Flow and Metabolism* 26(11):1407-1418.

Smith, D. H., J. A. Wolf, T. A. Lusardi, V. M. Lee, and D. F. Meaney. 1999. High tolerance and delayed elastic response of cultured axons to dynamic stretch injury. *Journal of Neuroscience* 19(11):4263-4269.

Sowell, E. R., P. M. Thompson, and A. W. Toga. 2004. Mapping changes in the human cortex throughout the span of life. *Neuroscientist* 10(4):372-392.

Spear, L. P. 2010. *The Behavioral Neuroscience of Adolescence.* New York: Norton.

Stålhammar, D. 1986. Experimental models of head injury. *Acta Neurochirurgica Supplementum (Wien)* 36:33-46.

Stålhammar, D. A. 1990. The mechanism of brain injuries. In *Handbook of Clinical Neurology, Vol. 13(57): Head Injury*, edited by R. Braakman. New York: Elsevier Science Publishers. Pp. 17-41.

Stojsih, S., M. Boitano, M. Wilhelm, and C. Bir. 2010. A prospective study of punch biomechanics and cognitive function for amateur boxers. *British Journal of Sports Medicine* 44(10):725-730.

Strich, S. J. 1956. Diffuse degeneration of the cerebral white matter in severe dementia following head injury. *Journal of Neurology, Neurosurgery, and Psychiatry* 19(3):163-185.

Strich, S. J., and D. M. Oxon. 1961. Shearing of nerve fibers as a cause of brain damage due to head injury: A pathological study of twenty cases. *Lancet* 278(7200):443-448.

Sullivan, S., S. H. Friess, J. Ralston, C. Smith, K. J. Propert, P. E. Rapp, and S. S. Margulies. 2013. Behavioral deficits and axonal injury persistence after rotational head injury are direction dependent. *Journal of Neurotrauma* 30(7):520-534.

Sutton, R. L., D. A. Hovda, P. D. Adelson, E. C. Benzel, and D. P. Becker. 1994. Metabolic changes following cortical contusion: Relationships to edema and morphological changes. *Acta Neurochirurgica* 60(Suppl):446-448.

Takhounts, E. G., S. A. Ridella, V. Hasiia, R. E. Tannous, J. Q. Campbell, D. Malone, K. Danelson, J. Stitzel, S. Rowson, and S. Duma. 2008. Investigation of traumatic brain injuries using the next generation of simulated injury monitor (SIMon) finite element head model. *Stapp Car Crash Journal* 52:1-31.

Terrell, T., R. Bostick, R. Abramson, D. Xie, W. Barfield, R. Cantu, M. Stanek, and T. Ewing. 2008. APOE, APOE promoter, and tau genotypes and risk for concussion in college athletes. *Clinical Journal of Sports Medicine* 18(1):10-17.

Terrell, T. R., R. M. Bostick, and J. T. Barth. 2012. Prospective cohort study of the association of genetic polymorphisms and concussion risk and postconcussion neurocognitive deficits in college athletes. *Clinical Journal of Sports Medicine* 22(2):172-208.

Terrell, T. R., R. M. Bostick, J. Barth, D. McKeag, R. C. Cantu, R. Sloane, L. Galloway, D. Erlanger, V. Valentine, and K. Bielak. 2013. Genetic polymorphisms, concussion risk, and post concussion neurocognitive deficits in college and high school athletes. *British Journal of Sports Medicine* 47(5):e1.

Thomas, S., M. L. Prins, M. Samii, and D. A. Hovda. 2000. Cerebral metabolic response to traumatic brain injury sustained early in development: A 2-deoxy-D-glucose autoradiographic study. *Journal of Neurotrauma* 17(8):649-665.

Tierney, R. T., M. R. Sitler, B. Swanik, K. Swanik, M. Higgins, and J. Torg. 2005. Gender differences in head-neck segment dynamic stabilization during head acceleration. *Medicine and Science in Sports and Exercise* 37(2):272-279.

Tierney, R. T., M. Higgins, S. V. Caswell, J. Brady, K. McHardy, J. B. Driban, and K. Davish. 2008. Sex differences in head acceleration during heading while wearing soccer headgear. *Journal of Athletic Training* 43(6):578-584.

Tierney, R. T., J. L. Mansell, M. Higgins, J. T. McDevitt, N. Toone, J. P. Gaughan, A. Mishra, and E. Krynetskiy. 2010. Apolipoprotein E genotype and concussion in college athletes. *Clinical Journal of Sport Medicine* 20(6):464-468.

Tong, W., T. Igarashi, D. M. Ferriero, and L. J. Noble. 2002. Traumatic brain injury in the immature mouse brain: Characterization of regional vulnerability. *Experimental Neurology* 176(1):105-116.

Tontisirin, N., S. Muangman, P. Suz, C. Pihoker, D. Fisk, A. Moore, A. M. Lam, and M. S. Vivilala. 2007. Early childhood gender differences in anterior and posterior cerebral blood flow velocity and autoregulation. *Pediatrics* 119(3):610-615.

Tsuru-Aoyagi, K., M. B. Potts, A. Trivedi, T. Pfankuch, J. Raber, M. Wendland, C. P. Claus, S. E. Koh, D. Ferriero, and L. J. Noble-Haeusslein. 2009. Glutathione peroxidase activity modulates recovery in the injured immature brain. *Annals of Neurology* 65(5):540-549.

Tyurin, V. A., Y. Y. Tyurina, G. G. Borisenko, T. V. Sokolova, V. B. Ritov, P. J. Quinn, M. Rose, P. Kochanek, S. H. Graham, and V. E. Kagan. 2000. Oxidative stress following traumatic brain injury in rats: Quantitation of biomarkers and detection of free radical intermediates. *Journal of Neurochemistry* 75(5):2178-2189.

Udomphorn, Y., W. M. Armstead, and M. S. Vavilala. 2008. Cerebral blood flow and autoregulation after pediatric traumatic brain injury. *Pediatric Neurology* 38(4):225-234.

Umile, E., M. Sandel, A. Alavi, C. Terry, and R. Plotkin. 2002. Dynamic imaging in mild traumatic brain injury: Support for the theory of medial temporal vulnerability. *Archive of Physical Medical Rehabilitation* 83(11):1506-1513.

Vagnozzi, R., A. Marmarou, B. Tavazzi, S. Signoretti, D. Di Pierro, F. del Bolgia, A. M. Amorini, G. Fazzina, S. Sherkat, and G. Lazzarino. 1999. Changes of cerebral energy metabolism and lipid peroxidation in rats leading to mitochondrial dysfunction after diffuse brain injury. *Journal of Neurotrauma* 16(10):903-913.

Vagnozzi, R., S. Signoretti, B. Tavazzi, A. Lucovici, S. Marziali, G. Tarascio, A. M. Amorini, V. DiPietro, R. Delfini, and G. Lazzorino. 2008. Temporal window of metabolic brain vulnerability to concussion: A pilot 1H-magnetic resonance spectropic study in concussed athletes—Part III. *Neurosurgery* 62(6):1286-1295.

Vavilala, M. S., L. A. Lee, and A. M. Lam. 2002a. Cerebral blood flow and vascular physiology. *Anesthesiology Clinics of North America* 20(2):247-264.

Vavilala, M. S., D. W. Newell, E. Junger, C. M. Douville, R. Aaslid, F. P. Rivara, and A. M. Lam. 2002b. Dynamic cerebral autoregulation in healthy adolescents. *Acta Anaesthesiologica Scandinavica* 46(4):393-397.

Vavilala, M. S., L. A. Lee, K. Boddu, E. Visco, D. W. Newell, J. J. Zimmerman, and A. M. Lam. 2004. Cerebral autoregulation in pediatric traumatic brain injury. *Pediatric Critical Care Medicine* 5(3):257-263.

Vavilala, M., M. Kincaid, S. Muangman, P. Suz, I. Rozet, and A. Lam. 2005. Gender differences in cerebral blood flow velocity and autoregulation between the anterior and posterior circulations in healthy children. *Pediatric Research* 58(3):574-578.

Vespa, P., M. Prins, E. Ronne-Engstrom, M. Caron, E. Shalmon, D. A. Hovda, N. A. Martin, and D. P. Becker. 1998. Increase in extracellular glutamate caused by reduced cerebral perfusion pressure and seizures after human traumatic brain injury: A microdialysis study. *Journal of Neurosurgery* 89(6):971-982.

Viano, D. C., A. Hamberger, H. Bolouri, and A. Saljo. 2012. Evaluation of three animal models for concussion and serious brain injury. *Annals of Biomedical Engineering* 40(1): 212-226.

Vink, R., P. G. Mullins, M. D. Temple, W. Bao, and A. I. Faden. 2001. Small shifts in craniotomy position in the lateral fluid percussion injury model are associated with differential lesion development. *Journal of Neurotrauma* 18(8):839-847.

Wada, K., K. Chatzipanteli, S. Kraydieh, R. Busto, and W. D. Dietrich. 1998. Inducible nitric oxide synthase expression after traumatic brain injury and neuroprotection with aminoguanidine treatment in rats. *Neurosurgery* 43(6):1427-1436.

Wall, W. J., and M. Shani. 2008. Are animal models as good as we think? *Theriogenology* 69(1):2-9.

Werner, C., and K. Engelhard. 2007. Pathophysiology of traumatic brain injury. *British Journal of Anaesthesia* 99(1):4-9.

Worley, G., J. M. Hoffman, S. S. Paine, S. L. Kalman, S. J. Claerhout, O. B. Boyko, R. S. Kandt, C. C. Santos, M. W. Hanson, and W. J. Oakes. 1995. 18-Flurodeoxyglucose positron emission tomography in children and adolescents with traumatic brain injury. *Developmental Medicine and Child Neurology* 37(3):213-220.

Xiong, Y., A. Mahmood, and M. Chopp. 2013. Animal models of traumatic brain injury. *Nature Reviews Neuroscience* 14(2):128-142.

Yakovlev, P. I., and A. R. Lecours. 1967. The myelogenetic cycles of regional maturation of the brain. In *Regional Development of the Brain in Early Life*, edited by A. Minkowski. Oxford: Blackwell Scientific. Pp. 3-70.

Yoshino, A., D. A. Hovda, T. Kawamata, Y. Katayama, and D. P. Becker. 1991. Dynamic changes in local cerebral glucose utilization following cerebral conclusion in rats: Evidence of a hyper- and subsequent hypometabolic state. *Brain Research* 561(1):106-119.

Yoshino, A., D. A. Hovda, T. Kawamata, Y. Katayama, and D. P. Becker. 1992. Hippocampal CA3 lesion prevents postconcussive metabolic dysfunction in CA1. *Journal of Cerebral Blood Flow and Metabolism* 12(6):996-1006.

Zemper, E. D. 2003. Two-year prospective study of relative risk of a second cerebral concussion. *American Journal of Physical Medicine and Rehabilitation* 82(9):653-659.

Zhou, C., S. A. Eucker, T. Durduran, G. Yu, J. Ralston, S. H. Friess, R. N. Ichord, S. S. Margulies, and A. G. Yodh. 2009. Diffuse optical monitoring of hemodynamic changes in piglet brain with closed head injury. *Journal of Biomedical Optics* 14(3):034015.

Zhu, Q., M. Prange, and S. Margulies. 2006. Predicting unconsciousness from a pediatric brain injury threshold. *Developmental Neuroscience* 28(4-5):388-395.

Zuckerman, S. L., Y. M. Lee, M. J. Odom, G. S. Solomon, J. A. Forbes, and A. K. Sills. 2012. Recovery from sports-related concussion: Days to return to neurocognitive baseline in adolescents versus young adults. *Surgical Neurology International* 3:130.

3

Concussion Recognition, Diagnosis, and Acute Management

One of the first challenges in responding to sports-related concussions is to recognize that a player may have sustained a concussion and therefore should be removed from the activity for further evaluation. As discussed in Chapter 1, although previous generations of athletes were encouraged to "shake it off" and return to play, current guidelines (Halstead et al., 2010; Harmon et al., 2013; McCrory et al., 2013b) and most state laws (NCSL, 2013) require athletes to be removed from competition or practice if a concussion is suspected so that a more formal evaluation can be completed. In this chapter, the committee responds to the portions of its charge concerning cognitive, affective, and behavioral changes that can occur during the acute phase of concussion; hospital- and non-hospital-based diagnostic tools; and the treatment and management of sports concussion. The chapter provides an overview of concussion screening and diagnosis, including sideline assessments at the time of injury, subsequent clinical evaluation, and the use of evaluation tools such as symptom checklists, and neuropsychological testing. The chapter also reviews the signs and symptoms of concussions and various considerations pertaining to the acute management of concussion, including the reintegration of concussed individuals into academic and athletic activities.

SIDELINE ASSESSMENT

The assessment of an injured player is facilitated by the presence of a certified athletic trainer, team physician, or other health care provider at the venue (e.g., field, gymnasium, or rink) where the injury occurred. However, the vast majority of young athletes practice and play in circumstances where trained personnel are not routinely available to make sideline injury assessments, and the responsibility for determining whether to remove an athlete from play falls on coaches, parents, players, and, perhaps, officials. A further impediment to identification is that symptoms may not become apparent for several hours after injury, and one result of this is that a large number of concussions are not identified until 24 hours or more after the injury (Duhaime et al., 2012; McCrory et al., 2013b). The Centers for Disease Control and Prevention (CDC) Heads Up campaign is designed to educate coaches, parents, and athletes about the prevention and recognition of and response to concussions (CDC, 2012a). A central feature of the campaign is the dissemination of information about the signs and symptoms of concussion (see Table 3-1) along with the message that players suspected of having sustained a concussion should be removed from play for the remainder of the day, referred to a health care provider for evaluation, and not permitted to return to play until they have been cleared by a health professional trained in concussion diagnosis and management (CDC, 2012a).

The sideline evaluation of a player's symptoms may be complicated by the tendency of athletes to underreport their symptoms (Anderson et al., 2013; Dziemianowicz et al., 2012; McCrea et al., 2004). A 2004 study

TABLE 3-1 Signs and Symptoms of Concussions Relevant to Sideline Assessment

Signs Observed	Symptoms Reported by Athlete
• Appears dazed or stunned (such as glassy eyes) • Is confused about assignment or position • Forgets an instruction or play • Is unsure of score or opponent • Moves clumsily or has poor balance • Answers questions slowly • Loses consciousness (even briefly) • Shows mood, behavior, or personality changes • Cannot recall events prior to hit or fall • Cannot recall events after hit or fall	• Headache or "pressure" in head • Nausea or vomiting • Balance problems or dizziness • Double or blurry vision • Sensitivity to light or noise • Feeling sluggish, hazy, foggy, or groggy • Concentration or memory problems • Confusion • Feeling more emotional, nervous, or anxious • Does not "feel right" or is "feeling down"

SOURCE: Based on CDC, 2012b.

of high school football players found that 41 percent of subjects reported not wanting to leave the game as their reason for not reporting a possible concussion, and 66 percent said they did not report their symptoms because they did not think their injury was serious enough to warrant medical attention (McCrea et al., 2004).[1] In a 2012 survey of high school football players, a majority indicated that it was "okay" to play with a concussion and said that they would "play through any injury to win a game," despite being knowledgeable about the symptoms and dangers of concussions (Anderson et al., 2013; see also Coyne, 2013; Kroshus et al., 2013; Register-Mihalik et al., 2013a,c; Torres et al., 2013). In addition, concussion signs and symptoms may develop and evolve over time, particularly within the first hours following injury (Duhaime et al., 2012; McCrory et al., 2013b). The mantra for laypersons faced with a potentially concussed athlete is "when in doubt, sit them out": If a player has received "a bump, blow, or jolt to the head or body" and exhibits or reports one or more of the signs or symptoms of concussion, the player may have sustained a concussion (CDC, 2012a).

Appropriately trained personnel have a number of tools available for use in the initial assessment of an individual for a possible concussion (see, e.g., Table 3-2; Appendix C). The Standardized Assessment of Concussion (SAC) and the Sport Concussion Assessment Tool (SCAT) 3 or Child SCAT3 were developed for the sideline evaluation of potentially concussed athletes. The Military Acute Concussion Evaluation (MACE) is a screening tool used to assess service members involved in a potentially concussive event. Such tools as well as balance tests (see Table 3-2) may be used either by trained responders as part of an acute sideline or in-field assessment or by health care providers during subsequent clinical evaluation. It is important to note, however, that because of the natural evolution of concussions, not all concussed athletes will be identified at the time of (presumed) injury even when personnel trained in concussion recognition are present (McCrory et al., 2013b). Duhaime and colleagues (2012) found that 50 percent of a sample of collegiate athletes who sustained a diagnosed concussion (with athletic trainers present for all games and practices) did not experience an "immediate or near immediate" onset of symptoms.

---

[1]The reasons for athletes not reporting concussion were not mutually exclusive. The subjects were asked to select all that applied.

TABLE 3-2 Sideline Concussion Screening Tools

Test	Function Assessed	Baseline Needed
Glasgow Coma Scale (GCS) (Teasdale and Jennett, 1974)	Degree of brain impairment	No
Standardized Assessment of Concussion (SAC) (McCrea, 2001; McCrea et al., 1998, 2000)	Memory and attention processes	Recommended
Sport Concussion Assessment Tool (SCAT) 3 and Child SCAT3 (McCrory et al., 2013a,c)	Compilation of: GCS, SAC, BESS, symptom checklist, and neck evaluation	Recommended
Military Acute Concussion Evaluation (MACE) (DVBIC, 2012)	Compilation of event history, symptom checklist, modified SAC, neurological screening	
Balance Error Scoring System (BESS) (Riemann et al., 1999)	Central integration of vestibular, visual, and somatosensory information	Normative data available but baseline recommended
Sensory Organization Test (SOT) (Neurocom, 2013)	Central integration of vestibular, visual, and somatosensory information	
King-Devick Test (Galetta et al., 2011)	Saccadic eye movements	Recommended
Clinical reaction time (RT_{clin}) (Eckner et al., 2010, 2013)	Reaction time	Yes

CLINICAL EVALUATION

Concussion Diagnosis

Given the absence of a diagnostic test or biomarker for concussion, the current cornerstone of concussion diagnosis is confirming the presence of a constellation of signs and symptoms after an individual has experienced a hit to the head or body. Symptoms are self-reported by the athlete, often using a symptom scale. Reliance on an athlete's self-report of symptoms as a fundamental part of diagnosing a concussion is complicated by the subjective nature of the assessment and by the possibility of an athlete under-reporting the symptoms (Anderson et al., 2013; Dziemianowicz et al., 2012; McCrea et al., 2004). Using multiple evaluation tools, such as symptom scales and checklists, balance testing, and neurocognitive assessments, may increase the sensitivity and specificity of concussion identification (Broglio et al., 2007b; Guskiewicz and Register-Mihalik, 2011; Harmon et al., 2013; Register-Mihalik et al., 2013b), and this is the current preferred method of diagnosing a concussion, although existing evidence is insufficient to determine the best combination of measures (Giza et al., 2013).

Traditional neuroimaging techniques, such as standard computed tomography (CT) and magnetic resonance imaging (MRI) (see Box 3-1), are

---

BOX 3-1
Imaging Techniques

A number of imaging techniques have evolved for measuring the structure, function, and connectivity of the developing human brain in vivo. The most commonly used techniques, which are briefly described below, vary in invasiveness (i.e., requirement of radioactive isotope, intravenous injection, or concentrated radiation).

Computed Tomography (CT) uses focused X-rays together with computer imaging technology to make three-dimensional pictures of the head and can detect skull fracture, hemorrhage, and swelling.

Diffusion tensor imaging (DTI) noninvasively measures axonal microstructure based on diffusion of water molecules that are impeded by the orientation, myelination, and regularity of fibers. The most common measures include water diffusion (*mean diffusivity*) and the directionality and strength of the diffusion (*fractional anisotropy*).

Functional magnetic resonance imaging (fMRI) noninvasively measures changes in blood oxygenation in the brain that are assumed to reflect changes in neural activity. Activity is measured either while the individual is performing a task (*task-based fMRI*) to link brain activity with cognitive performance or while at rest (*resting state fMRI*) to examine synchronous activity across brain regions.

Magnetic resonance imaging (MRI) uses a magnetic field and pulses of radio wave energy to perturb water molecules in the brain to generate images of different types of brain tissue. This noninvasive technique is used to measure regional and whole brain volume and to identify brain lesions and bleeds.

Magnetic resonance spectroscopy (MRS) uses signals from water molecules to measure concentrations of metabolites noninvasively.

Single-photon emission computed (SPECT) and *positron emission tomography (PET)* measure cerebral metabolism and blood flow using intravenous injections of radioactive isotopes to construct pictures of functional processes of the brain, including glucose metabolism and blood flow.

used to rule out more severe head and brain injuries, such as skull fractures and intracranial hemorrhages, as well as cerebral swelling that would require surgical intervention (Giza et al., 2013; McCrory et al., 2013b; Suskauer and Huisman, 2009). Because of its accessibility in the emergency room, CT is the most commonly used imaging technique for clinical assessment of head trauma (Belanger et al., 2007; Toledo et al., 2012). CT exposes the individual to radiation, which is an important consideration when evaluating youth. The American Academy of Neurology has recently recommended that CT not be used to evaluate suspected sports-related concussion in the absence of signs or symptoms of more serious traumatic brain injury (TBI) (Giza et al., 2013). Although MRIs avoid the use of ionizing radiation, instead using a magnetic field and pulses of radio wave energy to image different types of brain and body tissue, they too are of little diagnostic value for concussions per se, because structural imaging results are normal in concussions that are uncomplicated by skull fracture or hematoma.

Newer imaging techniques (see Box 3-1), such as magnetic resonance spectroscopy, positron emission tomography, single-photon emission computed tomography, functional magnetic resonance imaging, and diffusion tensor imaging—which all can be used to track metabolic, blood flow, and axonal changes—build on animal work and clinical outcome measures in mild traumatic brain injury (mTBI). Although such techniques may be useful in the future for assessing sports-related concussions, at present they have not been validated for clinical use (Cubon et al., 2011; DiFiori and Giza, 2010; Jantzen et al., 2004; Koerte et al., 2012; Lovell et al., 2007; Vagnozzi et al., 2010; Virji-Babul et al., 2013).

Signs and Symptoms

The signs and symptoms of concussion reported within 1 to 7 days post injury (see Table 3-3) typically fall into four categories—physical (somatic), cognitive, emotional (affective), and sleep—and patients will experience one or more symptoms from one or more categories. A study of high school athletes found that female athletes reported more somatic symptoms (drowsiness and sensitivity to noise) while their male counterparts reported more cognitive symptoms (amnesia and confusion/disorientation), although the number of symptoms reported did not differ by sex (Frommer et al., 2011). Kontos and colleagues (2012) have reported a revised factor structure—cognitive-migraine-fatigue, affective, somatic, and sleep. In their study, high school athletes reported lower levels of the sleep symptom factor than did college athletes, and female athletes reported higher levels of the affective symptom factor than did their male counterparts. There were no age or sex differences for the other factors, and the interaction between age and sex

TABLE 3-3 Concussion Symptoms by Category

Somatic	Cognitive	Emotional	Sleep
• Headache • Fuzzy or blurry vision • Dizziness • Fatigue • Drowsiness • Sensitivity to light • Sensitivity to noise • Balance problems • Nausea or vomiting (early on)	• Difficulty thinking clearly • Feeling slowed down • Difficulty concentrating • Difficulty remembering new information	• Irritability • Sadness • Feeling more emotional • Nervousness or anxiety	• Sleeping more than usual • Sleeping less than usual • Trouble falling asleep

SOURCE: CDC, 2013.

was not significant (Kontos et al., 2012). It should be noted that the symptoms reported differently by males and females in the Frommer study fell within a single factor in the structure presented by Kontos and colleagues.

Clinical Assessment

Because concussions can affect several aspects of brain function, a battery of tests is needed to assess and monitor a concussion. Relying on any one type of test for the ongoing monitoring of a concussed athlete and for making the decision to clear the athlete for activity risks an incomplete picture because the functions covered by each test recover at different rates (Ellemberg et al., 2009; Guskiewicz, 2011; Guskiewicz and Register-Mihalik, 2011).

A comprehensive concussion assessment includes symptom scores, objective measures of postural stability (Hunt et al., 2009), and cognitive testing as is often done with neuropsychological testing. Broglio and colleagues (2007b) found that a complete battery of tests, including assessment of neurocognitive functioning, self-reported symptom assessments, and postural control evaluation, was more sensitive to concussions than was each test individually. The sensitivity of the complete battery ranged from 89 to 96 percent, with the tests detecting no impairment in the other 4 to 11 percent of athletes diagnosed with concussion.

Register-Mihalik and colleagues (2013b) used a healthy sample of college football players to establish reliable change confidence intervals for common clinical concussion measures and applied the reliable change parameters to a sample of concussed players examined before and after injury. Outcome measures included symptom severity scores, Automated Neuropsychological Assessment Metrics (ANAM) computerized neuropsychological battery throughput scores, and SOT composite scores. Concussed athletes (n=132) were assessed within 5 days of injury. Based on the percentage of athletes with reliable change scores below or above various confidence interval cutoffs (80 percent, 90 percent, 95 percent), they calculated sensitivity and specificity based on the percent of cases that declined by more than the reliable change metric. At all three confidence intervals, individual tests and total battery scores exceeded 90 percent specificity, indicating that when there was either no change or an improvement, it was predictive of the athlete not having a concussion. On the other hand, a decline in the scores was not predictive of having a concussion. Although having at least one score decline across the entire battery improved sensitivity, the sensitivity was still at 50 percent. The authors emphasize the importance of using a total battery in the assessment of concussion. In this particular battery, score declines did not predict concussions any better than chance.

Symptom Assessment

An athlete who has had a concussion often will complete a post-concussion symptom scale at each visit with his or her health care provider. These self-reports of symptoms not only provide information pertinent to concussion diagnosis but also serve as the foundation of monitoring recovery and decision making about the individual's return to school and physical activity. A variety of symptom checklists are available and are usually completed by the athlete with each symptom graded using a Likert scale (e.g., 0 is "not experiencing" and 6 is "most severe"), although a few use a "yes/no" classification (Valovich McLeod and Leach, 2012). The variety and psychometric properties of several commonly used symptom scales and checklists are discussed later in the chapter (see also Appendix C).

Balance Testing

The dizziness and balance disturbances reported following an impact to the head or body may result from disruption of the central integration of vestibular, visual, and somatosensory information. Postural instability has been seen in patients following mild, moderate, and severe TBI (Geurts et al., 1996), while Guskiewicz (2001) found balance disturbances in college athletes within 2 days following a concussion. Other researchers have corroborated these results, and the equilibrium of the athlete is now objectively tested as a part of an acute concussion evaluation (Cavanaugh et al., 2005; Covassin et al., 2012a; McCrea et al., 2003; Register-Mihalik et al., 2008) carried out using a tool such as the BESS or SOT, described in Appendix C.

Neuropsychological Testing

Neuropsychological testing has become commonplace in the evaluation of concussed athletes. Traditionally neuropsychological tests have not been used to make diagnoses but rather to characterize cognitive function, testing memory, speed, and processing time. Although neuropsychological tests are able to detect cognitive changes in injured athletes, these tests are also sensitive to state effects which might include the symptoms associated with the injury (Fazio et al., 2007). A study by Van Kampen and colleagues (2006) demonstrated that neuropsychological testing improves diagnostic accuracy, particularly in ruling out a concussion if the test results are normal or typical relative to an appropriate individual or group norm (baseline). However, questions have been raised about whether the presence of ongoing cognitive deficits in the absence of symptoms actually predicts any risk for youth in terms of recurrent injury or long-term functional deficits or, conversely, whether the resolution of cognitive deficits on neuropsychological testing is helpful in predicting when it is safe for an athlete to return to full physical activity (Kirkwood et al., 2009). A full discussion of the use of neuropsychological testing in concussion diagnosis and management appears later in the chapter.

Electroencephalography

The electroencephalogram (EEG) provides a reading of the electrical activity on the scalp, which originates within the neurons (gray matter) that make up the surface of the brain. Quantitative EEG (QEEG) techniques record this EEG activity from large arrays of electrodes on the scalp and are effective in detecting changes in brain electrical processing following concussion (Gosselin et al., 2009) as well as after behavior deficits have disappeared (McCrea et al., 2010; Prichep et al., 2013). McCrea and colleagues (2010) compared performance and QEEG measures on 28 high school and college athletes who experienced sports-related concussions with those recorded from 28 matched, uninjured controls. All underwent pre-season baseline testing on QEEG measures as well as on measures of concussive symptoms, postural stability, and cognitive functioning. Controls were matched to injured players based on their baseline tests. Clinical testing and QEEG were performed on the day of injury and were repeated 8 days and 45 days after injury. Although both groups performed identically prior to injury, after injury the concussion group differed significantly from controls, exhibiting more severe levels of post-concussion behavior symptoms through day 3. Importantly, QEEG measures continued to show increasingly larger differences through day 8 even though no behavioral differences occurred after day 3, suggesting that abnormalities in brain function continued to increase for at least a week following injury, despite the absence of behavior impairments. Barr and colleagues (2012) reported similar results through 45 days post injury. QEEG was also much more effective in predicting when concussed athletes would be ready to return to play. Prichep and colleagues (2013) used a QEEG discriminant function algorithm based on frontal electrode sites to create a TBI Index of brain function that discriminated between those with mild (n=51) and those with moderate concussions (n=14) at 8 days and 45 days post injury. Only the QEEG index predicted return to play before 14 days post injury versus after 14 days post injury. Accuracy was 80 percent in both cases. Such results suggest that QEEG techniques could provide a more effective means to identify athletes with impairments following concussion and to predict when they might more safely return to play.

The event-related potential (ERP) is a portion of the continuous EEG signal, but it differs from the EEG in that the ERP is time-locked to the onset of a discrete stimulus. Upon onset, the EEG desynchronizes and produces an electrical waveform composed of a series of positive and negative voltage fluctuations that can differ in their amplitude (in μV, or millionths of a volt) and latency (in milliseconds). Under most conditions, the ERP continues for approximately 500 to 1,200 milliseconds before it returns to the baseline EEG signal (Molfese et al., 2001). Researchers report numerous instances in which information obtained using ERPs converges with functional findings from fMRI, magnetoencephalography, near-infrared and PET techniques. The advantage of the ERP measure over most other imaging techniques is that it provides very rapid temporal information about the order in which different neural and cognitive processes occur. As Broglio and colleagues (2011) note, this tool has been successful in identifying relationships between brain-behavior measures in concussed versus nonconcussed athletes. The most studied of the ERP components is the P300 or P3b component. Baillargeon and colleagues (2012) reported that this component is reliably smaller in children, adolescents, and adults who have experienced a concussion than in individuals who do not have a concussion. Importantly, as in the case of QEEG, ERP studies show that such differences may continue even after other indications of concussive injury—such as behavior tests and somatic complaints—suggest recovery, indicating that persistent abnormalities in the P3b could reflect suboptimal compensation in concussed athletes. Thériault and colleagues (2009) suggest that if such effects persist, they may indicate that a concussed athlete is at increased risk for future concussions. Subsequent concussions also appear to alter brain responses. Thériault and colleagues (2011) identified impairments of working memory storage capacity that correlated with athletes' history of concussions. Gosselin and colleagues (2012a) also recorded visual ERPs during a working memory task from 44 patients identified as having mTBI

(7 to 8 months post injury) and 40 control volunteers matched for age (19 to 41 years of age) and sex. They reported that the smaller amplitude ERPs correlated with slower reaction times and poorer working memory. Importantly, results did not differ for the type of injury (e.g., sports concussion versus motor vehicle).

There is some consensus in the literature that both QEEG and ERP procedures can detect differences in performance and neural responses in concussed versus non-concussed student athletes in high school and college even when behavior measures fail to do so. However, these findings are true for a relatively small set of tasks that assess a limited array of cognitive abilities. Use of a broader range of tasks that measure different aspects of cognitive processes is necessary to provide a comprehensive view of behaviors most likely affected and those more likely spared by concussion.

Serum Biomarkers

After a brain injury, proteins may leak from damaged cells into the cerebrospinal fluid, then cross the blood-brain barrier to enter into the bloodstream. Although research on serum brain biomarkers in adults with severe TBI dates back to the 1970s, research on serum biomarkers for milder TBI and in children has emerged in the last 15 years, and the literature on biomarkers for mTBI or concussion in the pediatric population is very limited (Berger and Zuckerbraun, 2012). Potential roles for serum biomarkers in the diagnosis and management of sports-related head injury include (1) distinguishing individuals with a concussion from those with non-concussion head injury; (2) identifying individuals who may have a skull fracture or more severe intracranial injury (e.g., intracranial hemorrhage, cerebral swelling); and (3) identifying those individuals who may be at risk for a prolonged recovery (Berger and Zuckerbraun, 2012). Three biomarkers in particular have emerged from the mTBI literature: S100B, neuron-specific enolase (NSE), and cleaved tau protein (CTP) (Berger and Zuckerbraun, 2012; Finnoff et al., 2011).

S100B is a protein that is found in the brain and also in cartilage and skin. It originates in the glial cells, and plays a role in neuronal proliferation, differentiation, regeneration, and apoptosis (Geyer et al., 2009). Geyer and colleagues (2009) examined S100B levels in 148 children ages 6 months to 15 years of age with either head injury alone or head injury accompanied by symptoms of mTBI. They found that S100B did not readily discriminate between the two groups. Other studies have found elevated S100B levels in uninjured adult marathon runners, adult ice hockey players, adult boxers, and adult basketball players, which suggests that S100B is increased by extracranial release due to exercise (Hasselblatt et al., 2004; Otto et al., 2000; Stålnacke et al., 2003), which may limit its usefulness as a biomarker for identifying sports-related concussion. In addition, the normal level of S100B varies with age and is particularly high in children under 2 years of age, indicating the need for age-specific normative values. S100B also has a short half-life, so the time a blood sample is obtained after injury is important (Berger and Zuckerbraun, 2012). All of these factors can lead to inadequate and confusing results, which limit the current utility of serum biomarkers (Filippidis et al., 2010).

S100B may have a role in the identification of individuals who require further assessment (e.g., neuroimaging) for intracranial injury. Adult studies have shown that S100B may be useful for identifying individuals with head injury who do not have intracranial injury thereby preventing unnecessary imaging procedures (Berger and Zuckerbraun, 2012). Castellani and colleagues (2009) studied 109 children and adolescents (0 to 18 years of age) diagnosed with mTBI who underwent CT. They found that normal S100B levels predicted the absence of intracranial injury and skull fracture with 100 percent accuracy. Another study of 152 children under 18 years of age with closed head trauma found higher levels of S100B in children with intracranial injury than in those without (Bechtel et al., 2009). However, the study included some patients with more severe TBI and was not designed to maximize sensitivity; the study demonstrated only a 90 percent negative predictive value for intracranial injury (Berger and Zuckerbraun, 2012).

NSE is found in neuron cytoplasm as well as in smooth muscle cells, adipose cells, red blood cells, and platelets. Because of the presence of NSE in red blood cells and platelets, hemolysis of blood samples, which is common in pediatric samples, may lead to false positive results when using NSE levels to evaluate mTBI (Berger and Zuckerbraun, 2012). The previously mentioned study by Geyer and colleagues (2009) showed that NSE was insensitive for distinguishing children and adolescents with head injury and symptoms of mTBI from those with head injury only. A study of 50 children and adolescents 0 to 18 years of age with blunt head trauma (not all mTBI) found that NSE levels in the acute phase following injury were neither sensitive nor specific for detecting the presence of intracranial injury; nearly 25 percent of patients identified with intracranial injury following CT scans would have been missed (Fridriksson et al., 2000). The study did not report the negative predictive value of a normal NSE level (Berger and Zuckerbraun, 2012).

Several pediatric TBI studies suggest that high levels of NSE and S100B and myelin-basic protein may be associated with poorer outcome (Bandyopadhyay et al., 2005; Beers et al., 2007; Berger et al., 2007), but none was limited to patients with mTBI (Berger and Zuckerbraun, 2012). CTP is a microtubule-associated protein in axons. No studies were found that looked at CTP use in pediatric concussions, but studies showed that

CTP had no diagnostic or prognostic value with adult mTBI (Bazarian et al., 2006; Finnoff et al., 2011).

There is little research on the use of serum biomarkers in the diagnosis and management of pediatric concussions. Although appropriately sensitive and specific serum biomarkers could be of great diagnostic and prognostic value in sports-related concussion sometime in the future, there currently is no evidence to support their use. There is some evidence, however, to suggest that normal levels of S100B following head injury may predict individuals who do *not* have intracranial injury.

Symptom Scales and Checklists

Concussion symptom checklists survey a broad range of symptoms that are considered to be pathognomonic of concussion. Of the approximately 20 different symptom scales commonly used to evaluate concussion, 14 are variations of 6 core scales,[2] which include symptoms associated with sports-related concussion, although the number of items on each scale varies (Alla et al., 2009; Valovich McLeod and Leach, 2012). A 2009 review of literature pertaining to the psychometric properties of these self-report concussion scales and checklists found that very few of them had been developed systematically or had published psychometric properties (Alla et al., 2009; Valovich McLeod and Leach, 2012). The recent American Academy of Neurology guideline states that "evidence indicates it is likely that [a symptom scale or checklist] will accurately identify concussion in athletes involved in an event during which biomechanical forces were imparted to the head" (Giza et al., 2013, p. 3). The guideline indicates that the sensitivity of such symptom reporting tools ranges from 64 to 89 percent and their specificity ranges from 91 to 100 percent (Giza et al., 2013).

A 2009 literature review of symptom scales used in the pediatric, adolescent, and young adult populations (ages 5 to 22 years) identified one research-based scale and four scales that were in clinical use; psychometric evidence for the scales was assessed for younger children (5 to 12 years) and for adolescents and young adults (13 to 22 years) (Gioia et al., 2009).[3] The psychometric evidence relating to symptom scales is stronger for ado-

---

[2]The core scales are the Pittsburgh Steelers Post-Concussion scale (17 items), Post-Concussion Symptom Assessment Questionnaire (10 items), Concussion Resolution Index post-concussion questionnaire (15 items), Signs and Symptoms Checklist (34 items), Sport Concussion Assessment Tool (SCAT) post-concussion symptom scale (25 items), and Concussion Symptom Inventory (12 items).

[3]The research-based scale is the Health and Behavior Inventory; the four clinical scales are the Post-Concussion Symptom Scale, Graded Symptom Checklist/Scale, Rivermead Post-Concussion Symptom Questionnaire, and Post-Concussion Symptom Inventory/Acute Concussion Evaluation (Gioia et al., 2009).

lescents than for younger children, and there is reasonable evidence to support the validity of the scales, although data on their reliability is limited and additional research is needed (Gioia et al., 2009). A more recent review by Janusz and colleagues (2012) discussed the psychometric properties of these same symptom scales as well as of the Concussion Symptom Inventory (CSI) (Randolph et al., 2009) and the Acute Concussion Evaluation (ACE) (Gioia et al., 2008a).

Randolph and colleagues (2009) analyzed a large set of data from three separate projects to develop the 12-item CSI, which is the first empirically derived symptom scale for concussion identification and short-term serial use following a sports-related concussion. The CSI was shown to be as effective as longer symptom inventories, such as the Graded Symptom Checklist, at recognizing concussions.

TABLE 3-4 Measures of Post-Concussion Symptomatology

Instrument	Age Range (years)	Parent Form
Health and Behavior Inventory (HBI) (Ayr et al., 2009)	8-15	Yes
Acute Concussion Evaluation (ACE) (Gioia and Collins, 2006; Gioia et al., 2008a)	3-18	Yes
Concussion Symptom Inventory (CSI) (Randolph et al., 2009)	High school–college	No
Graded Symptom Checklist/Scale (GSC/GSS) (Mailer et al., 2008; Piland et al., 2006)	≥ 13	No

The characteristics of the instruments and their psychometric properties are discussed in Appendix C and summarized in Table 3-4.

The Health Behavior Inventory and Post-Concussion Symptom Inventory (PCSI) are the only measures that are well studied in children under the age of 12 and have the advantage of having reports from parents and, in the case of the PCSI, teachers. Studies looking at the concordance of symptoms reported by 8- to 15-year-old patients and their parents found that mean symptom ratings tended to be higher for children as compared to their parents (Ayr et al., 2009; Hajek et al., 2011). Gioia has also found that the self-report of symptoms differs between athletes and their parents, with parent reports demonstrating better diagnostic utility than youth self-report (Gioia, 2013).

Description	Reliability	Validity
20 items, 4-point Guttman scale 3-factor structure (cognitive, somatic, emotional) (Ayr et al., 2009)	Internal consistency, parent-child correlation, no test-retest reliability	Discriminates head injury from orthopedic injuries; correlates with quality of life, family burden, educational, and social difficulties (Yeates et al., 2012)
22 items, 2-point Guttman scale	Test-retest and interrater reliability	Content validity, relationship to other measures, group discrimination, sensitivity to recovery
12 items, 7-point Guttman scale	No report	Sensitivity and specificity high via receiver operating characteristics (ROCs) curve analysis (Randolph et al., 2009)
GSC 16 items; GSS 17-20 items, 7-point Guttman scale 3-factor solution reported (cognitive, somatic, neurobehavioral) (Piland et al., 2006)	Internal consistency, test-retest reliability	Discriminates between patients who suffered blows of lower and higher impact (McCaffrey et al., 2007). Convergent validity with measures of balance, neurocognitive function, headaches (McCrea et al., 2003; Register-Mihalik et al., 2007)

continued

TABLE 3-4 Continued

Instrument	Age Range (years)	Parent Form
Post-Concussion Symptom Scale (PCSS) (Lovell and Collins, 1998)	≥12	No
Rivermead Post-Concussion Symptoms Questionnaire (RPCSQ) (King et al., 1995)	≥8	No
Post-Concussion Symptom Inventory (PCSI) (Gioia et al., 2008b, 2009)	5-18	Yes, also version for teachers

SOURCES: Based on Gioia et al., 2009; Janusz et al., 2012; Randolph et al., 2009.

NEUROPSYCHOLOGICAL TESTING

Introduction to Neuropsychological Testing

Neuropsychology is the study of brain-behavior relationships, that is, the ways in which specific neural (brain) structure and activity are reflected in cognitive and physical behavior. The terms "neuropsychological" and "cognitive" are often used interchangeably (as in neuropsychological testing, cognitive testing, and neurocognitive testing). For the purposes of this document, the terms can be understood as equivalent.

Tests such as Trail Making, Paced Auditory Serial Attention Test, Digit

Description	Reliability	Validity
22 items; in youth ages 13-22, 7-point Guttman scale; 4-factor structure score (cognitive-fatigue-migraine; affective, somatic, and sleep)	Test-retest reliability (pre-post season, ICC=0.55; test retest, r=0.65	Discriminates concussed from non-concussed athletes (Echemendia et al., 2001; Field et al., 2003; Iverson et al., 2003; Lovell et al., 2006; Schatz et al., 2006); greater abnormalities in those with multiple concussions (Collins et al., 1999). Convergent validity: correlates with neurocognitive performance and fMRI changes during working memory tasks (Collins et al., 2003b; Pardini et al., 2010)
16 items, 5-point Guttman scale; no reported factor structure	In adolescents, high internal consistency, low test-retest reliability (Iverson and Gaetz, 2004)	Discriminant validity between concussed and non-concussed youth (Wilde et al., 2008)
Age 5-7, 13 items, 3-point Guttman scale Age 8-12, 17 items, 3-point Gutmann scale Age 13-18, 20 items, 7-point Guttman scale Parent, 20 items, 7-point Guttman scale; focus on cognitive, emotional, sleep, and physical domains	Test-retest reliability for self-report; high interrater reliability and internal consistency (Schneider and Gioia, 2007; Vaughan et al., 2008); moderate (r=0.4-0.5) (Gioia et al., 2008b); agreement between reporters in one of two studies (Gioia et al., 2009)	Good predictive and discriminant validity (Diver et al., 2007; Vaughan et al., 2008)

Symbol Substitution, and Digit Span have long been used in documenting cognitive deficits in TBI. The earlier neuropsychological literature on TBI has documented several specific areas of typical deficit, with processing speed, attention and memory typically showing the most significant deficits. Sports concussions may have the following effects:

- Reduced planning and ability to switch mental set (Barth et al., 1983, 1989, 2000; Rimel et al., 1982)
- Impaired memory and learning (Gronwall and Wrightson, 1981; Guskiewicz et al., 2001; Lovell et al., 2003)

- Reduced attention and ability to process information (Maddocks et al., 1995)
- Slowed reaction times and increased variability in response (Collins et al., 2003b; Makdissi et al., 2001)

Although neuropsychological testing is recognized as a powerful tool for understanding the cognitive effects of brain injury, it has inherent limitations and factors that affect the resulting scores and interpretations.

In 2001, Grindel and colleagues reviewed the existing literature on sports concussions and commented on several important issues that needed to be addressed by the field (Grindel et al., 2001). These included the availability of baseline testing, the validity of the test battery, problems involving repeated testing, interpretation of the test, the costs of testing, the presence of severe or prolonged symptoms, the presence of multiple concussions, age, gender, and perhaps the athlete's level of play. Many of these issues have been addressed as newer tools and improved analyses have been published. Baseline testing has become prevalent with the advent of Web-based computerized tests; the validity of the tests themselves has been established, although confounding factors such as symptom load, test administration environment, and comorbid conditions continue to plague the field. Reliable change metrics have improved the problems with repeat testing, and the effects of multiple concussions have been recognized and often used as a covariate in group studies.

Randolph and colleagues (2005) reviewed the state of neuropsychological testing in sports-related concussion management and concluded that the (then) existing tests did not meet necessary standards for use. Issues of reliability and validity as well as poor psychometric controls were felt to render testing useless for this specified purpose. They opined that athletic trainers and sports medicine professionals would do just as well using standardized graded checklists.

In 2010, Comper and colleagues published a systematic review of the methodological features of research in sports concussion, focusing on studies that used neuropsychological tests. They concluded that the methodological quality of studies were highly variable (Comper et al., 2010). In a separate paper, they noted that no prospective studies using control groups had been done to validate the use of neuropsychological tests (Hutchison et al., 2011). Prospective studies with controls are difficult to complete, but there are now some studies with control groups and within-subjects designs that use baseline test performance and the amount of change relative to expectation as dependent variables.

In spite of these concerns, the use of neuropsychological testing in sports has proliferated, with ever more computerized batteries coming on the market, and professional, college, high school, and youth sports teams implementing some form of testing.

Factors Affecting Neuropsychological Testing

The influence of intrinsic and extrinsic factors on neuropsychological test performance has long been studied, and clinicians attempt to minimize the effects of these factors by using standardized procedures and testing environments. McCrory and colleagues (2005) listed a number of individual factors (e.g., genetics, general cognitive level of functioning, gender, ethnicity, mood) and methodological factors (e.g., testing environment, practice and learning effects, administrative expertise) that may influence test outcomes (see Figure 3-1). Other individual factors that may affect test outcomes include learning disabilities, attention deficit hyperactivity disorder, and color blindness. Symptom load as a state factor should also be considered as a factor that affects test performance (McCrory et al., 2005). Score interpretation depends on reliable administration and the proper consideration of all of these factors, some of which are reduced with computerized testing (McCrory et al., 2005).

Using trained test administrators and testing in appropriate environ-

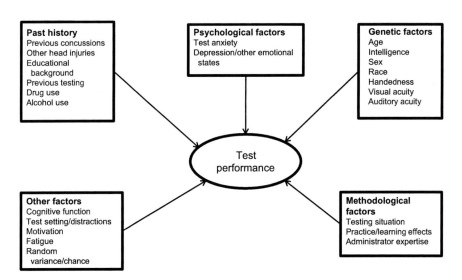

FIGURE 3-1 Factors that impact the results of neuropsychological tests.
SOURCE: McCrory et al., 2005, p. i61. Reproduced with permission from BMJ Group Ltd.

ments are fairly obvious requirements, but there are no data on the actual training or testing environments that are currently in use. Group testing, the way in which most baseline assessments are administered, appears to systematically lower scores compared to individualized administration (Moser et al., 2011).

Age and sex are well-known contributors to score differences in all educational and psychological tests. Test standardization requires validity studies that determine these differences and allow the presentation of separate norms (see AERA et al., 1999). Most published tests, including Immediate Post-Concussion Assessment and Cognitive Testing (ImPACT), CogSport, Concussion Resolution Index (CRI), and Automated Neuropsychological Assessment Metrics, provide age and gender normative standards or references. Unless tests have been shown to be insensitive to gender, they are expected to offer separate scoring parameters.

Higher academic achievement has been linked to higher computerized neuropsychological test scores. One study looked at neuropsychological test scores in more than 300 Division I NCAA schools. Athletes with the highest levels of academic achievement based on the Scholastic Aptitude Test (SAT) had higher scores on the ANAM test battery than did those athletes with lower SAT scores (Brown et al., 2007). Comorbid conditions such as attention deficit hyperactivity disorder, learning disabilities (Collins et al., 1999), and autism also may be reflected in test scores. Some medications can also affect scores, including anti-epileptic drugs and psycho-stimulants (see, e.g., Biederman et al., 2008).

Poor effort is somewhat more difficult to detect and control, but it is a factor that lowers scores. This has been documented in the general TBI literature (Green, 2007; Lange et al., 2010). A major concern in testing for sports-related concussions is the willful lowering of baseline scores in order to establish an easier threshold for "return to baseline" (Pennington, 2013). The ImPACT test has embedded validity indicators to help examiners determine atypically low scores on specific subtests. However, individuals with neurologic or developmental disorders or those who are under acute stress may legitimately score low on these indicators; thus, individual analysis is required before declaring a test invalid. There are also specific tests and profiles within neuropsychological tests that are used to detect poor effort, "malingering," or suboptimal performance.

Hunt and colleagues (2007) found that 11 percent of their sample of 199 high school athletes exhibited poor effort as indexed by the Dot Counting Test and the Rey 15-Item Test with recognition trial. Statistically significant differences existed between effort groups ($p < 0.05$) on several of the neuropsychological tests. By comparing a group with unusually low baseline scores versus post-injury scores at 1 week to a group with high baseline scores, Bailey and colleagues (2006) found significantly more improvement from baseline to post injury for athletes who reported "low motivation" on baseline testing. The authors concluded that low motivation exists and that it does affect test scores. However, Erdal (2012) found that it was difficult for athletes to purposely do poorly on the ImPACT test without tripping the validity indicators embedded in the ImPACT test. Nevertheless, the perceived secondary gain of lowering one's baseline test score is a concern when using the baseline-testing paradigm. In the case of large-scale baseline testing sessions, it is particularly difficult to know whether low scores are due to intrinsic factors or poor motivation.

In the clinical pediatric population, sleep debt does not appear to interfere with neuropsychological testing, although it is strongly implicated in poor school performance (see Beebe, 2012, for review). Although sleep does not appear to affect laboratory test performances, one small study indicated that the number of hours of sleep the night before baseline testing was related to higher non-sleep symptom scores (i.e., less sleep was related to higher non-sleep symptom totals; see Maerlender and Alt, 2012).

Mood and anxiety have long been known to affect neuropsychological test performance in clinical patients. Bailey and colleagues (2010) and Maerlender and colleagues (2010) presented data demonstrating that mood and anxiety scores on independent measures were related to specific test score patterns on ImPACT and on a paper-and-pencil neuropsychological battery. The Bailey study administered the Personality Assessment Inventory together with the CRI and found that a significant amount of variance in baseline scores was accounted for by mood and anxiety symptom load. Using the symptom scale that is part of the ImPACT battery, Covassin and colleagues (2012b) found that athletes with high levels of depression reported more concussion-like symptoms and had lower ImPACT test scores on baseline tests.[4] The ANAM battery has validated a mood scale and demonstrated its relationship to test scores (Johnson et al., 2008). Given the increased use of neuropsychological testing at baseline and post injury, it is important to understand the effect of these factors, and the potential effect of these factors on test results highlights the need for interpretation of the tests by experienced providers. There are several ways in which mood and anxiety can be related to neuropsychological performance in concussed athletes. It could be, for example, that both increased anxiety and decreased performance are the result of the same brain injury, or that the depression and anxiety symptoms are a response to the problems in the cognitive performance, or that depression and anxiety have negatively affected neurocognitive performance. Indeed, there is evidence to support

---

[4]High school athletes reported more somatic or migraine symptoms than did college athletes, whereas college athletes reported more emotional and sleep symptoms than did their high school counterparts.

each of these three possibilities (Chen et al., 2007; Pardini et al., 2010). Although most studies of athletes have used older samples and there are no systematic studies in athletes younger than high school age, there is no reason to believe that the state effects of anxiety, mood, or stress would be different in a younger population.

Pain has been shown to affect cognition in some groups of patients. A recent study by Gosselin and colleagues (2012b) compared groups of adolescents with mTBI (n=24, 50 percent of whom had sports-related injuries), non-injured controls (n=16), and athletes with orthopedic injuries (n=29). Levels of pain were the dependent measure and blood oxygen level-dependent activation during working memory task was the outcome. While results were somewhat complicated, the authors interpreted the results as demonstrating that behavioral performance and cerebral function were related to levels of pain.

The validity of neuropsychological tests for interpreting brain-behavior relationships rests on psychometric characteristics, including reliability. The use of the same test multiple times for tracking change or measuring injury (i.e., baseline to post injury) is compromised by several factors, most notably the practice effect of retaking the test. Although multiple forms (using different specific items) can reduce this, the effect of exposure to the procedure (directions, pacing, sequence of tasks) has a greater effect than the likelihood of memorizing specific responses (Heilbronner et al., 2010). To address this issue, several statistical procedures have been developed to account for practice effects, the tendency of scores to "regress to the mean," and differential pre-injury test scores (for review, see Hinton-Bayre, 2012). The American Academy of Clinical Neuropsychology has issued a position paper that outlines these concerns and discusses the recommended statistical procedures (reliable change indices, regression-based methods) (Bauer et al., 2012; Heilbronner et al., 2010). It recommends that such statistical adjustments be used any time tests are used in a serial fashion.

Neuropsychological Testing and Sports-Related Concussions

Jeffrey Barth and his colleagues are generally credited with originating the use of athletes and teams as a laboratory for studying the nature and outcomes of concussion through sports (the Sports as a Laboratory Assessment Model) and the baseline pre-season testing of athletes with brief neuropsychological batteries for later post-injury comparisons (Barth et al., 1989; Macciocchi et al., 1996). With the growing use of neuropsychological testing in the identification and management of sports-related concussions has come controversy and criticism about the methods and outcomes.

This section considers the following questions concerning neuropsychological assessment in sports-related concussions:

- Can neuropsychological testing assist in the diagnosis of sports-related concussions in youth?
- Does neuropsychological testing have a role in tracking recovery and informing management (e.g., return to school, return to play, return to work)?
- Are computerized tests valid and reliable?
- Does baseline testing improve the utility of neuropsychological testing in the diagnosis and management of sports-related concussion?

Can Neuropsychological Testing Assist in the Diagnosis of Sports-Related Concussions in Youth?

In the context of sports-related concussions, an important distinction must be made between the use of neuropsychological tests for diagnosis and their use for tracking recovery (McCrory et al., 2005). Studies of the ability of neuropsychological tests to provide accurate diagnoses of concussion typically involve tests administered within 72 hours of the injury. They include studies comparing group-level score changes in groups of concussed individuals versus groups of non-concussed individuals and studies looking at individual diagnostic accuracy. However, it should be noted that neuropsychological tests are traditionally not used to make diagnoses, but rather to characterize function. So it is a useful question to ask whether these tests can contribute to diagnosis.

An often unmentioned aspect of concussion research and practice is the variability in identification of concussion and the still-limited knowledge of the biological nature of concussions (i.e., the lack of biomarkers for diagnosis and recovery). Although studies typically rely on the identification of concussions by athletic trainers according to generally accepted standards, the validity of these diagnoses has never been established. In one study, 50 percent of diagnosed concussions were identified more than 24 hours after the incident, and 30 percent of this group had no identifiable biomechanical impacts on the day of the reported injury (based on accelerometer readings in the helmets) (Duhaime et al., 2012). Determinations of the diagnostic efficiency of a test will be affected by the validity of actual diagnoses. Thus variability in this process can produce conflicting or limited results in studies of the predictive ability of any tool.

Given the relatively rapid time-course of concussions, the temporal aspects of the injury are also significant factors in studying the phenomena. Indeed, studies have shown that the closer the assessment was to the time of injury, the more pronounced the effect of the biomechanical force on cognition was (Beckwith et al., 2013a,b; McAllister et al., 2012). Broglio and Puetz (2008) questioned whether comparing athletes who are assessed at different time-points from injury likely invalidates the findings.

As Hutchinson and colleagues (2011) found, the presence of pain can have an effect on test scores. Controlling for diagnosis and time of testing, baseline exposure to the tests, and other factors adds to the complexity of studying concussions at the group and individual levels, particularly in the immediate aftermath of the injury when symptoms are typically high. McCrory and colleagues (2005) also questioned whether the presence of symptoms could preclude accurate (valid) test results. Symptoms may interfere in test performance through any or all attention mechanisms, reducing arousal, orienting, focus, sustaining focus, and so on, or symptoms may make the individual feel too bad to participate (a type of motivational effect). Unfortunately, the actual evidence is limited, as few studies directly test the hypothesis that symptoms (either in total or individually) account for significant variance in test scores.

As a practical matter the test scores may reflect the overall status of the individual, but, because neuropsychological tests are designed to assess brain function, the inclusion of symptom-related error into the test score interferes in the psychometric accuracy of the test. In other words, poor performance on a neuropsychological test because one feels bad may obscure the test's ability to accurately measure brain function. Studies indirectly point to the correlation of symptoms and test scores (Collins et al., 2003a; Fazio et al., 2007), particularly immediately after injury, when symptoms tend to be highest. Thus, the mediating effect of symptoms on test scores in the immediate aftermath of the injury likely reduces the predictive power of tests alone. The evidence for diagnostic validity and utility comes from group studies and from studies of individual probability. Group studies have employed cross-sectional designs and within-subjects designs using baseline or multiple test points for comparisons. Group studies have been described in two meta-analytic studies (Belanger and Vanderploeg, 2005; Broglio and Puetz, 2008). There was considerable overlap in the groups of studies reviewed in the two analyses, but Broglio and Puetz were interested in the effect of using multimodal assessments, while Belanger and Vanderploeg were focused on neuropsychological assessments only.

Group studies have generally shown that a significant proportion of concussed athletes have neurocognitive decrements compared to controls (or compared to baseline performances) in the initial days following the injury, but scores are back to normal or baseline by 7 days post injury. Belanger and Vanderploeg (2005) analyzed 21 studies from 1994 to 2004. All had multiple assessment points using control groups tested at the same interval. They found significant acute effects (changes in scores reflecting worsening in the first 24 hours after injury) for most cognitive domains (delayed memory: $d=1.00$; memory acquisition: $d=1.03$; and global cognitive functioning: $d=1.42$). However, when analyzed across all studies, no group residual neuropsychological reductions were found when testing was completed beyond 7 days post injury.

The meta-analysis of Broglio and Puetz (2008) included 39 studies from 1970 to 2006 that met their inclusion criteria: studies of concussed athletes who were evaluated using symptom assessment, balance assessment, or neuropsychological/cognitive assessment. One post-injury assessment had to have been completed within 14 days of injury and compared with a baseline measure or control group. Three types of cognitive assessments were included: the SAC, paper-and-pencil batteries, and computerized batteries. They found significant effects of concussion on all three types of assessments immediately after injury. The type of cognitive assessment was determined to be a moderator effect, as was the time from injury to assessment. The largest effect was for the SAC administered immediately after injury.

The usefulness of tests to diagnose a disease entity (e.g., their ability to detect a person with disease or exclude a person without disease) is usually described by such terms as sensitivity, specificity, positive predictive value, and negative predictive value. These various measures describe how well the tests identify people who actually have the disease (or not) as diagnosed by some gold standard method. Sensitivity (the chance that a person with the disease is correctly identified as having it) and specificity (the chance that a person without the disease is correctly identified as being free of it) are the characteristics most reported for a diagnostic test because they reflect the characteristics of the test and not those of the group tested. However, the users of the test are likely to be more interested in the predictive values (the chance that a person identified by the test as concussed actually had a concussion—positive predictive value—and the chance that a person identified as not having a concussion was actually free of a recent concussion—negative predictive value). The predictive value changes depending on what fraction of the athletes tested truly had a concussion.

Van Kampen and colleagues (2006) tested the diagnostic value of adding neuropsychological testing to assessments of symptom load. One hundred twenty-two athletes diagnosed with concussion and 70 without a recent concussion were compared by looking at their post-injury symptoms and their ImPACT test scores. Concussed athletes were tested 2 days after injury. Ninety-three percent of athletes with a reliable increase in symptoms actually had a concussion—a positive predictive value (PPV) of 93 percent—but 41 percent of those without a reliable increase in symptoms also had a concussion—a negative predictive value (NPV) of 59 percent. When ImPACT was used in the absence of symptom data, 83 percent of those having at least one abnormal[5] neurocognitive test score had a concussion (PPV=83%) and 70 percent of those with no abnormal neurocognitive scores did not have a concussion (NPV=70%). However, when criteria for concussion classification were changed to require at least one abnormal ImPACT test *or* a reliable increase in symptoms, 81 percent of those who the tests indicated had a concussion actually did (PPV=81%) and 83 percent of those the tests indicated were free of concussion actually were (NPV=83%). These predictive values are based on 64 percent (122 of 192) of the athletes studied having a recent concussion. If the same diagnostic criteria were used to screen every football player after every game (prevalence under 1 percent), more than 97 percent of the athletes the test identified as having a recent concussion actually would be diagnosed in error.

Several other studies have demonstrated a strong diagnostic efficiency for neuropsychological tests. Schatz and colleagues (2006) obtained 82 percent sensitivity and 89 percent specificity comparing ImPACT tests scores (n=72) within 72 hours of injury to scores of non-concussed athletes (n=66). A similar approach was used by this group analyzing ImPACT data of 81 concussed athletes and 81 controls, ages 13 to 21 (Schatz and Sandel, 2013). High sensitivity (91 percent) and adequate specificity (69 percent) were obtained.

Summary Neuropsychological tests have the ability to detect cognitive changes in injured athletes, although cognition as indexed by test scores appears to improve for the vast majority of injuries within 2 weeks. There are mixed results of the diagnostic utility of neuropsychological testing immediately (within 48 hours) after injury, although significant differences between concussed and non-concussed individuals are more often found in group studies. There is general agreement that neuropsychological tests should not be used in isolation for diagnosis; symptom levels are the best predictor of diagnosis (i.e., concussion diagnosis is made based on symptom presentation). Although the presence of symptoms can influence test results, potentially obscuring the accurate measurement of brain function, neuropsychological testing is one of several tools (along with symptom assessment, clinical evaluation, and the like) that may aid in concussion diagnosis. It appears that high scores on neuropsychological tests, indicating good cognitive function, are predictive of *not* having a concussion.

---

[5]Abnormal here means a change from baseline to post-injury score outside the 80 percent confidence interval for reliable change: abnormal reliable change index. This does not necessarily imply clinical abnormality.

Does Neuropsychological Testing Have a Role in Tracking Recovery and Informing Management?

Neuropsychological testing has been used extensively in the rehabilitation setting to document and track cognitive recovery. In the area of sports-related concussions, the standard as promulgated by the Zurich statement and other consensus statements has been that recovery can be said to have taken place when symptoms, cognition, and balance have returned to the athlete's baseline (or typical) performance (Halstead et al., 2010; Harmon et al., 2013; McCrory et al., 2013b). Using that as the benchmark, studies have generally found neuropsychological testing to be a useful aid in determining when an athlete has recovered enough to return to competition. Although the methodological rigor of the studies varies (Comper et al., 2010), the ability of neuropsychological tests to detect subtle changes in cognitive function is well established.

Several studies have documented persistent declines in post-injury neuropsychological scores even after symptoms have resolved (Broglio et al., 2007a; Iverson et al., 2006; Peterson et al., 2003). These studies found improvements in cognitive scores, balance testing, and symptoms over time, with the cognitive scores taking longer to improve than the balance and symptom scores. Iverson and colleagues (2006) included a reliable change methodology and demonstrated that 37 percent of the concussed athletes continued to have at least two ImPACT composite scores significantly lower than expected after 10 days, even though the symptoms had resolved after 5 days. A more recent study using ANAM found that several subtest scores differentiated mild from moderate concussions on the day of injury but not at 8 days post injury (Prichep et al., 2013).

The two meta-analyses noted above also examined the ability of neuropsychological tests to measure changes in cognitive function through recovery. Belanger and Vanderploeg (2005) found significant improvement between days 7 and 10 for verbal memory retention scores only. Broglio and Puetz (2008) examined how the effects of concussion were manifested in three assessment modalities: the SAC, paper-and-pencil batteries, and computerized batteries. They found significant effects of concussion on the scores of all three assessment modalities immediately after injury as well as reduced but still large effects for the cognitive assessment at 14 days post injury interval. The type of cognitive assessment was determined to be a moderator effect, as was the time from the injury to the assessment. The largest effect was seen for the SAC immediately after injury, with the paper-and-pencil batteries having significantly greater effects than the SAC or computer batteries at 14 days.

Summary There is a long history of neuropsychological tests being used to track recovery from brain injury as they are thought to reflect functional cognitive recovery. Group studies of individuals with sports-related concussions have shown that neuropsychological test scores improve as the time from injury increases. Some studies have found continued cognitive declines on neuropsychological testing, even after individuals' concussion symptoms have resolved, although other studies show symptoms lasting longer than cognitive declines. The persistence of cognitive declines following symptom resolution in some individuals suggests there may be a role for neuropsychological testing in concussion management, for example, to help inform return-to-play decisions in these cases. Such a role for computerized neuropsychological testing has been criticized, however, on the grounds that there currently is no evidence to show that delaying an individual's return to full physical activity on the basis of residual neurocognitive deficits actually improves recovery outcomes or reduces the risk of subsequent injury (Kirkwood et al., 2009; Randolph and Kirkwood, 2009).

Are Computerized Tests Valid and Reliable?

All neuropsychological tests require standardized administration and expert interpretation of results. Assuming that these conditions are met, test effectiveness is typically determined by several factors: Is it reliable (does it produce consistent results each time it is administered), is it valid (do the test scores represent the construct of interest, e.g., working memory), and does it measure individuals with respect to the construct of interest (i.e., specific cognitive functions, diagnostic efficiency)? Test developers attempt to show that their tests meet these criteria, but a fourth aspect is also important: Does independent research obtain the same results as the test developers' research? Computerized test batteries are not unique to sports neuropsychology, but it is important to examine their role in concussions because of how extensively they are used.

A complete neuropsychological assessment of the multiple cognitive functions of an individual can take between 4 and 8 hours (Lezak et al., 2012). Screening tools that focus on functions typically affected by brain injuries were developed to reduce the length of the typical neuropsychological batteries and to focus on identifying acute cognitive dysfunction. Such targeted batteries also made larger-scale testing feasible, which in turn created the opportunity to implement the Sports as a Laboratory Assessment Model (SLAM) for sports-related concussion.

Collie and colleagues (2001) raised concerns about paper-and-pencil testing that centered on interrater reliability issues, the general lack of alternative forms, and the effect of practice in repeat testing. McCrory and colleagues (2005) noted that computerized testing offered advantages such as standardized and randomized presentation of stimuli, shorter administration time, central data storage, and more sensitive and accurate detection of reaction times. Furthermore, standard paper-and-pencil tests did not typically have normative standards developed specifically for athletes, and computerized tests allowed for easier repeat (serial) testing to track cognitive recovery. Indeed, an entire industry, with its corresponding potential financial conflicts of interest, has developed around providing baseline and serial post-injury testing to thousands of athletes. By 2003, the brief paper-and-pencil test battery was becoming replaced by computerized test batteries such as ImPACT, CogSport, ANAM, and CRI (see, e.g., Cernich et al., 2007; Collie et al., 2003; Collins et al., 2003b; Erlanger et al., 2003).

Between 1999 and 2002 there were 10 studies using paper-and-pencil batteries and only one using computer testing; between 2003 and 2008 there were 8 studies utilizing paper-and-pencil batteries and 15 using computer testing (Comper et al., 2010). Thus, in terms of research, there was a dramatic shift in focus. The shift in research focus also appears to have been mirrored by practice. In 2009, Covassin and colleagues reported that 95 percent of the 266 athletic trainers who participated in a survey said they administered baseline computerized neurocognitive testing to their athletes. However, only 51.9 percent examined the baseline test validity indices. The researchers concluded that the athletic trainers in the study appeared to rely more on symptoms than on neurocognitive test scores when making return-to-play decisions (Covassin et al., 2009). When Meehan and colleagues (2011) reviewed data from the High School RIO^{TM} database of athletic injuries for the 2009-2010 school year (1,056 sports-related concussions), they found that computerized neuropsychological testing was used for 41.2 percent of concussions. Although there are concerns with the use of such testing, it continues to represent a large portion of concussion management activity. At this point, all of the computerized tests have some peer-reviewed research to support their use.

Psychometric tests are judged on their reliability and validity as documented in their manuals and published studies. Reliability is usually assessed as a test-retest correlation or in terms of an intraclass correlation coefficient (ICC). A Pearson correlation can be a valid estimator of inter-rater reliability (i.e., test-retest reliability), but only when there are meaningful pairings between two and only two raters. A test of internal stability (Chronbach's alpha) is a test of the function of the number of test items and the average intercorrelation among the items (see Anastasi and Urbina, 1997). These are statistical tests that provide information about the ability of the test to maintain its performance and psychometric characteristics over time.

Evidence to support test interpretation (validity) may come from various forms: evidence based on test content, evidence based on response processes, evidence based on internal structure, evidence based on relations to other variables, and evidence based on the consequences of testing. Establishing validity is seen as a long-term process, and no one study can make that determination. Test development practice calls for documentation of some form of reliability and validity (see AERA et al., 1999). All of the major computerized tests have demonstrated some level of reliability and validity. Other aspects of their structure may make them more suitable for some situations than others, and practitioner preference, experience, and knowledge are important factors. It should be noted that the Department of Defense currently uses ANAM to assess post-concussion neurocognitive changes in service members in all branches of the military. Table 3-5 outlines the basic features of several of the currently available computerized tests.

Reliability of computerized tests The ability of a test to perform consistently is important to having confidence in its scores. Table 3-6 lists published reliability studies of several different computerized neuropsychological tests used in concussion management. Several approaches to reliability can be taken: Internal consistency can be measured using Chronbach's alpha test or one can examine the correlation between half of the items and the other half (split-half reliability). Test-retest reliabilities are used to determine consistency across test administration: a Pearson correlation or an ICC can be calculated. The ICC has become the preferred measure as it is a type of interrater reliability. However, there is no agreement on the minimum ICC value that is considered "acceptable" for computerized neuropsychological tests. Some authors find a minimum correlation of 0.60 to be acceptable (e.g., Baumgartner and Chung, 2001; Weir, 2005), while others employ a higher standard of 0.70 (e.g., Anastasi and Urbina, 2007) and still others may consider 0.80 or 0.90 to be the mark of a good, reproducible automated test.

As Table 3-6 demonstrates, ICCs for different composite scores within tests are quite variable, and low intraclass correlations are frequently found. If there is a trend across tests, it appears to be that speeded tests have better reliability than do tests of other functions such as memory. This may have to do with the inherent nature of computerized tests and the manner in which tasks must be presented in this format.

Reliability studies are quite variable, with some studies demonstrating adequate reliability and some indicating less than adequate reliability. There are many possible reasons for the variability, including different sample sizes, unknown testing conditions, and variable item pools. Most computerized tests produce multiple forms through a quasi-randomization of items. All of the commercial test batteries that were reviewed had some studies indicating acceptable reliability. Tests involving speed appear to be more reliable than those involving memory or accuracy. This may be due to computer-format constraints. Clinicians and researchers need to be aware of the variability in reliability studies with these tools.

Validity of computerized tests The presentation format of a computer-based test presents different limitations and strengths than those of paper-and-pencil testing. For instance, memory is a complex function and computerized tests of memory are limited to recognition formats. This format limitation may be one reason for the difficulty in isolating specific cognitive functions, as there may be overlap between (for example) processing speed and working memory (Maerlender et al., 2010). However, answering questions about identification and recovery may not require such construct specification.

As the previous sections document, a large number of studies have demonstrated the various aspects of validity of these computerized batteries. Table 3-7 lists published validity studies of several different computerized neuropsychological tests used in concussion management. Concurrent validity (comparing the scores from one test to those from another similar test) and criterion and predictive validity (predicting a criterion such as the diagnosis of concussion) are the most frequently cited methods of establishing validity. Construct validity attempts to establish the underlying cognitive mechanisms that the test is actually measuring (e.g., memory, attention). There is overlap in these types and methods for understanding validity.

Concurrent validity has been demonstrated for each of the batteries when compared with paper-and-pencil neuropsychological tests. Most studies show high correlations with tests thought to measure similar constructs. Only two studies mention the discriminating ability of the tests, that is, whether a particular test shows low correlations with other tests that it should not be highly correlated with. For example, although the ImPACT test has high correlations between the composite scores and similar paper-and-pencil tests (convergent construct validity), the same sample showed high correlations with dissimilar paper-and-pencil measures (Maerlender et al., 2010). On the other hand, Newman and colleagues (2013) found that the new Pediatric ImPACT test showed good discrimination between speed of processing and memory tests. Using a factor-analytic approach, Allen and Gfeller (2011) also demonstrated construct validity for ImPACT. ANAM (Bleiberg et al., 1997, 2000, 2004; Prichep et al., 2013), CogSport (Collie et al., 2003; Makdissi et al., 2010; Moriarity et al., 2012), and CRI (Erlanger et al., 2003) also have been shown to possess various types of validity.

In group studies, neuropsychological test scores have generally not been shown to predict prolonged recovery. Most recently, McCrea and colleagues

TABLE 3-5 Common Computerized Neuropsychological Tests

Test Name	Age Range	Time to Administer	Functions Assessed	Other
Automated Neuropsychological Assessment Metrics (ANAM) 4 Traumatic Brain Injury battery (Eonta et al., 2011; VistaLife Sciences, 2013)	Not given	20-25 minutes	Simple reaction time, code substitution, procedural reaction time, mathematical processing, matching to sample, code substitution delayed	Demographics, sleep scale, mood scale; pseudorandomized items; embedded effort measure included with the ANAM Performance Report
ANAM Sports battery (Cernich et al., 2007; Reeves et al., 2007)	17-65	20-25 minutes	Simple reaction time, code substitution learning, running memory continuous performance task, mathematical processing, delayed matching to sample, code substitution delayed memory test, spatial processing, Sternberg procedure, procedural reaction time	Demographics module, Modified Stanford Sleepiness Scale, pseudorandomized items; "throughput score" is a speed-versus-accuracy measure
CNS Vital Signs (CNS Vital Signs, 2013; Gualtieri and Johnson, 2006)	8-90	25-30 minutes (Brief Core battery)	Composite memory, verbal memory, visual memory, psychomotor speed, reaction time, complex attention, cognitive flexibility, processing speed, executive function, simple attention, motor speed	General purpose neuropsychological test developed for drug trials but used in neuropsychiatric clinics; no studies available that assess sports concussions, although materials indicate it is valid and reliable for that purpose; performance validity measure

Instrument	Age	Time	Domains measured	Additional features
Concussion Vital Signs (CNS Vital Signs, 2013; Concussion Vital Signs, 2013)	8-90	25-30 minutes	Verbal memory, visual memory, psychomotor speed, executive function, cognitive flexibility, continuous performance task correct responses, reaction time	Concussion version of CNS Vital Signs; performance validity measure
CogSport/Axon/Computerized Cognitive Assessment Tool (CCAT) (Axon Sports, 2013; Falleti et al., 2006)	Not given	15-20 minutes	Processing speed, attention, learning, working memory	Basic demographics
Concussion Resolution Index (CRI)/ Headminder (Erlanger et al., 2001, 2003)	13-35	25-30 minutes	Processing speed, simple reaction time, complex reaction time	Basic demographics and health history
Immediate Post-Concussion Assessment and Cognitive Testing (ImPACT) (ImPACT, 2013)	12-60	20-25 minutes	Composite scores: verbal memory, visual memory, visual-motor speed, reaction time	Background and basic health information; symptoms assessment; calculates post-injury change in reliable change index metrics; has baseline test validity indicators
Pediatric ImPACT (Gioia et al., 2013a; Newman et al., 2013)	5-12		Symptom scale, response speed, learning and memory accuracy	Validity indicators; regression-based reliable change metrics built in

TABLE 3-6 Reliability Studies on Common Neuropsychological Tests

Test	Study Author	N/population
Automated Neuropsychological Assessment Metrics (ANAM)	Segalowitz et al., 2007	29 adolescents, age 15
ANAM	Cernich et al., 2007	Review of previous tests; U.S. Military Academy cadets
ANAM4	Cole et al., 2013[a]	50 active duty military, predominantly male (83%); ages 19-59 (mean 34)
CogSport	Collie et al., 2003	60 healthy youth

Subtest	Statistic/Reliability	Test Intervals	Comment
Matching to Sample	ICC=.72 r=.72	2 times over 1-week	
Continuous		interval	
Performance	ICC=.65 r=.70		
Math Processing	ICC=.61 r=.71		
Code Substitution	ICC=.58 r=.81		
Simple Reaction			
Time	ICC=.44 r=.48		
Simple Reaction			
Time 2	ICC=.47 r=.50		
Code Substitution			
Delayed	ICC=.68 r=.67		
Matching to Sample	ICC=.66	166 days	
Continuous			
Performance	ICC=.58		
Math Processing	ICC=.87		
Simple Reaction			
Time	ICC=.38		
Spatial Processing	ICC=.60		
Sternberg Memory	ICC=.48		
Matching to Sample	r=.69; ICC=.67	21-42 days	Sample likely is
Procedural Reaction			not comparable
Time	r=.62; ICC=.51		to youth
Math Processing	r=.70; ICC=.70		athletics
Simple Reaction			
Time	r=.65; ICC=.60		
Simple Reaction			
Time repeated	r=.41; ICC=.40		
Code Substitution			
Learning	r=.79; ICC=.79		
Code Substitution			
Memory	r=.68; ICC=.59		
speed indices	ICC 1 hr.=.69,	1 hour, 1 week	
	1 week=.90		
accuracy indices	ICC 1 hr.=.08,		
	1 week=.51		

continued

TABLE 3-6 Continued

Test	Study Author	N/population
CogSport	Straume-Naesheim et al., 2005	232 male professional soccer players (Norwegian and Spanish) ages 17-35
Concussion Sentinel (CogSport)	Broglio et al., 2007c[b]	73 high school
CogSport	Faleti et al., 2006	45 adults, ages 18-40
CogState v5.6	Cole et al., 2013[a]	53 active duty military, predominantly male (83%); ages 19-59 (mean 34)

Subtest	Statistic/Reliability	Test Intervals	Comment
Simple Reaction Time	ICC=.73	Immediate	Sample is somewhat atypical for sports concussion management
Choice Reaction Time	ICC=.65		
Complex Reaction Time	ICC=.69		
Monitoring	ICC=.45		
1-back Monitoring	ICC=.71		
Matching	ICC=.69		
Learning	ICC=.79		
Working Memory	ICC 45 days=.65; 5 days later=.64	T1 to T2: 45 days; T2 to T3: 5 days	
Reaction Time	ICC 45 days=.60; 5 days later=.55		
Decision Making	ICC 45 days=.56; 5 days later=.63		
Attention	ICC 45 days=.43; 5 days later=.39		
Matching	ICC 45 days=.23; 5 days later=.66		
Simple Reaction Time	T1-2, T2-3, T3-4, T4-5 ICC>.73	T1, T2, T3, T4 at 10-minute intervals, T4-5 at 1 week interval	Model and form of ICC not provided. These ICCs are for the reaction times; very few ICCs were >.60 for accuracy measures
Choice Reaction Time	T3-4, T4-5 ICC>.71		
Complex Reaction Time	T2-3, T3-4, T4-5 ICC>.64		
Monitoring	T2-3, T3-4, ICC>.68		
1-back Monitoring	T1-2, T2-3, T3-4, T4-5 ICC>.62		
Matching	T1-2, T2-3, T3-4, T4-5 ICC>.71		
Incidental Learn	T3-4, T4-5 ICC>.60		
Associative Learn	T1-2, T2-3, T3-4, T4-5 ICC>.77		
Detection Speed	r=.77; ICC=.78	21-42 days	Sample is atypical for sports-related concussion management
Identification Speed	r=.78; ICC=.77		
One Card Learning Accuracy	r=.25; ICC=.22		
One Back Speed	r=.76; ICC=.74		
Composite	r=.80; ICC=.79		

continued

TABLE 3-6 Continued

Test	Study Author	N/population
Concussion Resolution Index (CRI)	Broglio et al., 2007c[b]	73 high school
CRI	Erlanger et al., 2003	414, ages 13-35
CRI	Erlanger et al., 2002	46-49, ages 18-29
Immediate Post-Concussion Assessment and Cognitive Testing (ImPACT)	Iverson et al., 2003	29 males and 27 females, average age 17.6 years
ImPACT	Elbin et al., 2011	369 high school varsity athletes
ImPACT	Miller et al., 2007	58 Division III college football

Subtest	Statistic/Reliability	Test Intervals	Comment
Simple Reaction Time Error	ICC 45 days =.15; 5 days later=.03	T1 to T2: 45 days; T2 to T3: 5 days	
Complex Reaction Time	ICC 45 days=.43; 5 days later=.66		
Complex Reaction Time Error	ICC 45 days=.26; 5 days later=.46		
Processing Speed Index	ICC 45 days=.66; 5 days later=.58		
Processing Speed	r=.82	2 week	Authors noted that reliabilities for the sample under 18 years were "with a trend of lower reliability scores in the sample under 18 years of age" (pp. 306-307)
Simple Reaction Time	r=.70		
Complex Reaction Time	r=.68		
Processing speed factor	r=.78	Random 1 to 110 days	Practice effects significant for Processing Speed only
Response speed factor	r=.80		
Memory factor	r=.68		
Attention factor	r=.74		
Verbal Memory	r=.70	1 week	Significant practice effects for Visual-Motor Speed
Visual Memory	r=.67		
Visual-Motor Speed	r=.89		
Reaction Time	r=.79		
Verbal Memory	ICC=.62	1.2 year	
Visual Memory	ICC=.76		
Visual-Motor Speed	ICC=.85		
Reaction Time	ICC=.76		
	Significant practice effects for Visual Memory and Visual-Motor Speed composites only	Preseason, mid-season, end of season	Raw scores at each time-point compared

continued

TABLE 3-6 Continued

Test	Study Author	N/population
ImPACT	Schatz, 2010	95 collegiate athletes
ImPACT	Broglio et al., 2007c[b]	73 high school
ImPACT	Schatz and Ferris, 2013	25 undergraduates, no concussion history
ImPACT	Cole et al., 2013[a]	44 active duty military predominantly male (83%); ages 19-59 (mean 34)
ImPACT	Register-Mihalik et al., 2012	20 high school, 20 college (male=female)

Subtest	Statistic/Reliability	Test Intervals	Comment
Verbal Memory	ICC=.46	2 year	
Visual Memory	ICC=.65		
Visual-Motor Speed	ICC=.74		
Reaction Time	ICC=.68		
Verbal Memory	ICC 45 days=.23; 5 days later=.40	T1 to T2: 45 days; T2 to T3: 5 days	Serial testing of three batteries, one after the other; few expected practice effects
Visual Memory	ICC 45 days=.32; 5 days later=.39		
Visual-Motor Speed	ICC 45 days=.38; 5 days later=.61		
Reaction Time	ICC 45 days=.39; 5 days later=.51		
Verbal Memory	ICC=.79; r=.66	4 weeks	Has a table comparing ICC and r across five studies. Only visual memory showed significant practice effects
Visual Memory	ICC=.60; r=.43		
Visual-Motor Speed	ICC=.88; r=.63		
Reaction Time	ICC=.77; r=.63		
Verbal Memory	r=.61; ICC=60	21-42 days	All showed improvement from T1 to T2, except RT; sample is atypical for sports-related concussion management
Visual Memory	r=.49; ICC=50		
Visual-Motor Speed	r=.86; ICC=.83		
Reaction Time	r=.53; ICC=.53		
Verbal Memory	ICC (T1-T2)=.29; r's T1-T2, T2-T3, NS; T1-&3 r p=.013	3 times each 24 hours apart	Significant practice effect for Visual-Motor Speed only, no age effects
Visual Memory	ICC (T1-T2)=.45; T1-T2, T2-T3 r p's <.002, T1-T3 r p=.023		
Visual-Motor Speed	ICC (T1-T2)=.71; all r p's <.001		
Reaction Time	ICC (T1-T2)=.60; all r p's <.001		
Impulse Control	ICC (T1-T2)=.6; all r p's <.05		

continued

TABLE 3-6 Continued

Test	Study Author	N/population
ImPACT	Resch et al., 2013	2 groups college n=45, n=46
Pediatric ImPACT	Gioia et al., 2013b	705, ages 5-12
CNS Vital Signs	Cole et al., 2013[a]	39 active duty military, predominantly male (83%); ages 19-59 (mean 34)

[a]Same study, different subjects; demographics for overall sample.
[b]Same study
NOTES: ICC = intraclass correlation coefficient, T = time.

(2013) analyzed data obtained from 570 high school and college athletes with concussions at several time-points after injury. The study divided the athletes into groups in which symptoms had resolved within 7 days (typical) and had lasted more than 7 days (prolonged recovery). Neuro-psychological test scores at less than 2 days post injury were not predictive of which recovery group an athlete would be in. This finding was similar to findings in the two meta-analytic studies described previously (Belanger and Vanderploeg, 2005; Broglio and Puetz, 2008). It should be noted that because in 90 percent of concussion cases the individuals recover by the end of 2 weeks (typical), group analyses may obscure the effects in those 10 percent of cases in which scores continue to suggest injury.

Subtest	Statistic/Reliability	Test Intervals	Comment
Verbal Memory	Both Groups, all intervals ICC<.59	Group 1: T1 to T2=7 days,	Used a one-way random effects
Visual Memory	Group 1 ICC.26, .53, .85; Group 2 ICC .52-.55	T2 to T3=7days, T1 to T3=14 days Group 2:	model (atypical)
Visual-Motor Speed	Both Groups, all intervals ICC>.66	T1 to T2=45 days, T2 to T3=5 days, T1 to T3=50 days	
Reaction Time	Group 1 all intervals >.78; Group 2 .57, .49, .71		
Response speed	r=.97		
Memory	r=.53; ICC=.54	21-42 days	Sample is
Verbal Memory	r=.34; ICC=.29		atypical for
Visual Memory	r=.48; ICC=.47		sports-related
Psychomotor Speed	r=.77; ICC=.72		concussion
Reaction Time	r=.78; ICC=.75		management
Complex Attention	r=.79; ICC=.79		
Cognitive Flexibility	r=.71; ICC=.62		
Processing Speed	r=.68; ICC=.63		
Executive Functioning	r=.73; ICC=.64		
Neurocognitive Index	r=.76; ICC=.70		

Summary All of the computerized neuropsychological test batteries present some evidence of concurrent validity with traditional paper-and-pencil tests. Direct comparisons between tests provide some strong relationships, typically for the speeded tests rather than the memory tests. Within-battery reliabilities tend to be better for speeded tests as well. The CRI does not include a memory component. CogSport has demonstrated good reliability for working memory speed, but not for accuracy.

The generally poorer performance of "memory" tasks is unfortunate because working memory has long been identified as a significant cognitive function that declines in all forms of TBI; the poorer performance may be a function of the computer presentation of the tests. The trend of speeded

TABLE 3-7 Validity Studies on Common Neuropsychological Tests

Test	Study Author	Age Range	Subjects (n)
Automated Neuropsychological Assessment Metrics (ANAM)	Bleiberg et al., 1997		6 concussed, 6 control
ANAM	Bleiberg et al., 2000	High school, college	122 high school and college
ANAM	Bleiberg et al., 2004	College	68 concussed of 729; 18 controls tested at same interval
ANAM	Prichep et al., 2013	15-23 years	65 concussed
ANAM	Register-Mihalik et al., 2013b	College	132 concussed
ANAM	Woodard et al., 2002	High school, non-concussed	

Type of Validity	Comparisons	Findings
Concurrent	ANAM with H-R plus other tests	Too few subjects for meaningful interpretation
Concurrent	Trail Making Test Part B, Auditory Consonant Trigrams total score, Paced Auditory Serial Addition test (PASAT), Hopkins Verbal Learning test, Stroop Color-Word test	PASAT r Mathematical Processing=.66; PASAT r with Sternberg Memory=.45; PASAT r with Spatial Processing=.33; Trails B r Matching to Sample=.50 //PASAT & Trails B correlated with Mathematical Processing, Sternberg Memory, Spatial processing, and Matching to Sample
Predictive	Test intervals: 0 to 23 hours, 1 to 2 days, 3 to 7 days, and 8 to 14	<24 hour: Spatial Processing p<.01; Mathematical Processing <.05; 1-2 d Spatial Processing <.05/ no other findings
Predictive	Moderate versus severe concussion	At the time of injury, athletes with moderate concussion performed significantly worse than athletes with mild concussion on ANAM Code Substitution-Delayed, Code Substitution, Matching to Sample, Simple Reaction Time and Simple Reaction Time 2 subtests (p<0.05)
Predictive	Percent exceeding reliable change index; reliable change index values based on separate healthy sample	Sensitivity at 80%, 90%, and 95% all <15%; specificity >90%
Concurrent	Healthy athletes ANAM and paper-and-pencil tests	Significant correlations between individual ANAM scores and Hopkins Verbal Learning test, Controlled Oral Word Association test, Digit Symbol Substitution test, Symbol Search

continued

TABLE 3-7 Continued

Test	Study Author	Age Range	Subjects (n)
CogSport	Collie et al., 2003		240 elite Australian rules football players
CogSport/Axon	Makdissi et al., 2010	16-35 years, median=22 years	88 concussed Australian rules football
CogSport/ Axon	Moriarity et al., 2012		Amateur boxers
CogSport	Schatz and Putz, 2006	18-23	30 college students
Immediate Post-Concussion Assessment and Cognitive Testing (ImPACT)	Iverson et al., 2005	Mean age 17 years	72 amateur
ImPACT	Iverson et al., 2004	None given	25 amateur

Type of Validity	Comparisons	Findings
Concurrent	Trails, Digit Symbol Substitution test; ICCs calculated from z-scores	ICCs stronger for Digit Symbol than Trails; speed scores better than accuracy
Predictive	Trails B, Digit Symbol, and CogSport; symptomatic versus asymptomatic at time of testing	Both CogSport and paper-and-pencil showed more reliable change index changes for symptomatic than asymptomatic; significantly more athletes showed reliable change index changes on CogSport than paper-and-pencil for both
Predictive	Baseline to post bout	2 of 96 had low scores but no concussion; not clear what the conclusion was; some took baseline tests in dorm room
Concurrent	Significant correlations (p<.05) Simple Reaction Time: no significant r; Complex Reaction Time to ImPACT Reaction Time r=.649; to Trails A r=.544; to Trails B r=.535; Memory to CogSport Learning r=.723	Complex Reaction Time correlated with paper-and-pencil and ImPACT
Concurrent	Tested within 21 days of concussion; correlated with Symbol Digit Modalities	All composites and symptom total significantly correlated with Symbol Digit Modalities
Concurrent-construct	Tested within 20 days of injury; Brief Visual Memory test, Trail Making, Symbol Digit Modalities	Symbol Digit Modalities and Brief Visual Memory tests delayed significantly correlated with all 4 ImPACT composites. Both Trails correlated with processing speed

continued

TABLE 3-7 Continued

Test	Study Author	Age Range	Subjects (n)
ImPACT	Schatz et al., 2006	High school	72 concussed athletes
ImPACT	Schatz and Putz, 2006	18-23	30 college students
ImPACT	Schatz and Sandel, 2013	High school and college	81 concussed symptomatic athletes; 37 concussed asymptomatic athletes, ages 13-21
ImPACT	Tsushima et al., 2013	High school	26 concussed versus 25 controls
ImPACT	Maerlender et al., 2010	College	54 non-concussed

Type of Validity	Comparisons	Findings
Predictive	72 concussed (within 72 hours of injury) compared to 66 controls	Significant differences between groups on all ImPACT composites and symptoms; 1 discriminant function included Visual Memory, Processing Speed, Impulse Control and symptom total: sensitivity=82%, specificity=89%
Concurrent	Significant correlations (p<.05) Complex Reaction Time to Headminder r=.407; to CogSport r=.649; to Trails A r=.641; to Trails B r=.442; to Digit Symbol r=−.455 Memory no significant r Processing Speed to Headminder r=−.373	Speed tests show correlations with paper-and-pencil and other computer tests; memory tests do not correlate (no memory tests in paper-and-pencil battery)
Predictive	81 concussed evaluated within hours of injury compared to 81 controls' baseline testing; also compared scores of 37 symptomatic athletes to asymptomatic athletes to 37 matched controls	Symptomatic athletes: Sensitivity=.75; specificity=.89; PPP=.91, NPP=.69; Asymptomatic: Sensitivity, Specificity, PPP, NPP=.97 (only 2 cases were misclassified) Sample was well characterized and clean (no learning disability, attention deficit hyperactivity disorder)
Criterion	Score comparisons at 6 days	No difference in test scores at 6 days, significant difference in symptoms; authors felt it replicated previous findings of no test score difference at 7 days (6) Very small n, no control for baseline, so amount of actual change may be obscured
Convergent, concurrent, construct	ImPACT to paper-and-pencil and to in-scanner behavioral tests	High correlations between similar measures for all 4 composites

continued

TABLE 3-7 Continued

Test	Study Author	Age Range	Subjects (n)
ImPACT	Maerlender et al., 2013	College	54 non-concussed (same sample as 2010 study)
ImPACT	Allen and Gfeller, 2011	College	100 non-concussed
Pediatric ImPACT	Newman et al., 2013	5-12 years	164 concussed
Pediatric ImPACT	Gioia et al., 2013a	5-12 years, <7 days post concussion	22 ages 5-7, 67 ages 8-12
Concussion Resolution Index (CRI)	Erlanger et al., 2003	13-35 years	414

Type of Validity	Comparisons	Findings
Discriminant, concurrent, construct	ImPACT to paper-and-pencil and to in-scanner behavioral tests	Poor discriminant validity for 3 or 4 composites–high correlations with dissimilar paper-and-pencil measures, except for reaction time
Construct	Factor analysis of ImPACT and paper-and-pencil battery	Five ImPACT factors accounted for 69 percent of variance; significant correlations between ImPACT composites and paper-and-pencil tests (except impulse control)
Concurrent, construct	Tested an average of 12 days from injury; correlations with paper-and-pencil and fluency tests	Response Speed Composite r: Digit Span, forward and backward, Auditory Consonant Trigrams, Symbol Digit memory; Response Speed Composite was more strongly associated with traditional speed measures than it was with the Learning and Memory Composite, indicating relative independence of the Response Speed and Learning and Memory Accuracy
Criterion, predictive	Response speed and symptoms by age	Response speed and symptoms together correctly classified by age
Concurrent	CRI factors correlated with paper-and-pencil tests (Processing Speed, Simple Reaction Time, Complex Reaction Time)	Symbol Digit Modalities and Grooved pegs (bilateral) correlated with all three factors; Trails A correlated with Simple and Complex Reaction Time; Trails B and Stroop interference correlated with Processing Speed; Digit Symbol (WAIS-III) correlated with Simple Reaction Time

continued

TABLE 3-7 Continued

Test	Study Author	Age Range	Subjects (n)
CRI	Erlanger et al., 2002	18-87 years	66 out of a larger sample
CRI/Head-minder	Schatz and Putz, 2006	18-23	30 college students

NOTES: ICC = intraclass correlation coefficient, NPP = negative predictive power, PPP = positive predictive power.

tests showing better performance than the accuracy measures may be reflecting the strengths of the computerized platform.

Does Baseline Testing Improve the Utility of Neuropsychological Testing in the Diagnosis and Management of Sports-Related Concussion?

Baseline testing has become commonplace and often is considered an invaluable part of sports concussion management as it allows for more accurate interpretation of post-injury scores (McCrory et al., 2005). In 2011, Congress mandated that the Department of Defense develop and implement a comprehensive policy on consistent neurological cognitive assessments of service members before and after deployment (P.L. 111-383, sec. 722). The Department of Defense now mandates pre-deployment baseline testing to be performed on all service members within 12 months of their deployment (DoD, 2013). Comparing a post-injury score to an individual's baseline allows a comparison that controls for many of the individual factors that can affect test performance, and several papers have called for its (continued) use (Barth et al., 1989; Gardner et al., 2012; Hinton-Bayre et al., 1997,

Type of Validity	Comparisons	Findings
Concurrent	4 factors identified (Response Speed, Processing Speed, Memory, Attention) and correlated with paper-and-pencil tests	Symbol Digit Modalities correlated with all four factors; Symbol Search and Digit Span correlated with Response Speed, Processing Speed, Reaction Time; Bushke Selective Reminding correlated with Response Speed, Memory, Attention; Trails A and B correlated with Response Speed
Concurrent	Significant correlations (p<.05) Simple Reaction Time to Trails A r=.428; to Digit Symbol r=−.526 Complex Reaction Time no significant r Processing Speed to Trails B r=.601; to Digit Symbol r=−.610; to ImPACT r=−.373	Simple Reaction Time and processing speed correlate with paper-and-pencil and ImPACT

1999; Lovell and Collins, 1998). Only a few empirical studies have examined the potential benefit of using baseline test scores instead of comparing post-injury scores to normative standards. Baseline testing is costly and, as indicated previously, is not without its logistical and administration problems, which can sometimes lead to questionable results. Furthermore, the use of baseline testing automatically presumes repeat testing; with that, appropriate statistical procedures are needed for interpreting results (Heilbronner et al., 2010; McCrory et al., 2005). Test scores are known to "regress to the mean" after multiple exposures, practice effects can inflate scores, and baseline scores on the extremes of the distribution will have different effects with repeat testing. Although having different "forms" of a test (different items) reduces the test taker's ability to memorize responses, the test procedures are the same, so practice increases test familiarity, which can enhance performance.

Schmidt and colleagues (2012) analyzed retrospective data for 1,060 collegiate athletes with baseline neuropsychological test (ANAM), balance, and symptom checklist results. The study used reliable-change methodology for the baseline comparisons and difference from mean baseline score for the normative comparison. An analysis of variance comparing the number of correct identifications between methods found that the baseline comparison was significantly better (fewer misidentifications) for a reaction time score, and the normative comparison was better for a mathematical reasoning score. The authors noted that individual differences in baseline performance on math processing may have caused the high rate of misidentifications. This is a drawback of the reliable-change method as opposed to a regression-based method. No other significant neuropsychological score disagreements were observed, nor were there any score disagreements for postural control or symptom severity.

Summary Baseline testing has been called for and recommended for many years. It was a cornerstone of Barth's original SLAM model and has been seen as an answer to the limitations of normative comparisons for detecting clinical change. However, very few studies have specifically examined the value of baseline testing, and establishing the validity of baseline testing is difficult. The consensus statement from the Fourth International Conference on Concussion in Sport held in Zurich has taken the lack of evidence for baseline testing as an indication that baseline testing should not be required (McCrory et al., 2013b). Baseline testing is a common practice in schools and programs for many sports (Covassin et al., 2009), and it has a theoretical foundation. On the other hand, there are drawbacks to conducting large-scale baseline assessments; as Moser and colleagues (2011) have pointed out, group testing has its disadvantages. In addition, baseline testing is expensive and time-consuming, and there is the question of whether the use of baseline testing in concussion management actually reduces risks of recurrent injury or long-term functional deficits.

Randolph and Kirkwood (2009) provided a comprehensive review of the evidence to that date regarding the use of different strategies in sports concussion management. They acknowledged that few prospective studies had been done regarding risks and means for minimizing them. Their review of the literature on football concussions (as the paradigmatic sport) noted potential risks of death or permanent disability, delayed recovery, same-season repeat concussion, and the late-life consequences of multiple concussions. They observed that catastrophic outcomes associated with sports-related concussion are extremely rare, and less serious short-term adverse outcomes also are rare and generally transient. In addition, they argued that current management strategies, including baseline testing, did not modify these risks. The same group followed up with a critique of baseline testing specifically. They argued that the utility of using baseline tests rests on the function (real-world) outcomes derived from the procedure. They note:

The primary justification for the baseline method is that it helps to ensure that athletes are fully recovered from a concussion and are therefore "safe" to [return to play]. At present, however, little to no empirical evidence is available to demonstrate that such testing actually reduces any known risk associated with concussive injury. (Kirkwood et al., 2009, p. 1410)

The 2013 position statement of the American Medical Society for Sports Medicine states that most concussions can be managed appropriately without neuropsychological testing and also notes the lack of evidence that use of baseline testing in the clinical management of concussions improves short- or long-term outcomes (Harmon et al., 2013).

Summary

Neuropsychological testing has been an important element of clinical practice in traumatic brain injury research and practice for many years. Its adoption into the sports concussion field is thus based on a considerable history. The temporal aspects of concussions, together with the potential consequences of improper behavior management, create the need for effective and efficient tools with strong psychometric foundations. However, these demands create challenges for tests and test interpretations. Furthermore, changes in knowledge and the development of newer tools have led to the need for more sophisticated analytic procedures and more nuanced interpretations. Although the quality of the studies varies, the tests reviewed here have some level of validity; reliability is even more variable, however, and users must be aware of the limitations that these studies imply. Even though computerized neuropsychological tests are easy to obtain and administer, the many factors that affect test interpretation along with the need for technical expertise in understanding test scores as they relate to individual cases together make it important that neuropsychologists or other professionals with training and expertise in neuropsychological testing and concussion management provide test interpretation.

Research on the effectiveness of neuropsychological tests in the identification and management of sports concussions is mixed. Some studies are challenged by the difficulty in establishing solid diagnostic criteria of what a concussion is, by confusion between statistical and clinical significance, by inappropriate analyses of multiple exposures to tests, and by questionable control of state-related and intrinsic subject factors. The universal "screening" approach of using baseline tests may be a significant improvement, but there are very few data on that issue, and it is not clear how one could determine if one approach is "better" than another (i.e., comparing post injury to one's own baseline or to normative standards).

Neuropsychological test scores appear to reflect the presence of a concussion, although, again, the complexity and associated factors make interpretation more difficult than it might seem on the surface. Neuropsychological testing may be of use in tracking recovery, although studies are emerging that question the presence of ongoing cognitive dysfunction when test results appear to be back to normal or baseline. The use of computerized batteries has allowed for easier test administration, but at the cost of what appears to be a loss of some specificity; that is, tests may be valid indicators of concussion in a broad sense, but they are less useful for saying what cognitive functions are actually affected. Although baseline testing is a common practice, studies provide mixed (and limited) evidence concerning the utility and cost-effectiveness of such testing.

ACUTE CONCUSSION MANAGEMENT

The time-course of the effects of a concussive blow or blows appears to take place on the order of minutes, hours, and days. Within the period of recovery, the brain is thought to be vulnerable to further injury, which can be more severe and may complicate recovery (Cantu, 1998; Cantu and Voy, 1995; Eisenberg et al., 2013; McCrory and Berkovic, 1998; Saunders and Harbaugh, 1984). Thus, although the initial injury may be mild, acute management is still needed to protect the individual from more significant harm.

In 80 to 90 percent of high-school- and college-age patients, concussion symptoms resolve within 2 weeks without any overt intervention (McClincy et al., 2006; McCrea et al., 2004, 2013). McCrea and colleagues (2013) examined 570 high school and college athletes with concussions[6] and 166 non-concussed athlete controls. Only 10 percent of the concussed athletes (n=57) took longer than 7 days to recover. In an earlier study, McCrea and colleagues (2004) reported on the recovery from concussions in 94 concussed college football players and 56 non-concussed controls. On average the athletes reverted to baseline by day 7, and there were no symptomatic or functional differences between the two groups by 3 months. This study also found that neuropsychological recovery tended to lag 2 to 3 days behind symptomatic recovery. McClincy and colleagues (2006) documented symptom and ImPACT test scores at baseline and at 2, 7, and 14 days post injury in 104 concussed high school and college athletes. They found significant differences in symptom and ImPACT scores through 7 days post injury, although the magnitude of differences dropped over time. There was no significant difference between symptom scores at baseline and at 14 days post injury. In addition, at day 14, only the verbal memory composite

---

[6]Of the injuries, 60.5 percent were in high school athletes, and 39.5 percent were in college athletes.

score of the ImPACT test was significantly different from baseline, although this suggests that at least some areas of neuropsychological recovery may persist in asymptomatic individuals. However, no adjustments for baseline scores or repeat testing were made. Makdissi and colleagues (2010) reported on the natural history of concussion in Australia elite junior and senior football players. The mean time to return to play was 4.8 days, with 18 percent showing symptoms for more than 7 days. Again, computerized neuropsychological testing revealed that abnormalities in neurocognitive performance persisted for 2 to 3 days after the athletes no longer were asymptomatic.

In a study comparing concussion recovery times of high school and college athletes through 7 days post injury, Field and colleagues (2003) found that high school athletes recovered more slowly within the first week after injury, but there was no difference in performance by 7 days in most areas tested. Unlike their college counterparts, high school athletes with a concussion still exhibited a significant decrease in memory performance at 7 days compared with controls (Field et al., 2003).

There is no body of literature on sports-related concussion recovery times for younger children (5 to 12 years). Eisenberg and colleagues (2013) found that concussion symptoms in children 11 to 13 years old presenting to the emergency department (ED) resolved more quickly than in those age 13 and older. It is important to note that the sample in the Eisenberg study was drawn from patients presenting to the ED with acute concussions, raising the possibility that participants may have experienced a more severe injury or a higher initial symptom load than did individuals with acute concussion who do not seek care in an ED. Almost 64 percent of those included in the study sustained their concussions playing sports, 22 percent experienced loss of consciousness, and 43 percent experienced amnesia.

In most studies, the majority of youth adjust well after an mTBI, but in studies that had a non-head-injury control group and good sample retention, around 10 to 13 percent were still symptomatic at 3 months and 1 year after the injury (Barlow et al., 2010; McCrea et al., 2013; Yeates et al., 2009, 2012). Chapter 4 includes recovery curves for reported symptoms, postural stability, and cognitive function (see Figures 4-1, 4-2, and 4-3).

In the acute phase of concussion management, in addition to symptom resolution, the goals include protecting the brain from additional injury and stress, avoiding potential long-term cognitive sequelae of repeated injury, and avoiding the risk of second impact syndrome. The current consensus statements put forth by the international Concussion in Sport Group (McCrory et al., 2013b), the American Medical Society for Sports Medicine (Harmon et al., 2012), the American Academy of Pediatrics (Halstead et al., 2010), and the American Academy of Neurology (Giza et al., 2013) state that athletes who sustain a concussion should not return to play on the same day as the injury. There is evidence that high school and college athletes may have a delayed onset in symptoms and demonstrate post-injury neuropsychological deficits that may not be apparent on the sideline of an athletic event, and therefore the athletes would benefit from immediate removal from play for their protection (Collins et al., 1999, 2003b; Duhaime et al., 2012; Guskiewicz et al., 2003; Lovell et al., 2003; McCrea et al., 2003). This suggests that same-day return would place that athlete at higher risk for adverse outcomes.

During the acute phase, clinical management strategies to limit physical and cognitive activity are emphasized. The more aggressive medical management of symptoms typically does not begin until 2 to 4 weeks post injury, when an athlete may be said to be experiencing prolonged recovery (see Chapter 4).

Physical Rest

Consensus opinion holds that athletes who have sustained a concussion should refrain from aerobic exercise, sport-specific training, and competition until symptoms resolve (Giza et al., 2013; Halstead et al., 2010; Harmon et al., 2013; McCrory et al., 2013b). Two issues underlie this consensus recommendation. First, concussed athletes are usually instructed to avoid any activity that will increase their heart rate, as this may worsen symptoms and potentially increase recovery time. Second, a premature return to contact or collision activities may increase the risk of repeat injury (Cantu, 1998; Cantu and Voy, 1995; Guskiewicz et al., 2003; McCrory and Berkovic, 1998; Saunders and Harbaugh, 1984). There is evidence in animals that additional concussive injury within a certain period of vulnerability following the initial injury has an additive effect (see Chapter 5). The period of vulnerability may be related to metabolic depression in the brain following the initial injury, but it is not yet known what the time frame is for this vulnerable period, how it varies across ages ranges, and how best to measure it.

Physical rest can range from bed rest to simply refraining from full contact athletic activity. It is important to distinguish between potentially concussive activities (e.g., contact sports or activities that carry a risk of head or body impact) and noncontact physical activity, which may or may not exacerbate symptoms.

Cognitive Rest

Cognitive rest is also recommended for the initial period following a concussion (Halstead et al., 2010; Harmon et al., 2013; McCrory et al., 2013b), although what cognitive rest entails has not been well defined, and its efficacy in promoting recovery has not been fully determined. Generally, cognitive rest is achieved by eliminating or decreasing activities that require concentration, including schoolwork (McCrory et al., 2009, 2013b) and mental stimulation, as these may exacerbate symptoms and prolong recovery. However, there is a suggestion in the literature that 1 to 2 weeks away from school and schoolwork may place students at academic risk (Allensworth and Easton, 2007).

Evidence for Physical and Cognitive Rest

There is limited evidence about the effects of physical and cognitive rest in youth recovering from sports-related concussion, although it is widely accepted that concussion symptoms are aggravated by both physical and mental exertion (Kissik and Johnston, 2005), and, as previously mentioned, there is evidence of a period of vulnerability during which the brain is more susceptible to secondary injury and during which it is prudent to avoid activities that may lead to additional impacts. In a prospective, nonrandomized study of 635 high school and college athletes with concussion, McCrea and colleagues (2009) found that the more time that elapsed between an athlete's injury and return to play, the less likely the athlete was to have a repeat concussion during the same season. In addition to the adverse effects of concussion on physical and cognitive function in the acute post-concussion period, there is evidence that the brain is recovering from metabolic changes, as described in Chapter 2. Physical and cognitive activities may increase energy demands on an already overtaxed system. Evidence from a study of voluntary exercise in rats suggests that an initial period of physical and cognitive rest is therapeutic after concussive injury (Griesbach et al., 2004). A retrospective cohort study of 95 high school athletes found that individuals engaging in high levels of activity (school and full athletic participation) after a concussion did not perform as well on neurocognitive testing as those with moderate levels of activity (school and moderate physical activity—light jogging, mowing the lawn) (Majerske et al., 2008). In another study, high school and college athletes who completed at least 1 week of cognitive and physical rest after injury showed significant improvement on concussion symptom scale ratings and neurocognitive scores, even when rest was prescribed weeks or months following a concussion (Moser et al., 2012).

Other studies, however, suggest little or no beneficial effect of physical rest on length of recovery. The same study by McCrea and colleagues (2009) found no difference in concussion outcomes at 45 and 90 days post injury between athletes who returned to play while symptomatic or immediately following symptom resolution and those who observed at least a 1- to 7-day wait following symptom resolution before returning to play.

Another study showed that rest (defined as no mental or physical exertion, but continued activities of daily living) as a treatment for mTBI was ineffective (see Willer and Leddy, 2006). A randomized human trial of patients presenting to the ED with mTBI showed that complete bed rest for 6 days after presentation was ineffective in reducing symptoms at 2 weeks and 6 months post injury (de Kruijk et al., 2002).

The expert consensus opinion is that an individualized treatment plan including physical and cognitive rest is beneficial for recovery from concussion, although current research is insufficient to identify the level and duration of physical and cognitive rest needed to promote recovery. Randomized controlled trials or other appropriately designed studies on the management of concussion in youth are needed in order to develop empirically based clinical guidelines; this includes studies to determine the efficacy of physical and cognitive rest following concussion and the optimal level and duration of rest.[7]

Return to Physical Activity

The return of an individual to physical activity following a concussion is typically governed by his or her symptom load. Consensus opinion (McCrory et al., 2013b) and practice guidelines (Giza et al., 2013; Halstead et al., 2010; Harmon et al., 2013) state that individuals who have sustained a concussion should avoid physical activity during the acute phase of recovery until they are symptom-free at rest and without medication (see also Buzzini and Guskiewicz, 2006; Canadian Academy of Sport Medicine Concussion Committee, 2000; Herring et al., 2011; Hunt and Asplund, 2010; Kutcher and Eckner, 2010; Lee, 2006; Moser et al., 2007; Poirier, 2003; Purcell and Canadian Paediatric Society, 2012; Putukian et al., 2009). Before returning to activity, individuals should also be back to either their own baseline or the appropriate population norm with regard to neuropsychological/cognitive functioning (McCrory et al., 2013b). When this is measured or obtained by computerized testing, it is important that interpreting providers consider reliable change in test scores rather than exclusively focusing on the numbered scores or percentile scores.

The Department of Defense requires that all deployed service members who are diagnosed with their first concussion observe a mandatory minimum 24-hour recovery period, which may be extended on the basis of

---

[7]The report reflects information that was available at the time it went to press. A prospective study of the effect of cognitive activity level on the duration of symptoms following sports-related concussions in 335 youth ages 8 to 23 years subsequently was published in January 2014 (Brown et al., 2014).

subsequent clinical evaluation (DoD, 2012).[8] Similar concussion management policies are being developed for concussed service members in the non-deployed setting as well (Tsao, 2013).

During the period when the patient denies symptoms but when metabolic changes presumably are still in effect, symptoms may be induced by rigorous exercise. Therefore, team physicians and athletic trainers may use exercise as a "symptom stress test" to determine whether a player is ready to return to play. Furthermore, evidence that the resolution of neurocognitive impairment following concussion may take longer than the resolution of physical symptoms (Broglio et al., 2007a; Iverson et al., 2006; Peterson et al., 2003; Sandel et al., 2012) and that moderate exercise may induce cognitive declines in athletes who are asymptomatic and have returned to neurocognitive baseline following concussion (McGrath et al., 2013) highlight the importance of appropriately managing an individual's return to physical activity.

Once individuals are symptom-free, it is frequently recommended that they follow a graded return-to-play protocol (see Table 3-8), progression through which is governed in part by recurrence of symptoms (Canadian Academy of Sport Medicine Concussion Committee, 2000; Halstead et al., 2010; Herring et al., 2011; McCrory et al., 2013b). The protocol calls for individuals to proceed to the next level if they remain asymptomatic at the current stage. If concussion symptoms reappear, the athlete should revert back to the previous asymptomatic stage and resume the progression after 24 hours (Canadian Academy of Sport Medicine Concussion Committee, 2000). The Department of Defense is also in the process of developing a gradual return-to-duty guideline (personal communication with Jack W. Tsao, October 8, 2013).

However, aside from evidence supporting refraining from activities that risk additional injury or re-injury during the temporally undefined "window of cerebral vulnerability" following a concussion, there is little empirical evidence to support the timing of return to physical activity or the use of graded approaches for doing so.

Return to Cognitive Activity

The resumption of cognitive activity, including returning to school, is a primary concern for the majority of the age groups under consideration in this report. Individualized academic adjustments are often needed and are

---

[8]Service members who receive a second concussion diagnosis within 12 months are not returned to full duty for 7 days following symptom resolution (DoD, 2012). Individuals who sustain 3 or more concussions within 12 months are required to undergo a "recurrent concussion evaluation," which is used in determining return-to-duty status (DoD, 2012).

TABLE 3-8 Graded Return-to-Play Protocol

Step	Rehabilitation Stage	Functional Exercise at Each Stage of Rehabilitation	Objective of Each Stage
1	No activity	Complete cognitive and physical rest.	Recovery
2	Light aerobic exercise	Walking, swimming, or stationary cycling, keeping intensity <70% maximum predicted heart rate. No resistance training.	Increase heart rate
3	Sport-specific activity	Skating drills in ice hockey, running drills in soccer. No head impact activities.	Add movement
4	Non-contact training drills	Progression to more complex training drills, e.g., passing drills in football and ice hockey. May start load progressive resistance training.	Exercise, coordination, and cognitive
5	Full contact practice	Following medical clearance, participate in normal training activities.	Restore confidence and assess functional skills by coaching staff
6	Return to play	Normal game play.	

SOURCE: Based on Canadian Academy of Sport Medicine Concussion Committee, 2000.

guided by the individual's experience of symptoms (Halstead et al., 2010; McCrory et al., 2013b). Some students may be unable to participate in full days of school or work, may need a reduced amount of classwork and homework, or may require additional time to take tests and accomplish other tasks (McGrath, 2010; Popoli et al., 2013; Sady et al., 2011). It is also important to note that students who are limited should specifically not be allowed to participate in physical education classes.

Evidence that the resolution of neurocognitive impairment following concussion may take longer than the resolution of physical symptoms (see, e.g., McClincy et al., 2006) highlights the importance of appropriately managing the return to cognitive activity. Academic work demands focus, memory, processing speeds, and concentration, which are the processes that are affected by a concussion (McCrory et al., 2004). In addition, cognitive stress may elicit or exacerbate concussive symptoms. Indeed, at 1 month post injury, individuals noted more symptoms with cognitive stress than with physical stress (Gioia et al., 2010). The ImPACT test has a post-test symptom checklist that in effect documents the effect of mental exertion on neurocognitive testing.

Although the majority of concussions resolve within 2 weeks, missing school for even a portion of that time can be detrimental to student performance. Assuming a standard school year of approximately 180 days, a 2-week absence for concussion translates into missing 5 percent of the school year. Minimizing time lost from school without compromising the recovery and academic performance of a student recovering from concussion is a challenge. Allensworth and Easton (2007) found that only 63 percent of students in the Chicago school system who missed 5 to 9 days of school in 1 year graduated in 4 years, compared to 87 percent of students who missed less than 1 week. As is the case with a return to physical activity, however, there is little evidence to support protocols for returning students to school following a concussion.

Nationally there are currently two categories of accommodations for disabled students, including those with TBI: the individualized educational plan (IEP) and the 504 plan. The details of each vary by state. In general, IEPs are designed to address long-term cognitive disabilities and ensure that qualified elementary or secondary school students receive individually appropriate specialized instruction, including modified curricula, and related services. A 504 plan is designed to accommodate those individuals with a disability under the Americans with Disabilities Act. This refers to specific laws that protect students who need accommodations in order to have a "level playing field" while pursuing the typical school curriculum—for example, ensuring that a blind student is provided with audio or Braille textbooks or a student with severe dyslexia is permitted additional time on timed assessments.

Although a concussed student, with limitations in memory and processing speeds, may qualify for accommodations under a 504 plan, in practice the time it often takes to determine eligibility and implement the plan makes this an impractical approach for meeting the needs of students who recover within the typical 2-week time frame (Popoli et al., 2013). In addition, a parental request for academic accommodations via a 504 plan or IEP obligates the school to act upon the request, which poses real costs to the school district, both financial and in terms of staff time. Because most concussions resolve within a few weeks, short-term school-based accommodations often can be arranged without the need for a 504 plan (Popoli et al., 2013). Longer-term accommodations may be considered in cases when concussive symptoms persist much longer (e.g., 3 months or more).

Several states, including Arizona (Barrow Concussion Network, 2013), Maine (Maine Department of Education, 2012), New Jersey (P.L.

2013, Ch. 71 [June 27, 2013]), New York (New York State Department of Education, 2012), and Oregon (Oregon Department of Education, 2010), have implemented formal systems to help educate educators on the effects of concussion and to manage the return of students with concussions to academic activity through the use of concussion management teams or other mechanisms. A number of other states provide links to informational material for parents and educators. A common element of the formal school-based concussion management policies is the inclusion of accommodations to permit a gradual return to academic activity (e.g., a shortened school day or extra time to make up assignments and tests).

The Brain Injury Association of Pennsylvania (BIAP), with input from the Pennsylvania Department of Education, has developed a model policy to provide guidance for Pennsylvania schools with respect to concussion and mTBI (BIAP, 2013). The BIAP—with additional funding from the Pennsylvania Departments of Health and Education—has developed a program called BrainSTEPS, which offers school districts trained assistance in reintegrating concussed students into school (BIAP, 2013; Brown, 2013). This work in Pennsylvania illustrates the potential for collaboration among government entities (e.g., Departments of Health and Education) and between government and the private sector to develop infrastructures for addressing issues associated with concussion in youth.

FINDINGS

The committee identified the following findings on concussion recognition, diagnosis, and management:

- Currently concussion diagnosis is based primarily on symptoms reported by the individual rather than on objective diagnostic markers, which might also serve as objective markers of recovery.
- The signs and symptoms of concussion typically fall into four categories—physical, cognitive, emotional, and sleep—with patients experiencing one or more symptoms from one or more categories.
- The use of multiple evaluation tools, such as symptom scales and checklists, balance testing, and neurocognitive testing, may increase the sensitivity and specificity of concussion identification, although existing evidence is insufficient to determine the best combination of measures.
- Traditional neuroimaging techniques, such as computerized tomography and magnetic resonance imaging, are of little diagnostic value for concussions per se, because structural imaging results are normal in the case of concussions uncomplicated by skull fracture or hematoma.

- Newer imaging techniques, such as magnetic resonance spectroscopy, positron emission tomography, single-photon emission computed tomography, functional magnetic resonance imaging, and diffusion tensor imaging may be useful in the future for assessing sports-related concussions, but at present they have not been validated for clinical use.

- There is some consensus in the literature that both quantitative electroencephalograph and event-related potential procedures can detect differences in performance and neural responses in concussed versus non-concussed student athletes in high school and college even when behavior measures fail. However, these findings are true for a relatively small set of tasks that assess a limited array of cognitive abilities. Use of a broader range of tasks that measure different aspects of cognitive processes is necessary to provide a comprehensive view of behaviors most likely affected and those more likely spared by concussion.

- There is little research on the use of serum biomarkers in pediatric concussion. Although appropriately sensitive and specific serum biomarkers could be of great diagnostic and prognostic value in sports-related concussion, there currently is no evidence to support their use. There is some evidence, however, to suggest that normal levels of S100B following head injury may predict individuals who do *not* have intracranial injury.

- Neuropsychological testing has a long tradition in measuring cognitive function after traumatic brain injury and is one of several tools (along with symptom assessment, clinical evaluation, and the like) that may aid in the diagnosis and management of concussions in youth. Studies of the effectiveness of these tests to predict diagnosis and track recovery have had mixed results, and the performance of individuals on neuropsychological tests can be influenced by many factors, including effort and the presence of concussion symptoms (e.g., fatigue resulting from sleep disturbance). It appears that high scores on neuropsychological tests, indicating good cognitive function, are predictive of *not* having a concussion. In group studies these tests have been shown to be useful for tracking cognitive recovery for up to 2 weeks post injury, with a majority of concussions considered to be resolved by that time. There are no data on the effectiveness of monitoring recovery in individuals whose symptoms persist beyond the typical recovery period.

- Reliability studies for computerized neuropsychological tests are quite variable, with some studies demonstrating adequate reliability and some indicating less than adequate reliability. There are many possible reasons for the variability, including different sample sizes, unknown testing conditions, and variable item pools. Most computerized tests produce multiple forms through a quasi-randomization of items. All commercial test batteries reviewed had some studies indicating acceptable reliability.

- Expert consensus opinion is that an individualized treatment plan including physical and cognitive rest is beneficial for recovery from concussion. There is little empirical evidence to indicate the optimal degree and duration of physical rest needed to promote recovery or the best timing and approach for returning to full physical activity, including the use of graded return-to-play protocols. However, there is evidence that the brain is more susceptible to injury while recovering; thus, common sense dictates reducing the risks of a repeat injury. Similarly, there is little evidence regarding the efficacy of cognitive rest following concussion or to inform the best timing and approach for return to cognitive activity following concussion, including protocols for returning students to school.
- Randomized controlled trials or other appropriately designed studies on the management of concussion youth are needed in order to develop empirically based clinical guidelines, including studies to determine the efficacy of physical and cognitive rest following concussion, the optimal period of rest, and the best protocol for returning individuals to full physical activity as well as to inform the development of evidence-based protocols and appropriate accommodations for students returning to school.

REFERENCES

AERA (American Educational Research Association), American Psychological Association, and National Council on Measurement in Education. 1999. *Standards for Educational and Psychological Testing.* Washington, DC: American Educational Research Association.

Alla, S., S. J. Sullivan, L. Hale, and P. McCrory. 2009. Self-report scales/checklists for the measurement of concussion symptoms: A systematic review. *British Journal of Sports Medicine* 43(suppl 1):i3–i12.

Allen, B. J., and J. D. Gfeller. 2011. The Immediate Post-Concussion Assessment and Cognitive Testing battery and traditional neuropsychological measures: A construct and concurrent validity study. *Brain Injury* 25(2):179-191.

Allensworth, E. M., and J. Q. Easton. 2007. *What Matters for Staying On-Track and Graduating in Chicago Public High Schools: A Close Look at Course Grades, Failures, and Attendance in the Freshman Year.* Chicago: University of Chicago, Consortium on Chicago School Research.

Anastasi, A., and S. Urbina, 1997. *Psychological Testing*, Seventh edition. Upper Saddle River, NJ: Prentice Hall.

Anderson, B. L., W. J. Pomerantz, J. K. Mann, and M. A. Gittelman. 2013. "I can't miss the big game": High school (HS) football players' knowledge and attitudes about concussions. Presented at the Pediatric Academic Societies Annual Meeting, Washington, DC, May 6.

Axon Sports. 2013. Doctor/trainer FAQs. http://www.axonsports.com/index.cfm?pid=88&page Title=Doctor/Trainer-FAQs (accessed October 8, 2013).

Ayr, L. K., K. O. Yeates, H. G. Taylor, and M. Browne. 2009. Dimensions of postconcussive symptoms in children with mild traumatic brain injuries. *Journal of the International Neuropsychological Society* 15(1):19-30.

Bailey, C. M., R. J. Echemendia, and P. A. Arnett. 2006. The impact of motivation on neuropsychological performance in sports-related mild traumatic brain injury. *Journal of the International Neuropsycholological Society* 12(4):475-484.

Bailey, C. M., H. L. Samples, D. K. Broshek, J. R. Freeman, and J. T. Barth. 2010. The relationship between psychological distress and baseline sports-related concussion testing. *Clinical Journal of Sport Medicine* 20(4):272-277.

Baillargeon, A., M. Lassonde, S. Leclerc, and D. Ellemberg. 2012. Neuropsychological and neurophysiological assessment of sport concussion in children, adolescents and adults. *Brain Injury* 26(3):211-220.

Bandyopadhyay, S., H. Hennes, M. H. Gorelick, R. G. Wells, and C. M. Walsh-Kelly. 2005. Serum neuron-specific enolase as a predictor of short-term outcome in children with closed traumatic brain injury. *Academic Emergency Medicine* 12(8):732-738.

Barlow, K. M., S. Crawford, A. Stevenson, S. S. Sandhu, F. Belanger, D. Dewey. 2010. Epidemiology of postconcussion syndrome in pediatric mild traumatic brain injury. *Pediatrics* 126(2):e374-e381.

Barr, W. B., L. S. Prichep, R. Chabot, M. R. Powell, and M. McCrea. 2012. Measuring brain electrical activity to track recovery from sport-related concussion. *Brain Injury* 26(1):58-66.

Barrow Concussion Network. 2013. Barrow Concussion Network. http://www.aiaonline.org/story/uploads/BCN_FAQ_1368640958.pdf (accessed September 23, 2013).

Barth, J. T., S. N. Macciocchi, B. Giordani, R. N. Rimel, J. A. Jane, and T. J. Boll. 1983. Neuropsychological sequelae of minor head injury. *Neurosurgery* 13(5):529-533.

Barth, J. T., W. M. Alves, T. V. Ryan, S. N. Macciocchi, R. W. Rimel, J. A. Jane, and W. E. Nelson. 1989. Mild head injury in sports: Neuropsychological sequelae and recovery of function. In *Mild Head Injury*, edited by H. S. Levin, H. M. Eisenberg, and A. L. Benton. New York: Oxford University Press, pp. 257-275.

Barth, J. T., J. R. Freeman, and J. E. Winters. 2000. Management of sports-related concussions. *Dental Clinics of North America* 44(1):67-83.

Bauer, R. M., G. L. Iverson, A. N. Cernich, L. M. Binder, R. M. Ruff, and R. I. Naugle. 2012. Computerized neuropsychological assessment devices: Joint position paper of the American Academy of Clinical Neuropsychology and the National Academy of Neuropsychology. *Archives of Clinical Neuropsychology* 27(3):362-373.

Baumgartner, T. A., and H. Chung. 2001. Confidence limits for intraclass reliability coefficients. *Measurement in Physical Education and Exercise Science* 5(3):179-188.

Bazarian, J. J., F. P. Zemlan, S. Mookerjee, and T. Stigbrand. 2006. Serum S-100B and cleaved-tau are poor predictors of long-term outcome after mild traumatic brain injury. *Brain Injury* 20(7):759-765.

Bechtel, K., S. Frasure, C. Marshall, J. Dziura, and C. Simpson. 2009. Relationship of serum S100B levels and intracranial injury in children with closed head trauma. *Pediatrics* 124(4):e697-e704.

Beckwith, J. G., R. M. Greenwald, J. J. Chu, J. J. Crisco, S. Rowson, S. M. Duma, S. P. Broglio, T. W. McAllister, K. M. Guskiewicz, J. P. Mihalik, S. Anderson, B. Schnebel, P. G. Brolinson, and M. W. Collins. 2013a. Head impact exposure sustained by football players on days of diagnosed concussion. *Medicine and Science in Sports and Exercise* 45(4):737-746.

Beckwith, J. G., R. M. Greenwald, J. J. Chu, J. J. Crisco, S. Rowson, S. M. Duma, S. P. Broglio, T. W. McAllister, K. M. Guskiewicz, J. P. Mihalik, S. Anderson, B. Schnebel, P. G. Brolinson, and M. W. Collins. 2013b. Timing of concussion diagnosis is related to head impact exposure prior to injury. *Medicine and Science in Sports and Exercise* 45(4):747-754.

Beebe, D. W. 2012. A brief primer on sleep for pediatric and child clinical neuropsychologists. *Child Neuropsychology* 18(4):313-338.

Beers, S. R., R. P. Berger, and P. D. Adelson. 2007. Neurocognitive outcome and serum biomarkers in inflicted versus non-inflicted traumatic brain injury in young children. *Journal of Neurotrauma* 24(1):97-105.

Belanger, H. G., and R. D. Vanderploeg. 2005. The neuropsychological impact of sports-related concussion: A meta-analysis. *Journal of the International Neuropsychological Society* 11(4):345-357.

Belanger, H. G., R. D. Vanderploeg, G. Curtiss, and D. L. Warden. 2007. Recent neuroimaging techniques in mild traumatic brain injury. *Jounal of Neuropsychiatry and Clinical Neurosciences* 19(1):5-20.

Berger, R. P., and N. Zuckerbraun. 2012. Biochemical markers. In *Mild Traumatic Brain Injury in Children and Adolescents: From Basic Science to Clinical Management*, edited by M. W. Kirkwood and K. O. Yeates. New York: Guilford Press. Pp. 145-161.

Berger, R. P., S. R. Beers, R. Richichi, D. Wiesman, and P. D. Adelson. 2007. Serum biomarker concentrations and outcome after pediatric traumatic brain injury. *Journal of Neurotrauma* 24(12):1793-1801.

BIAP (Brain Injury Association of Pennsylvania). 2013. BIAPA offers assistance to Pennsylvania schools. http://www.biapa.org/site/apps/nlnet/content2.aspx?c=iuLZJbMMKrH&b=1843921&ct=11590269&notoc=1 (accessed October 7, 2013).

Biederman, J., L. J. Seidman, C. R. Petty, R. Fried, A. E. Doyle, D. R. Cohen, D. C. Kenealy, and S. V. Faraone. 2008. Effects of stimulant medication on neuropsychological functioning in young adults with attention-deficit/hyperactivity disorder. *Journal of Clinical Psychiatry* 69(7):1150-1156.

Bleiberg, J., W. Garmoe, E. Halpern, D. Reeves, and J. Nadler. 1997. Consistency of within-day and across-day performance after mild brain injury. *Neuropsychiatry, Neuropsychology, and Behavioral Neurology* 10(4):247-253.

Bleiberg, J., R. L. Kane, D. L. Reeves, W. S. Garmoe, and E. Halpern. 2000. Factor analysis of computerized and traditional tests used in mild brain injury research. *Clinical Neuropsycholgist* 14(3):287-294.

Bleiberg J., A. Cernich, K. Cameron, W. Sun, K. Peck, J. Ecklund, D. Reeves, J. Uhorchak, M. B. Sparling, and D. L. Warden. 2004. Duration of cognitive impairment after sports concussion. *Neurosurgery* 54(5):1073-1078; discussion 1078-1080.

Broglio, S. P., and T. W. Puetz. 2008. The effect of sport concussion on neurocognitive function, self-report symptoms and postural control: A meta-analysis. *Sports Medicine* 38:53-67.

Broglio, S. P., S. N. Macciocchi, and M. S. Ferrara. 2007a. Neurocognitive performance of concussed athletes when symptom free. *Journal of Athletic Training* 42(4):504-508.

Broglio, S. P., S. N. Macciocchi, and M. S. Ferrara. 2007b. Sensitivity of the concussion assessment battery. *Neurosurgery* 60(6):1050-1057; discussion 1057-1058.

Broglio, S. P., M. S. Ferrara, S. N. Macciocchi, T. A. Baumgartner, and R. Elliott. 2007c. Test-retest reliability of computerized concussion assessment programs. *Journal of Athletic Training* 42(4):509-514.

Broglio, S. P., R. D. Moore, and C. H. Hillman. 2011. A history of sport-related concussion on event-related brain potential correlates of cognition. *International Journal of Psychophysiology* 82(1):16-23.

Brown, B. E. 2013. *Concussion: Return to Learning: How Schools Can Accommodate Concussed Youth Athletes & the Role of Schools in Recovery.* Presentation before the committee, Washington, DC, February 25.

Brown, C. N., K. M. Guskiewicz, and J. Bleiberg. 2007. Athlete characteristics and outcome scores for computerized neuropsychological assessment: A preliminary analysis. *Journal of Athletic Training* 42(4):515-523.

Brown, N. J., R. C. Mannix, M. J. O'Brien, D. Gostine, M. W. Collins, and W. P. Meehan III. 2014. Effect of cognitive activity level on duration of post-concussion symptoms. *Pediatrics* (January 6). [Epub ahead of print.] doi: 10.1542/peds.2013-2125.

Buzzini, S. R., and K. M. Guskiewicz. 2006. Sport-related concussion in the young athlete. *Current Opinion in Pediatrics* 18(4):376-382.

Canadian Academy of Sport Medicine Concussion Committee. 2000. Guidelines for assessment and management of sport-related concussion. *Clinical Journal of Sport Medicine* 10(3):209-211.

Cantu, R. C. 1998. Second-impact syndrome. *Clinics in Sports Medicine* 17(1):37-44.

Cantu, R. C., and R. Voy. 1995. Second impact syndrome a risk in any contact sport. *Physician and Sportsmedicine* 23(6):27-34.

Castellani, C., P. Bimbashi, E. Ruttenstock, P. Sacherer, T. Stojakovic, and A. M. Weinberg. 2009. Neuroprotein S-100B: A useful parameter in paediatric patients with mild traumatic brain injury? *Acta Paediatrica* 98(10):1607-1612.

Cavanaugh, J. T., K. M. Guskiewicz, C. Giuliani, S. Marshall, V. Mercer, and N. Stergiou. 2005. Detecting altered postural control after cerebral concussion in athletes with normal postural stability. *British Journal of Sports Medicine* 39(11): 805-811.

CDC (Centers for Disease Control and Prevention). 2012a. Heads up: Concussion in youth sports. http://www.cdc.gov/concussion/HeadsUp/youth.html (accessed April 3, 2013).

CDC. 2012b. Heads up: Concussion in youth sports. A fact sheet for coaches. http://www.cdc.gov/concussion/pdf/coaches_engl.pdf (accessed October 6, 2013).

CDC. 2013. Injury prevention and control: Traumatic brain injury. Concussion. http://www.cdc.gov/concussion/signs_symptoms.html (accessed September 16, 2013).

Cernich, A., D. Reeves, W. Y. Sun, and J. Bleiberg. 2007. Automated Neuropsychological Assessment Metrics sports medicine battery. *Archives of Clinical Neuropsychology* 22(1):S101-S114.

Chen, J. K., K. M. Johnston, A. Collie, P. McCrory, and A. Ptito. 2007. A validation of the Post Concussion Symptom Scale in the assessment of complex concussion using cognitive testing and functional MRI. *Journal of Neurology, Neurosurgery, and Psychiatry* 78(11):1231-1238.

CNS Vital Signs. 2013. CNS Vital Signs. http://www.cnsvs.com (accessed October 7, 2013).

Cole, W. R., J. P. Arrieux, K. Schwab, B. J. Ivins, F. M. Qashu, and S. C. Lewis. 2013. Test-retest reliability of four computerized neurocognitive assessment tools in an active duty military population. *Archives of Clinical Neuropsychology* (July 12). [Epub ahead of print.]

Collie, A., D. Darby, and P. Maruff. 2001. Computerised cognitive assessment of athletes with sports related head injury. *British Journal of Sports Medicine* 35(5):297-302.

Collie, A., P. Maruff, M. Makdissi, P. McCrory, M. McStephen, and D. Darby. 2003. CogSport: Reliability and correlation with conventional cognitive tests used in postconcussion medical evaluations. *Clinical Journal of Sport Medicine* 13(1):28-32.

Collins, M. W., S. H. Grindel, M. R. Lovell, D. E. Dede, D. J. Moser, B. R. Phalin, S. Nogle, M. Wasik, D. Cordry, K. M. Daugherty, S. F. Sears, G. Nicolette, P. Indelicato, and D. B. McKeag. 1999. Relationship between concussion and neuropsychological performance in college football players. *JAMA* 282(10):964-970.

Collins, M., M. Field, M. Lovell, G. Iverson, K. M. Johnston, J. Maroon, F. H. Fu. 2003a. Relationship between postconcussion headache and neuropsychological test performance in high school athletes. *American Journal of Sports Medicine* 31(2):168-173.

Collins, M. W., G. L. Iverson, M. R. Lovell, D. B. McKeag, J. Norwig, and J. Maroon. 2003b. On-field predictors of neuropsychological and symptom deficit following sports-related concussion. *Clinical Journal of Sport Medicine* 13(4):222-229.

Comper, P., M. Hutchison, S. Magrys, L. Mainwaring, and D. Richards. 2010. Evaluating the methodological quality of sports neuropsychology concussion research: A systematic review. *Brain Injury* 24(11):1257-1271.

Concussion Vital Signs. 2013. Concussion Vital Signs. http://www.concussionvitalsigns.com/About.html (accessed October 7, 2013).

Covassin, T., R. J. Elbin, III, J. L. Stiller-Ostrowski, and A. P. Kontos. 2009. Immediate Post-Concussion Assessment and Cognitive Testing (ImPACT) practices of sports medicine professionals. *Journal of Athletic Training* 44(6):639-644.

Covassin, T., R. J. Elbin, III, W. Harris, T. Parker, and A. Kontos. 2012a. The role of age and sex in symptoms, neurocognitive performance, and postural stability in athletes after concussion. *American Journal of Sports Medicine* 40(6):1303-1312.

Covassin, T., R. J. Elbin, III, E. Larson, and A. Kontos. 2012b. Sex and age differences in depression and baseline sport-related concussion neurocognitive performance and symptoms. *Clinical Journal of Sport Medicine* 22(2):98-104.

Coyne, C. 2103. Experiencing Concussion in Youth Sports: An Athlete's Perspective. Presentation before the committee, Seattle, WA, April 15.

Cubon, V. A., M. Putukian, C. Boyer, and A. Dettwiler. 2011. A diffusion tensor imaging study on the white matter skeleton in individuals with sports-related concussion. *Journal of Neurotrauma* 28(2):189-201.

de Kruijk, J. R., P. Leffers, S. Meerhoff, J. Rutten, and A. Twijnstra. 2002. Effectiveness of bed rest after mild traumatic brain injury: A randomised trial of no versus six days of bed rest. *Journal of Neurology, Neurosurgery, and Psychiatry* 73(2):167-172.

DiFiori, J. P., and C. C. Giza. 2010. New techniques in concussion imaging. *Current Sports Medicine Reports* 9(1):35-39.

Diver, T., G. Gioia, and S. Anderson. 2007. Discordance of symptom report across clinical and control groups with respect to parent and child. *Journal of the International Neuropsychological Society* 13(Suppl 1):63. [Poster presentation to the Annual Meeting of the International Neuropsychological Society, Portland, OR.]

DoD (Department of Defense). 2012. Instruction number 6490.11. DoD policy guidance for management of mild traumatic brain injury/concussion in the deployed setting. Issued September 18, 2012. http://www.dtic.mil/whs/directives/corres/pdf/649011p.pdf (accessed September 22, 2013).

DoD. 2013. Instruction number 6490.13. Comprehensive policy on neurocognitive assessments by the military services. Issued June 4, 2013. http://www.dtic.mil/whs/directives/corres/pdf/649013p.pdf (accessed September 21, 2013).

Duhaime, A-C., J. G. Beckwith, A. C. Maerlender, T. W. McAllister, J. J. Crisco, S. M. Duma, P. G. Brolinson, S. Rowson, L. A. Flashman, J. J. Chu, and R. M. Greenwald. 2012. Spectrum of acute clinical characteristics of diagnosed concussions in college athletes wearing instrumented helmets. *Journal of Neurosurgery* 117(6):1092-1099.

DVBIC (Defense and Veterans Brain Injury Center). 2012. MACE: Military Acute Concussion Evaluation. https://www.jsomonline.org/TBI/MACE_Revised_2012.pdf (accessed October 6, 2013).

Dziemianowicz, M., M. P. Kirschen, B. A. Pukenas, E. Laudano, L. J. Balcer, and S. L. Galetta. 2012. Sports-related concussion testing. *Current Neurology and Neuroscience Reports* 12(5):547-559.

Echemendia, R. J., M. Putukian, R. S. Mackin, L. Julian, and N. Shoss. 2001. Neuropsychological test performance prior to and following sports-related mild traumatic brain injury. *Clinical Journal of Sport Medicine* 11(1):23-31.

Eckner, J. T., J. S. Kutcher, and J. K. Richardson. 2010. Pilot evaluation of a novel clinical test of reaction time in National Collegiate Athletic Association Division I football players. *Journal of Athletic Training* 45(4):327-332.

Eckner, J. T., J. S. Kutcher, S. P. Broglio, and J. K. Richardson. 2013. Effect of sport-related concussion on clinically measured simple reaction time. *British Journal of Sports Medicine*. Published online first: January 11, doi:10.1136/bjsports-2012-0915792013.

Eisenberg, M. A., J. Andrea, W. Meehan, and R. Mannix. 2013. Time interval between concussions and symptom duration. *Pediatrics* 132(1):8-17.

Elbin, R. J., P. Schatz, and T. Covassin. 2011. One-year test-retest reliability of the online version of ImPACT in high school athletes. *American Journal of Sports Medicine* 39(11):2319-2324.

Ellemberg, D., L. C. Henry, S. N. Macciocchi, K. M. Guskiewicz, and S. P. Broglio. 2009. Advances in sport concussion assessment: From behavioral to brain imaging measures. *Journal of Neurotrauma* 26(12):2365-2382.

Eonta, S. E., W. Carr, J. J. McArdle, J. M. Kain, C. Tate, N. J. Wesensten, J. N. Norris, T. J. Balkin, and G. H. Kamimori. 2011. Automated Neuropsychological Assessment Metrics: Repeated assessment with two military samples. *Aviation, Space, and Environmental Medicine* 82(1):34-39.

Erdal, K. 2012. Neuropsychological testing for sports-related concussion: How athletes can sandbag their baseline testing without detection. *Archives of Clinical Neuropsychology* 27(5):473-479.

Erlanger, D., E. Saliba, J. Barth, J. Almquist, W. Webright, and J. Freeman. 2001. Monitoring resolution of postconcussion symptoms in athletes: Preliminary results of a Web-based neuropsychological test protocol. *Journal of Athletic Training* 36(3):280-287.

Erlanger, D. M., T. Kaushik, D. Broshek, J. Freeman, D. Feldman, and J. Festa. 2002. Development and validation of a web-based screening tool for monitoring cognitive status. *Journal of Head Trauma Rehabilitation* 17(5):458-476.

Erlanger, D., D. Feldman, K. Kutner, T. Kaushik, H. Kroger, J. Festa, J. Barth, J. Freeman, and D. Broshek. 2003. Development and validation of a web-based neuropsychological test protocol for sports-related return-to-play decision-making. *Archives of Clinical Neuropsychology* 18(3):293-316.

Falleti, M. G., P. Maruff, A. Collie, and D. G. Darby. 2006. Practice effects associated with the repeated assessment of cognitive function using the CogState battery at 10-minute, one week and one month test-retest intervals. *Journal of Clinical and Experimental Neuropsychology* 28(7):1095-1112.

Fazio, V. C., M. R. Lovell, J. E. Pardini, and M. W. Collins. 2007. The relation between post concussion symptoms and neurocognitive performance in concussed athletes. *NeuroRehabilitation* 22:207-216.

Field, M., M. W. Collins, M. R. Lovell, and J. Maroon. 2003. Does age play a role in recovery form sports-related concussion? A comparison of high school and collegiate athletes. *Journal of Pediatrics* 142(5):546-553.

Filippidis, A. S., D. C. Papadopoulos, E. Z. Kapsalaki, and K. N. Fountas. 2010. Role of the S100B serum biomarker in the treatment of children suffering from mild traumatic brain injury. *Neurosurgical Focus* 29(5):E2.

Finnoff, J. T., E. J. Jelsing, and J. Smith. 2011. Biomarkers, genetics, and risk factors for concussion. *PM & R* 3(10 Suppl 2):S452-S459.

Fridriksson, T., N. Kini, C. Walsh-Kelly, and H. Hennes. 2000. Serum neuron-specific enolase as a predictor of intracranial lesions in children with head trauma: A pilot study. *Academic Emergency Medicine* 7(7):816-820.

Frommer, L. J., K. K. Gurka, K. M. Cross, C. D. Ingersoll, R. D. Comstock, and S. A. Saliba. 2011. Sex differences in concussion symptoms of high school athletes. *Journal of Athletic Training* 46(1):76-84.

Galetta, K. M., L. E. Brandes, K. Maki, M. S. Dziemianowicz, E. Laudano, M. Allen, K. Lawler, B. Sennett, D. Wiebe, S. Devick, L. V. Messner, S. L. Galetta, and L. J. Balcer. 2011. The King-Devick test and sports-related concussion: Study of a rapid visual screening tool in a collegiate cohort. *Journal of the Neurological Sciences* 309(1-2):34-39.

Gardner, A., E. A. Shores, J. Batchelor, and C. A. Honan. 2012. Diagnostic efficiency of Im-PACT and CogSport in concussed rugby union players who have not undergone baseline neurocognitive testing. *Applied Neuropsychology Adult* 19(2):90-97.

Geurts A. C., G. M. Ribbers, J. A. Knoop, and J. van Limbeek. 1996. Identification of static and dynamic postural instability following traumatic brain injury. *Archives of Physical Medicine and Rehabilitation* 77(7):639-644.

Geyer, C., A. Ulrich, G. Gräfe, B. Stach, and H. Till. 2009. Diagnostic value of S100B and neuron-specific enolase in mild pediatric traumatic brain injury. *Journal of Neurosurgery Pediatrics* 4:339-344.

Gioia, G. 2013. Perspectives on Management of Students' Return to School. Presentation before the committee, Washington, DC, February 25.

Gioia, G., and M. Collins. 2006. *Acute Concussion Evaluation (ACE): Physician/Clinician Office Version.* http://www.cdc.gov/concussion/headsup/pdf/ace-a.pdf (accessed August 23, 2013).

Gioia, G., M. Collins, and P. K. Isquith. 2008a. Improving identification and diagnosis of mild traumatic brain injury with evidence: Psychometric support for the Acute Concussion Evaluation. *Journal of Head Trauma Rehabilitation* 23(4):230-242.

Gioia, G., J. Janusz, P. Isquith, and D. Vincent. 2008b. Psychometric properties of the parent and teacher Post-Concussion Symptom Inventory (PCSI) for children and adolescents. [Abstract.] *Journal of the International Neuropsychologcical Society* 14(Suppl 1):204.

Gioia, G. A., J. C. Schneider, C. G. Vaughan, and P. K. Isquith. 2009. Which symptom assessments and approaches are uniquely appropriate for paediatric concussion? *British Journal of Sports Medicine* 43(Suppl 1):i13-i22.

Gioia, G. A., C. G. Vaughan, J. Reesman, C. McGill, E. McGuire, L. Gathercole, H. Padia, K. Nichols, P. Allen, and C. Wells. 2010. Characterizing post-concussion exertional effects in the child and adolescent. [Abstract.] *Journal of the International Neuropsychological Society* 16(Suppl 1):178.

Gioia, G., P. Isquith, and C. Vaughan. 2013a. Classification analyses of pediatric concussion assessment battery. [Abstract.] *British Journal of Sports Medicine* 47(5):e1.

Gioia, G. A., C. G. Vaughan, and P. K. Isquith. 2013b. *Professional manual for Pediatric Immediate Post-Concussion Assessment and Cognitive Testing (ImPACT).* Odessa, FL: Psychological Assessment Resources.

Giza, C. C., J. S. Kutcher, S. Ashwal, J. Barth, T. S. D. Getchius, G. A. Gioia, G. S. Gronseth, K. Guskiewicz, S. Mandel, G. Manley, D. B. McKeag, D. J. Thurman, and R. Zafonte. 2013. *Evidence-Based Guideline Update: Evaluation and Management of Concussion in Sports.* Report of the Guideline Development Subcommittee of the American Academy of Neurology. American Academy of Neurology.

Gosselin, N., M. Lassonde, D. Petit, S. Leclerc, V. Mongrain, A. Collie, and J. Montplaisir. 2009. Sleep following sport-related concussions. *Sleep Medicine* 10(1):35-46.

Gosselin, N., C. Bottari, J. K. Chen, S. C. Huntgeburth, L. De Beaumont, M. Petrides, B. Cheung, and A. Ptito. 2012a. Evaluating the cognitive consequences of mild traumatic brain injury and concussion by using electrophysiology. *Neurosurgical Focus* 33(6):E7:1-7.

Gosselin, N., J. K. Chen, C. Bottari, M. Petrides, T. Jubault, S. Tinawi, E. de Guise, and A. Ptito. 2012b. The influence of pain on cerebral functioning after mild traumatic brain injury. *Journal of Neurotrauma* 29(17):2625-2634.

Green, P. 2007. The pervasive influence of effort on neuropsychological tests. *Physical Medicine Rehabilitation Clinics of North America* 18(1):43-68.

Griesbach, G. S., D. A. Hovda, R. Molteni, A. Wu, and F. Gomez-Pinilla. 2004. Voluntary exercise following traumatic brain injury: Brain-derived neurotrophic factor upregulation and recovery of function. *Neuroscience* 125(1):129-139.

Grindel, S. H., M. R. Lovell, M. W. Collins. 2001. The assessment of sport-related concussion: The evidence behind neuropsychological testing and management. *Clinical Journal of Sport Medicine* 11(3):134-143.

Gronwall, D., and P. Wrightson. 1981. Memory and information processing capacity after closed head injury. *Journal of Neurology, Neurosurgery, and Psychiatry* 44(10):889-895.

Gualtieri, C. T., and L. G. Johnson. 2006. Reliability and validity of a computerized neurocognitive test battery, CNS Vital Signs. *Archives of Clinical Neuropsychology* 21(7):623-643.

Guskiewicz, K. M. 2001. Postural stability assessment following concussion: One piece of the puzzle. *Clinical Journal of Sport Medicine* 11(3):182-189.

Guskiewicz, K. M. 2011. Balance assessment in the management of sport-related concussion. *Clinics in Sports Medicine* 30(1):89-102, ix.

Guskiewicz, K. M., and J. K. Register-Mihalik. 2011. Postconcussive impairment differences across a multifaceted concussion assessment protocol. *PM & R* 3(10 Suppl 2):S445-S451.

Guskiewicz, K. M., S. E. Ross, and S. W. Marshall. 2001. Postural stability and neuropsychological deficits after concussion in collegiate athletes. *Journal of Athletic Training* 36(3):263-273.

Guskiewicz, K. M., M. McCrea, S. W. Marshall, R. C. Cantu, C. Randolph, W. Barr, J. A. Onate, and J. P. Kelly. 2003. Cumulative effects associated with recurrent concussion in collegiate football players: The NCAA Concussion Study. *JAMA* 290(19):2549-2555.

Hajek, C. A., K. O. Yeates, H. G. Taylor, B. Bangert, A. Dietrich, K. E. Nuss, J. Rusin, and M. Wright. 2011. Agreement between parents and children on ratings of postconcussive symptoms following mild traumatic brain injury. *Child Neuropsychology* 17(1):17-33.

Halstead, M. E., K. D. Walter, and American Academy of Pediatrics, Council on Sports Medicine and Fitness. 2010. Sport-related concussion in children and adolescents. *Pediatrics* 126(3):597-615.

Harmon, K. G., J. Drezner, M. Gammons, K. Guskiewicz, M. Halstead, S. Herring, J. Kutcher, A. Pana, M. Putukian, W. Roberts, and American Medical Society for Sports Medicine. 2013. American Medical Society for Sports Medicine position statement: Concussion in sport. *British Journal of Sports Medicine* 47(1):15-26.

Hasselblatt, M., F. C. Mooren, N. von Ahsen, K. Keyvani, A. Fromme, K. Schwarze-Eicker, V. Senner, and W. Paulus. 2004. Serum S100beta increases in marathon runners reflect extracranial release rather than glial damage. *Neurology* 62(9):1634-1636.

Heilbronner, R. L., J. J. Sweet, D. K. Attix, K. R. Krull, G. K. Henry, and R. P. Hart. 2010. Official position of the American Academy of Clinical Neuropsychology on serial neuropsychological assessments: The utility and challenges of repeat test administrations in clinical and forensic contexts. *Clinical Neuropsychologist* 24(8):1267-1278.

Herring, S. A., R. C. Cantu, K. M. Guskiewicz, M. Putukian, W. B. Kibler, J. A. Bergfeld, L. A. Boyajian-O'Neill, R. R. Franks, P. A. Indelicato, and the American College of Sports Medicine. 2011. Concussion (mild traumatic brain injury) and the team physician: A consensus statement—2011 update. *Medicine and Science in Sports and Exercise* 43(12):2412-2422.

Hinton-Bayre, A. D. 2012. Choice of reliable change model can alter decisions regarding neuropsychological impairment after sports-related concussion. *Clinical Journal of Sport Medicine* 22(2):105-108.

Hinton-Bayre, A. D., G. Geffen, and K. McFarland. 1997. Mild head injury and speed of information processing: A prospective study of professional rugby league players. *Journal of Clinical and Experimental Neuropsychology* 19(2):275-289.

Hinton-Bayre, A. D., G. M. Geffen, L. B. Geffen, K. A. McFarland, and P. Friis. 1999. Concussion in contact sports: Reliable change indices of impairment and recovery. *Journal of Clinical and Experimental Neuropsychology* 21(1):70-86.

Hunt, T., and C. Asplund. 2010. Concussion assessment and management. *Clinics in Sports Medicine* 29(1):5-17.

Hunt, T. N., M. S. Ferrara, L. S. Miller, and S. N. Macciocchi. 2007. The effect of effort on baseline neuropsychological test scores in high school football athletes. *Archives of Clinical Neuropsychology* 22(5):615-621.

Hunt, T. N., M. S. Ferrara, R. A. Bornstein, and T. A. Baumgartner. 2009. The reliability of the Modified Balance Error Scoring System. *Clinical Journal of Sport Medicine* 19(6):471-475.

Hutchison, M., P. Comper, L. Mainwaring, and D. Richards. 2011. The influence of musculoskeletal injury on cognition: Implications for concussion research. *American Journal of Sports Medicine* 39(11):2331-2337.

ImPACT (Immediate Post-Concussion Assessment and Cognitive Testing). 2013. The ImPACT test. http://www.impacttest.com/about/?The-ImPACT-Test-4 (accessed October 8, 2013).

Iverson, G. L., and M. Gaetz. 2004. Practical consideration for interpreting change following brain injury. In *Traumatic Brain Injury in Sports: An International Neuropsychological Perspective*, edited by M. R. Lovell, R. J. Echemendia, J. T. Barth, and M. W. Collins. Exton, PA: Swets & Zeitlinger. Pp. 323-356.

Iverson, G. L., M. R. Lovell, and M. W. Collins. 2003. Interpreting change in ImPACT following sport concussion. *Clinical Neuropsychologist* 17(4):460-467.

Iverson, G. L., M. D. Franzen, M. R. Lovell, and M. W. Collins. 2004. Construct validity of impact in athletes with concussions. [Abstract.] *Archives of Clinical Neuropsychology* 19(7):961-962.

Iverson, G. L., M. R. Lovell, and M. W. Collins. 2005. Validity of ImPACT for measuring processing speed following sports-related concussion. *Journal of Clinical and Experimental Neuropsychology* 27(6):683-689.

Iverson, G. L., B. L. Brooks, M. W. Collins, and M. R. Lovell. 2006. Tracking neuropsychological recovery following concussion in sport. *Brain Injury* 20(3):245-252.

Jantzen, K. J., B. Anderson, F. L. Steinberg, and J. A. Kelso. 2004. Prospective functional MR imaging study of mild traumatic brain injury in college football players. *American Journal of Neuroradiology* 25(5):738-745.

Janusz, J. A., M. D. Sady, and G. A. Gioia. 2012. Postconcussion symptom assessment. In *Mild Traumatic Brain Injury in Children and Adolescents: From Basic Science to Clinical Management*, edited by M. W. Kirkwood and K. O. Yeates. New York: Guilford Press. Pp. 241-263.

Johnson, D. R., A. S. Vincent, A. E. Johnson, K. Gilliland, and R. E. Schlegel. 2008. Reliability and construct validity of the Automated Neuropsychological Assessment Metrics (ANAM) mood scale. *Archives of Clinical Neuropsychology* 23(1):73-85.

King, N. S., S. Crawford, F. J. Wenden, N. E. Moss, and D. T. Wade. 1995. The Rivermead Post Concussion Symptoms Questionnaire: A measure of symptoms commonly experienced after head injury and its reliability. *Journal of Neurology* 242(9):587-592.

Kirkwood, M. W., C. Randolph, and K. O. Yeates. 2009. Returning pediatric athletes to play after concussion: The evidence (or lack thereof) behind baseline neuropsychological testing. *Acta Paediatrica* 98(9):1409-1411.

Kissick, J., and K. M. Johnston. 2005. Return to play after concussion: Principles and practice. *Clinical Journal of Sport Medicine* 15(6):426-431.

Koerte, I. K., D. Kaufmann, E. Hartl, S. Bouix, O. Pasternak, M. Kubicki, A. Rauscher, D. K. Li, S. B. Dadachanji, J. A. Taunton, L. A. Forwell, A. M. Johnson, P. S. Echlin, and M. E. Shenton. 2012. A prospective study of physician-observed concussion during a varsity university hockey season: White matter integrity in ice hockey players. Part 3 of 4. *Neurosurgical Focus* 33(6):E3:1-7.

Kontos, A. P., R. J. Elbin, P. Schatz, T. Covassin, L. Henry, J. Pardini, and M. W. Collins. 2012. A revised factor structure for the Post-Concussion Symptom Scale: Baseline and postconcussion factors. *American Journal of Sports Medicine* 40(10):2375-2384.

Kroshus, E., D. H. Daneshvar, C. M. Baugh, C. J. Nowinski, and R. C. Cantu. 2013. NCAA concussion education in ice hockey: An ineffective mandate. *British Journal of Sports Medicine*, in press. doi: 10.1136/bjsports-2013-092498.

Kutcher, J. S., and J. T. Eckner. 2010. At-risk populations in sports-related concussion. *Current Sports Medicine Reports* 9(1):16-20.

Lange, R. T., G. L. Iverson, B. L. Brooks, and V. L. Rennison. 2010. Influence of poor effort on self-reported symptoms and neurocognitive test performance following mild traumatic brain injury. *Journal of Clinical and Experimental Neuropsychology* 32(9):961-972.

Lee, M. A. 2006. Adolescent concussions—Management recommendations: A practical approach. *Connecticut Medicine* 70(6):377-380.

Lezak, M. D., D. B. Howieson, E. D. Bigler, and D. Tranel. 2012. *Neuropsychological Assessment*, Fifth edition. Oxford University Press.

Lovell, M. R., and M. W. Collins. 1998. Neuropsychological assessment of the college football player. *Journal of Head Trauma Rehabilitation* 13(2):9-26.

Lovell, M. R., M. W. Collins, G. L. Iverson, M. Field, J. C. Maroon, R. Cantu, K. Podell, J. W. Powell, M. Belza, and F. H. Fu. 2003. Recovery from mild concussion in high school athletes. *Journal of Neurosurgery* 98(2):296-301.

Lovell, M. R., G. L. Iverson, M. W. Collins, K. Podell, K. M. Johnston, D. Pardini, J. Pardini, J. Norwig, and J. C. Maroon. 2006. Measurement of symptoms following sports-related concussion: Reliability and normative data for the Post-Concussion Scale. *Applied Neuropsychology* 13(3):166-174.

Lovell, M. R., J. E. Pardini, J. Welling, M. W. Collins, J. Bakal, N. Lazar, R. Roush, W. F. Eddy, and J. T. Becker. 2007. Functional brain abnormalities are related to clinical recovery and time to return-to-play in athletes. *Neurosurgery* 61(2):352-359.

Macciocchi, S. N., J. T. Barth, W. Alves, R. W. Rimel, and J. A. Jane. 1996. Neuropsychological functioning and recovery after mild head injury in collegiate athletes. *Neurosurgery* 39(3):510-514.

Maddocks, D. L., G. D. Dicker, and M. M. Saling. 1995. The assessment of orientation following concussion in athletes. *Clinical Journal of Sports Medicine* 5(1):32-35.

Maerlender, A., and A. Alt. 2012. The effect of sleep the night before on baseline neuropsychological screening and symptom reporting. [Abstract.] *Journal of the International Neuropsychological Society* 18(Suppl 1):165.

Maerlender, A., L. Flashman, A. Kessler, S. Kumbhani, R. Greenwald, T. Tosteson, and T. McAllister. 2010. Examination of the construct validity of ImPACT™ computerized test, traditional, and experimental neuropsychological measures. *Clinical Neuropsychologist* 24(8):1309-1325.

Maerlender, A., L. Flashman, A. Kessler, S. Kumbhani, R. Greenwald, T. Tosteson, and T. McAllister. 2013. The discriminant construct validity of ImPACT™: A companion study. *Clinical Neuropsychologist* 27(2):290-299.

Mailer, B. J., T. C. Valovich-McLeod, and R. C. Bay. 2008. Healthy youth are reliable in reporting symptoms on a graded symptom scale. *Journal of Sport Rehabilitation* 17(1):11-20.

Maine Department of Education. 2012. Management of concussion and other head injuries model policy. https://www.maine.gov/education/sh/concussion/model-policy.html (accessed September 23, 2013).

Majerske, C. W., J. P. Mihalik, D. Ren, M. W. Collins, C. C. Reddy, M. R. Lovell, and A. K. Wagner. 2008. Concussion in sports: Postconcussive activity levels, symptoms, and neurocognitive performance. *Journal of Athletic Training* 43(3):265-274.

Makdissi, M., A. Collie, P. Maruff, D. G. Darby, A. Bush, P. McCrory, and K. Bennell. 2001. Computerised cognitive assessment of concussed Australian Rules footballers. *British Journal of Sports Medicine* 35(5):354-360.

Makdissi, M., D. Darby, P. Maruff, A. Ugoni, P. Brukner, and P. R. McCrory. 2010. Natural history of concussion in sport: Markers of severity and implications for management. *American Journal of Sports Medicine* 38(3):464-471.

McAllister, T. W., L. A. Flashman, A. Maerlender, R. M. Greenwald, J. G. Beckwith, T. D. Tosteson, J. J. Crisco, P. G. Brolinson, S. M. Duma, A. C. Duhaime, M. R. Grove, J. H. Turco. 2012. Cognitive effects of one season of head impacts in a cohort of collegiate contact sport athletes. *Neurology* 78(22):1777-1784.

McCaffrey, M. A., J. P. Mihalik, D. H. Crowell, E. W. Shields, and K. M. Guskiewicz. 2007. Measurement of head impacts in collegiate football players: Clinical measures of concussion after high- and low-magnitude impacts. *Neurosurgery* 61(6):1236-1243.

McClincy, M. P., M. R. Lovell, J. Pardini, M. W. Collins, and M. K. Spore. 2006. Recovery from sports concussion in high school and collegiate athletes. *Brain Injury* 20(1):33-39.

McCrea, M. 2001. Standardized mental status testing on the sideline after sport-related concussion. *Journal of Athletic Training* 36(3):274-279.

McCrea, M., J. P. Kelly, C. Randolph, J. Kluge, E. Bartolic, G. Finn, and B. Baxter. 1998. Standardized Assessment of Concussion (SAC): On-site mental status evaluation of the athlete. *Journal of Head Trauma Rehabilitation* 13(2):27-35.

McCrea, M., J. P. Kelly, and C. Randolph. 2000. *Standardized Assessment of Concussion (SAC): Manual for Administration, Scoring and Interpretation*, Second edition. Waukesha, WI: CNS Inc.

McCrea, M., K. M. Guskiewicz, S. W. Marshall, W. Barr, C. Randolph, R. C. Cantu, J. A. Onate, J. Yang, and J. P. Kelly. 2003. Acute effects and recovery time following concussion in collegiate football players: The NCAA Concussion Study. *JAMA* 290(19):2556-2563.

McCrea, M., T. Hammeke, G. Olsen, P. Leo, K. Guskiewicz. 2004. Unreported concussion in high school football players: Implications for prevention. *Clinical Journal of Sport Medicine* 14(1):13-17.

McCrea, M., K. Guskiewicz, C. Randolph, W. B. Barr, T. A. Hammeke, S. W. Marshall, and J. P. Kelly. 2009. Effects of a symptom-free waiting period on clinical outcome and risk of reinjury after sport-related concussion. *Neurosurgery* 65(5):876-882; discussion 882-883.

McCrea, M., L. Prichep, M. Powell, R. Chabot, W. Barr. 2010. Acute effects and recovery after sport-related concussion: A neurocognitive and quantitative brain electrical activity study. *Journal of Head Trauma Rehabilitation* 25(4):283-292.

McCrea, M., K. Guskiewicz, C. Randolph, W. B. Barr, T. A. Hammeke, S. W. Marshall, M. R. Powell, K. Woo Ahn, Y. Wang, and J. P. Kelly. 2013. Incidence, clinical course, and predictors of prolonged recovery time following sport-related concussion in high school and college athletes. *Journal of the Inernational Neuropsychological Society* 19(1):22-33.

McCrory, P. R., and S. F. Berkovic. 1998. Second impact syndrome. *Neurology* 50(3):677-683.

McCrory, P., A. Collie, V. Anderson, and G. Davis. 2004. Can we manage sport related concussion in children the same as in adults? *British Journal of Sports Medicine* 38(5):516-519.

McCrory, P., M. Makdissi, G. Davis, and A. Collie. 2005. Value of neuropsychological testing after head injuries in football. *British Journal of Sports Medicine* 39(Suppl 1):i58-i63.

McCrory, P., W. Meeuwisse, K. Johnston, J. Dvořák, M. Aubry, M. Molloy, and R. Cantu. 2009. Consensus statement on concussion in sport: The 3rd International Conference on Concussion in Sport held in Zurich, November 2008. *British Journal of Sports Medicine* 43(Suppl 1):i76-i84.

McCrory, P., W. H. Meeuwisse, M. Aubry, B. Cantu, J. Dvořák, R. J. Echemendia, L. Engebretsen, K. Johnston, J. S. Kutcher, M. Raftery, A. Sills, B. W. Benson, G. A. Davis, R. G. Ellenbogen, K. Guskiewicz, S. A. Herring, G. L. Iverson, B. D. Jordan, J. Kissick, M. McCrea, A. S. McIntosh, D. Maddocks, M. Makdissi, L. Purcell, M. Putukian, K. Schneider, C. H. Tator, and M. Turner. 2013a. Child-SCAT3. *British Journal of Sports Medicine* 47(5):263-266.

McCrory, P., W. H. Meeuwisse, M. Aubry, B. Cantu, J. Dvořák, R. J. Echemendia, L. Engebretsen, K. Johnston, J. S. Kutcher, M. Raftery, A. Sills, B. W. Benson, G. A. Davis, R. G. Ellenbogen, K. Guskiewicz, S. A. Herring, G. L. Iverson, B. D. Jordan, J. Kissick, M. McCrea, A. S. McIntosh, D. Maddocks, M. Makdissi, L. Purcell, M. Putukian, K. Schneider, C. H. Tator, and M. Turner. 2013b. Consensus statement on concussion in sport: The 4th International Conference on Concussion in Sport held in Zurich, November 2012. *British Journal of Sports Medicine* 47(5):250-258.

McCrory, P., W. H. Meeuwisse, M. Aubry, B. Cantu, J. Dvořák, R. J. Echemendia, L. Engebretsen, K. Johnston, J. S. Kutcher, M. Raftery, A. Sills, B. W. Benson, G. A. Davis, R. G. Ellenbogen, K. Guskiewicz, S. A. Herring, G. L. Iverson, B. D. Jordan, J. Kissick, M. McCrea, A. S. McIntosh, D. Maddocks, M. Makdissi, L. Purcell, M. Putukian, K. Schneider, C. H. Tator, and M. Turner. 2013c. SCAT3. *British Journal of Sports Medicine* 47(5):259-262.

McGrath, N. 2010. Supporting the student-athlete's return to the classroom after a sport-related concussion. *Journal of Athletic Training* 45(5):492-498.

McGrath, N., W. M. Dinn, M. W. Collins, M. R. Lovell, R. J. Elbin, and A. P. Kontos. 2013. Post-exertion neurocognitive test failure among student-athletes following concussion. *Brain Injury* 27(1):103-113.

Meehan, W. P., III, P. d'Hemecourt, C. L. Collins, and R. D. Comstock. 2011. Assessment and management of sport-related concussions in United States high schools. *American Journal of Sports Medicine* 39(11):2304-2310.

Miller, J. R., G. J. Adamson, M. M. Pink, and J. C. Sweet. 2007. Comparison of preseason, midseason, and postseason neurocognitive scores in uninjured collegiate football players. *American Journal of Sports Medicine* 35(8):1284-1288.

Molfese, D. L., V. J. Molfese, and S. Kelly. 2001. The use of brain electrophysiology techniques to study language: A basic guide for the beginning consumer of electrophysiology information. *Learning Disabilities Quarterly* 24(3):177-188.

Moriarity, J. M., R. H. Pietrzak, J. S. Kutcher, M. H. Clausen, K. McAward, and D. G. Darby. 2012. Unrecognised ringside concussive injury in amateur boxers. *British Journal of Sports Medicine* 46(14):1011-1015.

Moser, R. S., G. L. Iverson, R. J. Echemendia, M. R. Lovell, P. Schatz, F. M. Webbe, R. M. Ruff, J. T. Barth, and National Academy of Neuropsychology Policy and Planning Committee: D. K. Broshek, S. S. Bush, S. P. Koffler, C. R. Reynolds, and C. H. Silver. 2007. Neuropsychological evaluation in the diagnosis and management of sports-related concussion. *Archives of Clinical Neuropsychology* 22(8):909-916.

Moser, R. S., P. Schatz, K. Neidzwski, and S. D. Ott. 2011. Group versus individual administration affects baseline neurocognitive test performance. *American Journal of Sports Medicine* 39(11):2325-2330.

Moser, R. S., C. Glatts, and P. Schatz. 2012. Efficacy of immediate and delayed cognitive and physical rest for treatment of sports-related concussion. *Journal of Pediatrics* 161(5):922-926.

NCSL (National Conference of State Legislatures). 2013. *Traumatic Brain Injury Legislation.* http://www.ncsl.org/issues-research/health/traumatic-brain-injury-legislation.aspx (accessed March 28, 2013).

Neurocom. 2013. Sensory organizing test. http://resourcesonbalance.com/neurocom/protocols/sensoryImpairment/SOT.aspx (accessed September 23, 2013).

New York State Department of Education. 2012. Guidelines for concussion management in the school setting. http://www.p12.nysed.gov/sss/schoolhealth/ConcussionManage Guidelines.pdf (accessed September 23, 2013).

Newman, J. B., J. H. Reesman, C. G. Vaughan, and G. A. Gioia. 2013. Assessment of processing speed in children with mild TBI: A "first look" at the validity of pediatric ImPACT. *Clinical Neuropsychologist* 27(5):779-793.

Oregon Department of Education. 2010. Max's law: Concussion management implementation guide for school administrators. http://www.ode.state.or.us/teachlearn/subjects/pe/ocampguide.pdf (accessed September 23, 2013).

Otto, M., S. Holthusen, E. Bahn, N. Söhnchen, J. Wiltfang, R. Geese, A. Fischer, and C. D. Reimers. 2000. Boxing and running lead to a rise in serum levels of S-100B protein. *International Journal of Sports Medicine* 21(8):551-555.

Pardini, J. E., D. A. Pardini, J. T. Becker, K. L. Dunfee, W. F. Eddy, M. R. Lovell, and J. S. Welling. 2010. Postconcussive symptoms are associated with compensatory cortical recruitment during a working memory task. *Neurosurgery* 67(4):1020-1027; discussion 1027-1028.

Pennington, B. 2013. Flubbing a baseline test on purpose is often futile. *New York Times* (May 6):D7. http://www.nytimes.com/2013/05/06/sports/sandbagging-first-concussion-test-probably-wont-help-later.html?_r=0 (accessed July 17, 2013).

Peterson, C. L., M. S. Ferrara, M. Mrazik, S. Piland, and R. Elliott. 2003. Evaluation of neuropsychological domain scores and postural stability following cerebral concussion in sports. *Clinical Journal of Sport Medicine* 13(4):230-237.

Piland, S. G., R. W. Motl, K. M. Guskiewicz, M. McCrea, and M. S. Ferrara. 2006. Structural validity of a self-report concussion-related symptom scale. *Medicine and Science in Sports and Exercise* 38(1):27-32.

Poirier, M. P. 2003. Concussions: Assessment, management, and recommendations for return to activity. *Clinical Pediatric Emergency Medicine* 4(3):179-185.

Popoli, D. M., T. G. Burns, W. P. Meehan, III, and A. Reisner. 2013. CHOA concussion consensus: Establishing a uniform policy for academic accommodations. *Clinical Pediatrics* (August 19). [Epub ahead of print.]

Prichep, L. S., M. McCrea, W. Barr, M. Powell, and R. J. Chabot. 2013. Time course of clinical and electrophysiological recovery after sport-related concussion. *Journal of Head Trauma Rehabilitation* 28(4):266-273.

Purcell, L. K., and Canadian Paediatric Society, Healthy Active Living and Sports Medicine Committee. 2012. Evaluation and management of children and adolescents with sports-related concussion. *Paediatrics & Child Health* 17(1):36-37.

Putukian, M., M. Aubry, and P. McCrory. 2009. Return to play after sports concussion in elite and non-elite athletes? *British Journal of Sports Medicine* 43(Suppl 1):i28-i31.

Randolph, C., and M. W. Kirkwood. 2009. What are the real risks of sport-related concussion, and are they modifiable? *Journal of the International Neuropsychological Society* 15 15(4):512-520.

Randolph, C., M. McCrea, and W. B. Barr. 2005. Is neuropsychological testing useful in the management of sport-related concussion? *Journal of Athletic Training* 40(3):139-152.

Randolph, C., S. Mills, W. B. Barr, M. McCrea, K. M. Guskiewicz, T. A. Hammeke, and J. P. Kelly. 2009. Concussion Symptom Inventory: An empirically-derived scale for monitoring resolution of symptoms following sports-related concussion. *Archives of Clinical Neuropsychology* 24(3):219-229.

Reeves, D. L., K. P. Winter, J. Bleiberg, and R. L. Kane. 2007. ANAM® genogram: Historical perspectives, description, and current endeavors. *Archives of Clinical Neuropsychology* 22(Suppl 1):S15-S37.

Register-Mihalik, J., K. M. Guskiewicz, J. D. Mann, and E. W. Shields. 2007. The effects of headache on clinical measures of neurocognitive function. *Clinical Journal of Sport Medicine* 17(4):282-288.

Register-Mihalik, J. K., J. P. Mihalik, and K. M. Guskiewicz. 2008. Balance deficits after sports-related concussion in individuals reporting posttraumatic headache. *Neurosurgery* 63(1):76-80; discussion 80-82.

Register-Mihalik J. K., D. L. Kontos, K. M. Guskiewicz, J. P. Mihalik, R. Conder, and E. W. Shields. 2012. Age-related differences and reliability on computerized and paper-and-pencil neurocognitive assessment batteries. *Journal of Athletic Training* 47(3):297-305.

Register-Mihalik, J. K., K. M. Guskiewicz, T. C. Valovich McLeod, L. A. Linnan, F. O. Mueller, and S. W. Marshall. 2013a. Knowledge, attitude, and concussion-reporting behaviors among high school athletes: A preliminary study. *Journal of Athletic Training* 48(5):645-653.

Register-Mihalik, J. K., K. M. Guskiewicz, J. P. Mihalik, J. D. Schmidt, Z. Y. Kerr, and M. McCrea. 2013b. Reliable change, sensitivity, and specificity of a multidimensional concussion assessment battery: Implications for caution in clinical practice. *Journal of Head Trauma Rehabilitation* 28(4):274-283.

Register-Mihalik, J. K., L. A. Linnan, S. W. Marshall, T. C. Valovich McLeod, F. O. Mueller, and K. M. Guskiewicz. 2013c. Using theory to understand high school aged athletes' intentions to report sport-related concussion: Implications for concussion education initiatives. *Brain Injury* 27(7-8):878-886.

Resch, J., A. Driscoll, N. McCaffrey, C. Brown, M. S. Ferrara, S. Macciocchi, T. Baumgartner, and K. Walpert. 2013. ImPACT test-retest reliability: Reliably unreliable? *Journal of Athletic Training* 48(4):506-511.

Riemann, B. L., K. M. Guskiewicz, and E. Shields. 1999. Relationship between clinical and forceplate measures of postural stability. *Journal of Sport Rehabilitation* 8(2):71-82.

Rimel, R. W., B. Giordani, J. T. Barth, and J. A. Jane. 1982. Moderate head injury: Completing the clinical spectrum of brain trauma. *Neurosurgery* 11(3):344-351.

Sady, M. D., C. G. Vaughan, and G. A. Gioia. 2011. School and the concussed youth: Recommendations for concussion education and management. *Physical Medicine and Rehabilitation Clinics of North America* 22(4):701-719.

Sandel, N. K., M. R. Lovell, N. Kegel, M. W. Collins, and A. P. Kontos. 2012. The relationship of symptoms and neurocognitive performance to perceived recovery from sports-related concussion among adolescent athletes. *Applied Neuropsychology: Child* 2(1):64-99.

Saunders, R. L., and R. E. Harbaugh.1984. Second impact in catastrophic contact-sports head trauma. *JAMA* 252(4):538-539.

Schatz, P. 2010. Long-term test-retest reliability of baseline cognitive assessments using ImPACT. *American Journal of Sports Medicine* 38(1):47-53.

Schatz, P., and C. S. Ferris. 2013. One-month test-retest reliability of the ImPACT test battery. *Archives of Clinical Neuropsychology* 28(5):499-504.

Schatz, P., and B. O. Putz. 2006. Cross-validation of measures used for computer-based assessment of concussion. *Applied Neuropsychology* 13(3):151-159.

Schatz, P., and N. Sandel. 2013. Sensitivity and specificity of the online version of ImPACT in high school and collegiate athletes. *American Journal of Sports Medicine* 41(2):321-326.

Schatz, P., J. Pardini, M. R. Lovell, M. W. Collins, and K. Podell. 2006. Sensitivity and specificity of the ImPACT Test Battery for concussion in athletes. *Archives of Clinical Neuropsychology* 21(1):91-99.

Schmidt, J. D., J. K. Register-Mihalik, J. P. Mihalik, Z. Y. Kerr, and K. M. Guskiewicz. 2012. Identifying impairments after concussion: Normative data versus individualized baselines. *Medicine & Science in Sports & Exercise* 44(9):1621-1628.

Schneider, J., and G. Gioia. 2007. Psychometric properties of the Post-Concussion Symptom Inventory (PCSI) in school age children. [Abstract.] *Developmental Neurorehabilitation* 10(4):282.

Segalowitz, S., P. Mahaney, D. Santesso, L. MacGregor, J. Dywan, and B. Willer. 2007. Retest reliability in adolescents of a computerized neuropsychological battery used to assess recovery from concussion. *NeuroRehabilitation* 22(3):243-251.

Stålnacke, B. M., Y. Tegner, and P. Sojka. 2003. Playing ice hockey and basketball increases serum levels of S100B in elite players: A pilot study. *Clinical Journal of Sport Medicine* 13:292-302.

Straume-Naesheim, T. M., T. E. Andersen, and R. Bahr. 2005. Reproducibility of computer based neuropsychological testing among Norwegian elite football players. *British Journal of Sports Medicine* 39(Suppl 1):i64-i69.

Suskauer, S. J., and T. A. Huisman. 2009. Neuroimaging in pediatric traumatic brain injury: Current and future predictors of functional outcome. *Developmental Disabilities Research Review* 15(2):117-123.

Teasdale, G., and B. Jennett. 1974. Assessment of coma and impaired consciousness: A practical scale. *Lancet* 2(7872):81-84.

Thériault, M., L. De Beaumont, N. Gosselin, M. Filipinni, and M. Lassonde. 2009. Electrophysiological abnormalities in well functioning multiple concussed athletes. *Brain Injury* 23(11):899-906.

Thériault, M., L. De Beaumont, S. Tremblay, M. Lassonde, and P. Jolicoeur. 2011. Cumulative effects of concussions in athletes revealed by electrophysiological abnormalities on visual working memory. *Journal of Clinical and Experimental Neuropsychology* 33(1):30-41.

Toledo, E., A. Lebel, L. Becerra, A. Minster, C. Linnman, N. Maleki, D. W. Dodick, and D. Borsook. 2012. The young brain and concussion: Imaging as a biomarker for diagnosis and prognosis. *Neuroscience and Biobehavioral Review* 3(6):1510-1531.

Torres, D. M., K. M. Galetta, H. W. Phillips, E. M. S. Dziemianowicz, J. A. Wilson, E. S. Dorman, E. Laudano, S. L. Galetta, and L. J. Balcer. 2013. Sports-related concussion: Anonymous survey of a collegiate cohort. *Neurology Clinical Practice* 3(4):279-283.

Tsao, J. W. 2013. Navy and Marine Corps TBI Efforts. Presentation before the committee, Washington, DC, February 25.

Tsushima, W. T., N. Shirakawa, and O. Geling. 2013. Neurocognitive functioning and symptom reporting of high school athletes following a single concussion. *Applied Neuropsychology: Child* 2(1):13-16.

Vagnozzi, R., S. Signoretti, L. Cristofori, F. Alessandrini, R. Floris, E. Isgro, A. Ria, S. Marziale, G. Zoccatelli, B. Tavazzi, F. Del Bolgia, R. Sorge, S. P. Broglio, T. K. McIntosh, and G. Lazzarino. 2010. Assessment of metabolic brain damage and recovery following mild traumatic brain injury: A multicentre, proton magnetic resonance spectroscopic study in concussed patients. *Brain* 133(11):3232-3242.

Valovich McLeod, T. C., and C. Leach. 2012. Psychometric properties of self-report concussion scales and checklists. *Journal of Athletic Training* 47(2):221-223.

Van Kampen, D. A., M. R. Lovell, J. E. Pardini, M. W. Collins, and F. H. Fu. 2006. The "value added" of neurocognitive testing after sports-related concussion. *American Journal of Sports Medicine* 34(10):1630-1635.

Vaughan, C., G. A. Gioia, and D. Vincent. 2008. Initial examination of self-reported post-concussion symptoms in normal and mTBI children ages 5 to 12. [Abstract.] *Journal of the International Neuropsychological Society* 14(Suppl 1):207.

Virji-Babul, N., M. R. Borich, N. Makan, T. Moore, K. Frew, C. A. Emery, and L. A. Boyd. 2013. Diffusion tensor imaging of sports-related concussion in adolescents. *Pediatric Neurology* 48(1):24-29.

VistaLifeSciences. 2013. ANAM4 FAQs. http://www.vistalifesciences.com/anam-faq.html (accessed September 23, 2013).

Weir, J. P. 2005. Quantifying test-retest reliability using the intraclass correlation coefficient and the SEM. *Journal of Strength and Conditioning Research* 19(1):231-240.

Wilde, E. A., S. R. McCauley, J. V. Hunter, E. D. Bigler, Z. Chu, Z. J. Wang, G. R. Hanten, M. Troyanskaya, R. Yallampalli, X. Li, J. Chia, and H. S. Levin. 2008. Diffusion tensor imaging of acute mild traumatic brain injury in adolescents. *Neurology* 70(12):948-955.

Willer, B., and J. J. Leddy. 2006. Management of concussion and post-concussion syndrome. *Current Treatment Options in Neurology* 8(5):415-426.

Woodard, J., C. Marker, F. Tabanico, S. Miller, E. Corsett, L. Cox, F. Gould, and J. Bleiberg. 2002. A validation study of the Automated Neuropsychological Assessment Metrics (ANAM) in non-concussed high school players. [Abstract.] *Journal of the International Neuropsychological Society* 8(2):175.

Yeates, K. O., H. G. Taylor, J. Rusin, B. Bangert, A. Dietrich, K. Nuss, M. Wright, D. S. Nagin, and B. L. Jones. 2009. Longitudinal trajectories of postconcussive symptoms in children with mild traumatic brain injuries and their relationship to acute clinical status. *Pediatrics* 123(3):735-743.

Yeates, K. O., E. Kaizar, J. Rusin, B. Bangert, A. Dietrich, K. Nuss, M. Wright, and H. G. Taylor. 2012. Reliable change in postconcussive symptoms and its functional consequences among children with mild traumatic brain injury. *Archives of Pediatrics and Adolescent Medicine* 166(7):615-622.

4

Treatment and Management of Prolonged Symptoms and Post-Concussion Syndrome

Most young people who sustain a concussion during active play or sports naturally progress from the injury event through a period of symptom resolution, followed by a return to full normal activities. As discussed in Chapter 3, in 80 to 90 percent of cases, individuals' symptoms resolve within 2 weeks (Makdissi et al., 2010; McClincy et al., 2006; McCrea et al., 2009, 2013; McCrory et al., 2013), although recovery within that period appears to be somewhat slower for adolescents ages 13 years through high school than for college-age athletes (Covassin et al., 2010; Eisenberg et al., 2013; Field et al., 2003; McClincy et al., 2006). In 10 to 20 percent of individuals, however, concussive symptoms persist for a number of weeks, months, or even years. These individuals may be said to be experiencing post-concussion syndrome (PCS). This chapter reviews the diagnostic definitions of PCS, potential early predictors of prolonged recovery, and the symptomatology and management of individuals with prolonged recovery or PCS. The chapter addresses those areas described in the statement of task that pertain to risk factors for PCS; the cognitive, affective, and behavioral changes that may occur during the subacute and chronic posttraumatic phases; and the treatment and management of PCS. The committee's charge did not include the development or recommendation of specific clinical practice guidelines. Given that, the chapter is limited to a review and discussion of the available literature on the treatment and management of individuals experiencing prolonged recovery from a concussion.[1]

---

[1]A number of groups are engaged in the ongoing development of practice guidelines for concussion (Giza et al., 2013; Harmon et al., 2013; McCrory et al., 2013).

DIAGNOSTIC DEFINITION

Post-concussion syndrome is the persistence of a constellation of physical, cognitive, emotional, and sleep symptoms beyond the usual recovery period after a concussion. The World Health Organization's *International Classification of Diseases*, 10th revision (ICD-10), defines PCS[2] as

> a syndrome that occurs following head trauma (usually sufficiently severe to result in loss of consciousness) and includes a number of disparate symptoms such as headache, dizziness, fatigue, irritability, difficulty in concentration and performing mental tasks, impairment of memory, insomnia, and reduced tolerance to stress, emotional excitement, or alcohol. (WHO, 2010, F07.2)

The *Diagnostic and Statistical Manual of Mental Disorders* (DSM) no longer contains a specific entry for "postconcussional disorder." Instead, the fifth edition of the DSM captures persistent concussive symptoms under "neurocognitive disorder due to traumatic brain injury" (APA, 2013, pp. 624ff). The diagnostic criteria specify that the neurocognitive disorder must persist "past the acute post-injury period." There is concern that the symptoms associated with the diagnostic criteria for PCS are nonspecific and that they frequently occur in the absence of head injury and in conjunction with other psychiatric conditions (Ruff, 2011).

SHORT-TERM PREDICTORS OF A PROLONGED SYMPTOMATIC PERIOD POST CONCUSSION

Several studies have looked at different approaches to predicting which athletes will be most likely to have a prolonged recovery (typically more than 2 weeks post injury). A study of high school and college athletes with concussions found that loss of consciousness, posttraumatic and retrograde amnesia, and greater symptom severity (an increase of 20 points or more on the Graded Symptom Checklist) within the first 24 hours following injury were associated with longer recoveries (7 or more days) (McCrea et al., 2013). The researchers also found that demographic variables, competition level (high school versus college), player position, mechanism of injury, concussion history, and acute scores on the Standardized Assessment of Concussion (SAC) and the Balance Error Scoring System (BESS) tests were not predictive of a longer recovery time (McCrea et al., 2013).

Chrisman and colleagues (2013) used High School RIO™ data to identify predictors of prolonged symptoms, defined as lasting 7 or more days, in high school athletes. Presenting with four or more symptoms

---

[2]The ICD-10 uses the term "postconcussional syndrome."

of concussion doubled the risk of prolonged symptoms. A history of prior concussion doubled the risk for prolonged symptoms in football players only. Symptoms of drowsiness, nausea, and concentration problems were associated with prolonged symptoms in all athletes, while sensitivity to light and noise was associated with prolonged symptoms only in non-football players. Amnesia was a risk factor only in males, and, contrary to the findings of McCrea and colleagues (2013), loss of consciousness was not a predictor of prolonged symptoms.

Iverson (2007) studied 114 concussed high school football players and found that slower-to-recover concussed athletes (those taking more than 10 days to recover) were more likely to have low scores on three neuropsychological tests (visual memory, reaction time, and processing speed). Lau and colleagues (2011b) examined 107 male high school football athletes who experienced a concussion and were divided into those with rapid (defined as ≤7 days) or prolonged (≥21 days) recovery. On-field dizziness was associated with a 6.3-fold increase in the odds of a prolonged recovery.

Related reports on the same sample that compared those with short (≤14 days) and prolonged (>14 days) recovery found that abnormal scores on both Immediate Post-Concussion Assessment and Cognitive Testing (ImPACT) neurocognitive testing and the Post-Concussion Symptom Scale (PCSS) at 2 days after injury could identify those who would have a prolonged recovery (Lau et al., 2011a, 2012). In an attempt to quantify the predictive value of symptoms and test scores for identifying protracted recovery, Lau and colleagues (2011a) followed 108 male high school football players from the time of their first post-injury evaluation (median of 2 days) until they returned to play. The athletes were classified as having a protracted recovery (>14 days; n=50) or a short recovery (≤14 days; n=58). Symptom clusters and neurocognitive composite scores used together had the highest sensitivity (65.22 percent), specificity (80.36 percent), positive predictive value (73.17 percent), and negative predictive value (73.80 percent) in predicting protracted recovery. Neither the symptom clusters nor the cognitive test scores alone provided adequate discriminating power. There was a net 24.41 increase in sensitivity when using neurocognitive testing and symptom clusters together compared with using total symptoms on PCSS alone.

A study of concussion in Australia elite football players found that delayed return to sport (i.e., more than 7 days) was associated with greater symptom load, headaches lasting more than 60 hours, and self-reported fatigue and fogginess (Makdissi et al., 2010). Youth with a history of multiple concussions also are at greater risk for prolonged recovery and PCS (Collins et al., 2002; Eisenberg et al., 2013; Guskiewicz et al., 2003; Kerr et al., 2012; Schatz et al., 2011; Zemper, 2003).

Recent imaging studies have begun to examine the role of depressive symptoms in predicting clinical outcome and brain abnormalities in individuals with mild traumatic brain injury (mTBI) (Chen et al., 2008; Maller et al., 2010; Rao et al., 2012). Functional and structural brain differences were examined between a group of 40 male athletes in their 20s and 30s who had a history of three or more concussions, on average, and a control group of male athletes, none of whom had had a concussion in the past 12 months (Chen et al., 2008). The results showed no performance differences between the groups on a working memory task. However, those individuals with symptoms of both concussion and depression showed the greatest reduction in activity in their prefrontal regions, an area of the brain previously implicated in working memory ability. Furthermore, there was a negative association between activity in this region and depressive symptoms. In contrast, activity in regions previously implicated in emotion and mood disorders (e.g., the cingulate, orbitofrontal cortex and hippocampus) was positively correlated with depressive symptoms. A voxel-based morphometry analysis showed gray matter loss within the cingulate that negatively correlated with depressive symptoms. Finally, depressive symptoms correlated with post-concussive symptoms. These findings suggest that post-concussive symptoms often co-occur with depression and have a shared pathology.

A systematic review of 15 prospective studies of sports concussion and mTBI found that predictors of persistent post-concussive symptoms included being older (adolescent versus child) and having had initial symptoms of headache and loss of consciousness. There also was some evidence to support premorbid conditions as contributing to symptom persistence (e.g., previous concussions, learning difficulties, psychiatric difficulties) (Zemek et al., 2013). The most comprehensive prospective study of sports concussion in youth found that prolonged symptoms were predicted by loss of consciousness, posttraumatic amnesia, and high initial levels of symptomatology (McCrea et al., 2013). A recent emergency department-based prospective study found that previous concussions, high levels of initial symptoms, ages greater than 13 years, and an absence of loss of consciousness predicted symptom persistence (Eisenberg et al., 2013). In that study, there was a dose-response relationship between the number of concussions (two or more versus one or fewer concussions) and how long the symptoms lasted, and a prior concussion that occurred within the previous year was associated with an increased risk for prolonged symptoms (Eisenberg et al., 2013).

SYMPTOMATOLOGY IN PROLONGED RECOVERY
AND POST-CONCUSSION SYNDROME

Aside from their duration, the symptoms experienced by individuals with prolonged recovery or PCS are the same as those experienced in the acute phase of the injury (e.g., physical, cognitive, emotional, and sleep), and the same symptom scales and checklists are used to assess and monitor individuals with persistent symptoms (see Chapter 3). There has been one carefully conducted, controlled prospective study of sports concussions in high school and college athletes, with high school students making up about two-thirds of the concussed athletes (n=570) and of the non-concussed athlete controls (n=166) (McCrea et al., 2013). Athletes had been given baseline, preseason testing with respect to symptoms using the Graded Symptom Checklist (GSC), postural stability using the BESS, and cognitive function using the SAC and paper-and-pencil neuropsychological testing. Symptom, cognitive, and postural recovery were assessed at baseline, the time of injury, 2 to 3 hours post injury, several times during the first week following injury, and at 45 or 90 days post injury.[3] Neuropsychological testing was done at baseline, 1 to 2 days and 1 week post injury, and at day 45 or 90 post injury. The athletes were divided into prolonged recovery (PR), typical recovery (TR), and non-concussed (NC) groups. Athletes were assigned to the TR group if their total GSC change score from baseline to post-injury day 7 was with within the 95th percentile of change score for the NC over the same period of time (i.e., a change score on the GSC of 5 or less). Athletes were assigned to the PR group if they had a change score on the GSC of 6 or greater between baseline and post-injury day 7.

Based on these criteria, 10 percent of the concussed athletes were assigned to the PR group. There were no baseline differences among the groups with respect to demographics, prior concussion history, or baseline testing in the symptomatic, cognitive, postural, or neuropsychological domains. The PR group had higher levels of symptoms at all assessment points, while the TR group's GSC scores were higher than those of the NC group at day 3, but not beyond that point (see Figure 4-1). Cognitive testing using the SAC showed that the PR group demonstrated differences from the other two groups through day 7, while the TR group had normalized by day 2 (see Figure 4-2). The trajectories of postural stability converged after the 3-hour point and at no point differentiated the PR from the TR groups (see Figure 4-3). The vast majority of neuropsychological measures did not discriminate across recovery groups, and none discriminated between recovery groups and controls at any time-points.

---

[3]Over the course of the 10-year study, the remote recovery assessment point changed from 90 to 45 days.

Predictors of prolonged recovery included loss of consciousness (odds ratio=4.2, 95% confidence interval, 2.1-8.2); retrograde amnesia (odds ratio=2.2, 95% confidence interval, 1.2-4.1); and posttraumatic amnesia (odds ratio=1.8, 95% confidence interval, 1-3.3). Also, an increase in the GSC of 20 or more from baseline to either the 2- to 3-hour assessment or day 1, conferred a nearly threefold increased risk of a prolonged recovery. At 45 or 90 days following injury, 23 percent of the PR group versus only 5 percent of the TR group had symptoms higher than the control recovery trajectory. In a companion study, the same research group showed that post-concussion migraine was associated with increased symptoms through day 7 but not beyond (Mihalik et al., 2013). Interestingly, although females were more likely to experience posttraumatic migraine, a history of previous migraine was rare in this sample and not contributory to risk.

Another study, which included youth with sports-related concussion as well as other types of mTBI, described the phenomenology and trajectory of different symptom clusters. The study, which looked at PCS symptomatology across four categories (cognitive, somatic, emotional, and behavioral) in children ages 8 to 15 years with mTBI, found that children experiencing prolonged recovery consistently self-reported the presence of symptoms in the somatic and cognitive categories, while parents reported the observation of emotional as well as somatic and cognitive symptoms in their children (Ayr et al., 2009). Although the majority of participants in the study had sports- or recreation-related injuries, 10 percent had Glasgow Coma Scale scores of less than 15; 39 percent experienced a loss of consciousness (for a median time of 1 minute, with a range of 0 to 15 minutes); and abnormalities on neuroimaging, which are indicative of more severe injury than that generally associated with sports-related concussion, did not exclude individuals from the study.

Evaluation of PCS symptoms poses a number of challenges. The experience of and reporting of symptoms are, by nature, subjective; the symptoms associated with PCS are not specific for the condition; and the symptoms are prevalent among the general pediatric population. In some cases, persistent symptoms appear to be an extension of symptoms experienced during the acute phase of the injury that are taking longer than usual to resolve; in other cases, because preexisting conditions or a prior history of problems (e.g., sleep, headache, attentional problems) are predictors of prolonged recovery, a concussion may trigger a recurrence of symptoms or exacerbate an ongoing problem (Leddy et al., 2012). The lack of comprehensive longitudinal studies of sports concussions makes it difficult to more precisely delineate the predictors and symptomatic correlates of recovery and persistence of post-concussive symptoms.

The interrelationship among PCS symptoms poses another challenge for evaluating the condition. Research has shown disturbed sleep to be re-

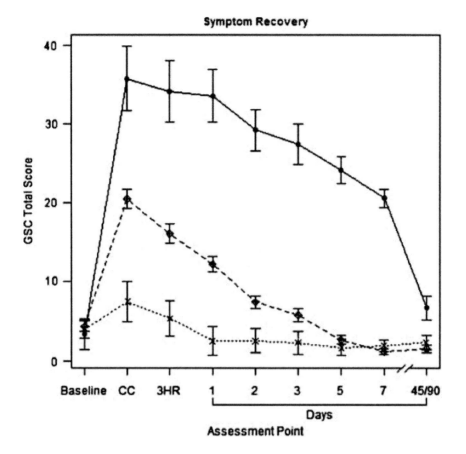

FIGURE 4-1 Symptom recovery curve.
NOTES: Figure compares typical recovery (dashed line), prolonged recovery (solid line), and normal control (dotted line) groups. Group × time interaction, p<.001. Higher scores indicate more severe symptoms on the GSC. Error bars indicate 95 percent confidence interval.
3HR = 3 hours post injury; CC = time of concussion; GSC = Graded Symptom Checklist.
SOURCE: McCrea et al., 2013, p. 26. Copyright © 2012 The International Neuropsychological Society. Reprinted with the permission of Cambridge University Press.

lated to poorer functional outcomes and pain (Milroy et al., 2008; Tham et al., 2012). There is also growing evidence that sleep insufficiency or impairment negatively affects children's learning and behavior (Archbold et al., 2004; Blunden et al., 2001; Gozal and O'Brien, 2004; Sadeh et al., 2003). Pain, particularly chronic headache, is very common in cases of traumatic

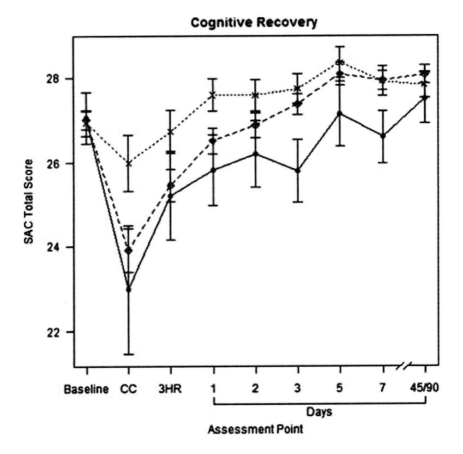

FIGURE 4-2 Cognitive recovery curve.
NOTES: Figure compares typical recovery (dashed line), prolonged recovery (solid line), and normal control (dotted line) groups. Group × time interaction, p<.001. Lower scores indicate poorer cognitive test performance on the SAC. Error bars indicate 95 percent confidence interval.
3HR = 3 hours post injury; CC = time of concussion; SAC = Standardized Assessment of Concussion.
SOURCE: McCrea et al., 2013, p. 26. Copyright © 2012 The International Neuropsychological Society. Reprinted with the permission of Cambridge University Press.

brain injury (TBI), and it is actually more common in those with mTBI than in those with moderate or severe TBI (Blume et al., 2012; Nampiaparampil, 2008). Concussed high school athletes with headaches 7 days following an injury performed more poorly on neurocognitive testing than did those without headaches (Collins et al., 2003).

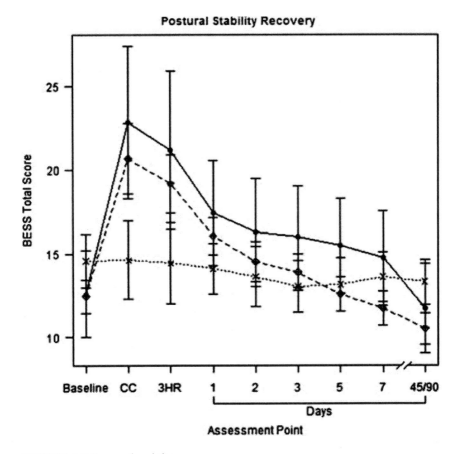

FIGURE 4-3 Postural stability recovery curve.
NOTES: Figure compares typical recovery (dashed line), prolonged recovery (solid line), and normal control (dotted line) groups. Group × time interaction, p<.001. Higher scores indicate poorer balance test performance on the BESS. Error bars indicate 95 percent confidence interval.
3HR = 3 hours post injury; BESS = Balance Error Scoring System; CC = time of concussion.
SOURCE: McCrea et al., 2013, p. 26. Copyright © 2012 The International Neuropsychological Society. Reprinted with the permission of Cambridge University Press.

Depression has also been associated with concussions up to 14 days post injury in high school and collegiate athletes and has been related to lower neurocognitive performance (Kontos et al., 2012). Researchers using functional imaging and diffusion tensor imaging (DTI) have begun to examine commonalities in the brain circuitry implicated in depression and in mTBI. In a review of 57 DTI studies (40 of TBI and 17 of depression), none of which examined depressive symptoms following TBI, common white matter irregularities were identified in frontotemporal regions of the brain, the internal capsule, and the corpus callosum (Maller et al., 2010). Subsequently a longitudinal study of 14 individuals ages 18 to 65 years with mTBI and no history of previous major depression or previous brain injury was completed. DTI measures were attained within 1 month of injury to examine the predictive validity of DTI for later depression. The results showed an association between Hamilton D ratings of depression over the course of the 1-year follow-up and microstructural abnormalities (lower fractional anisotropy and higher mean diffusivity) in frontotemporal regions of the brain within 1 month of the injury (Rao et al., 2012). Together these findings suggest an overlapping neural circuitry of depression and brain injury with frontotemporal neural circuitry that may increase the risk for depression following brain injury. Depressive symptoms following concussions may be associated with structural and functional brain changes, which may inform the treatment of depression and improve outcomes following brain injury.

Recently much attention has been paid to the long-term relationships between sports-related concussions and suicide, but there has been almost no focus on the risk for depression and suicidal behavior during the immediate (e.g., first week) and subsequent post-concussion recovery period. Only one study was identified that has examined the prevalence of suicidal ideation in athletes undergoing preseason testing (Bailey et al., 2010). In this study, 47 collegiate football players ages 17 to 19 were screened as part of preseason testing with the Concussion Resolution Index—a computerized neurocognitive test (see Chapter 3)—and the Personality Assessment Inventory. Significant correlations were found for subscales of the Personality Assessment Inventory with neurocognitive testing. Specifically, suicidal ideation was correlated with slower simple and complex reaction times. Although 23 percent of the sample had had a previous concussion, the relationship between concussion history and suicidal ideation was not assessed. There are no data to evaluate the short-term risk of suicide or suicidal behavior following sports-related concussions, in part because the extant longitudinal studies have primarily focused on post-concussion symptom inventories, which do not assess suicidal ideation or neurocognitive performance.

A study of the emotional responses of collegiate athletes following concussion or musculoskeletal injury found that the emotional profile of the concussed athletes exhibited significantly elevated fatigue and decreased vigor, while athletes with musculoskeletal injuries exhibited significant increases in anger, which resolved to a pre-injury level within 2 weeks (Hutchison et al., 2009).

CLINICAL MANAGEMENT OF PROLONGED SYMPTOMS AND POST-CONCUSSION SYNDROME

There are few interventions available for addressing prolonged recovery or PCS following concussion. Individuals experiencing prolonged symptoms following concussion may be prescribed pharmacologic or other interventions for the treatment of specific symptoms, but the research on such interventions as well as on more general rehabilitative interventions for prolonged recovery following concussion is limited, especially for youth, as is research on the appropriate time to begin interventions.

Role of Exercise in Management of Persistent Symptoms

There is some evidence that noncontact aerobic exercise may play a role in the rehabilitation of individuals experiencing a prolonged recovery or PCS. As long as the individual avoids additional impacts during the window of vulnerability for repeat injury (see Chapters 2, 3, and 5), it appears that exercise will not negatively affect outcomes in youth recovering from sports-related concussion (McCrea et al., 2009). Although there are no randomized controlled trials (RCTs) studying the effects of exercise in youth with a prolonged recovery following sports-related concussion, studies in animals suggest that the use of exercise may be beneficial in the management of individuals with a prolonged recovery and warrants further research.

Animal studies suggest that exercise increases brain chemicals that promote neuroplasticity and neurogenesis; decreases oxidative stress, which can impair brain cell function and lead to cell death; and reduces neuro-inflammation and cognitive dysfunction (Carro et al. 2001; Cotman and Berchtold, 2002; Ding et al., 2004, 2006; Griesbach et al., 2004; Neeper et al., 1995; Piao et al., 2013). In addition, exercise appears to have a beneficial effect on depression in adults (Rimer et al., 2012) and also appears to help prevent depression and anxiety in children and adolescents (Larun et al., 2006), but little is known about the role it might play in the prevention or treatment of post-concussive symptoms. Preliminary studies of the use of exercise to help reduce persistent symptoms following a concussion show there may be a positive effect (Gagnon et al., 2009; Leddy et al., 2010, 2013; Schneider et al., 2013).

The only experimental study of exercise and post-concussive symptoms that has been performed to date examined the impact of exercise on 12 adults with refractory PCS (6 athletes, 6 non-athletes) using a randomized, cross-over design. The exercise condition was associated with a reduction in symptoms of PCS, and that decline was correlated with peak exercise heart rate (Leddy et al., 2010). One additional suggestive study used functional magnetic resonance imaging (fMRI) to observe three groups of four subjects each—adults with PCS who engaged in aerobic exercise treatment, PCS patients treated with "flexibility training," and normal controls—as they performed a cognitive task (Leddy et al., 2013). The PCS exercise group showed fewer symptoms at follow-up than did the PCS "flexibility" group, and the exercise group's fMRI during the cognitive task normalized, whereas the PCS "flexibility" group did not. Although both of these studies are much too small to be definitive, they do suggest that it would be valuable to conduct further studies of the role of exercise in facilitating recovery in pediatric patients with PCS.

Symptom Management

The literature reports various interventions for the management of persistent symptoms of concussion and PCS, although the data to support the efficacy of these interventions in individuals, especially children and adolescents, with sports-related concussions are limited, with virtually no data stemming from RCTs (Giza et al., 2013; Makdissi et al., 2013; Management of Concussion/mTBI Working Group, 2009; Petraglia et al., 2012; Schneider et al., 2013). No RCTs have been conducted to assess the effectiveness of symptom-specific interventions in managing difficulties with sleep, emotional issues (e.g., depression, anxiety), problems with cognition, or headaches in children and adolescents suffering from persistent symptoms of concussion or PCS, and therefore there are insufficient data to show that any intervention enhances recovery or prevents long-term sequelae (Pangilinan et al., 2010). The evidence base underlying post-concussive symptom management in youth includes (1) a quasi-experimental study targeting cognitive symptoms in concussed adolescents with amantadine (Reddy et al., 2013) and open trials in adults with posttraumatic headache following either sports concussion or mTBI (Makdissi et al., 2013; McBeath and Nanda, 1994; Packard, 2000; Weiss et al., 1991); (2) RCTs using cognitive behavior therapy for PCS in adults with mild to moderate TBI, which have been suggestive of a beneficial effect, although all of the studies have had methodological limitations (reviewed in Al Sayegh et al., 2010); and (3) RCTs for symptoms similar to PCS in children and adolescents without a history of concussion, as discussed in the following paragraph.

There are RCTs for the management of such difficulties in non-concussed pediatric populations, but it is currently not known whether these medications and psychotherapeutic interventions would be as effective in concussed youth. For example, cognitive behavioral therapy (CBT) and melatonin have been demonstrated to be efficacious for the management of insomnia in non-concussed youth (Bendz and Scates, 2010; Clarke and Harvey, 2012; Cortesi et al., 2012; Galland et al., 2012; Gradisar et al.,

2011; Hollway and Aman, 2011; Paine and Gradisar, 2011; Quach et al., 2011); cognitive behavioral therapy and selective serotonin reuptake inhibitors have been shown to be efficacious for depression and anxiety (Birmaher et al., 2007; Strawn et al., 2012; Walkup et al., 2008); stimulants have been shown to be helpful for attention and concentration difficulties (Vaughan and Kratovil, 2012); and modest evidence supports the use of certain anti-epileptic and calcium channel agents for pediatric migraine (Eccleson et al., 2012; Papetti et al., 2010). It is logical to consider these agents for testing in concussed youth who present with post-concussive symptoms.

Cognitive and psychoeducational interventions early in the course of mTBI, including in pediatric populations, have been shown to decrease symptomatology upon follow-up, but no studies have been done in concussed youth. Ponsford and colleagues (2001) randomized youth with mTBI (but with more severe injuries than most sports concussions, because their Glasgow Coma Scale scores were 13 to 15) to either receiving an educational booklet describing expectable course and coping procedures or treatment as usual. At 3-month follow-up, the youth whose parents received the intervention were less symptomatic than were those in the control group. In adults with mTBI, both unselected and in those deemed to be at "high risk" for PCS, those who received CBT intervention delivered shortly after the injury reported a faster and more complete recovery (Mittenberg et al., 1996; Silverberg et al., 2013). Multifaceted approaches to rehabilitation following a concussion may aid in recovery by addressing the individual's physical, social, and psychological well-being (Bloom et al., 2004; Gagnon et al., 2009; Johnston et al., 2004).

EFFECTS OF PROLONGED RECOVERY ON FAMILY

It is important to note the potential effects of prolonged recovery from concussion on the injured person's family as well. Pediatric TBI, particularly of greater severity, is associated with significant family burden, which in turn can influence child outcomes (Peterson et al., 2013; Rivara et al., 1996). But even the symptoms associated with concussions can disrupt family patterns (Snedaker, 2013). Parents may need to take time off from work to care for a concussed child, who in turn may, if an adolescent, suddenly find him- or herself in need of care at a time when he or she is otherwise becoming increasingly independent. Conversely, siblings may receive disproportionately less time and attention from parents (Snedaker, 2013). Wade and colleagues (2006a,b) reported improvements in behavior in children with moderate to severe TBI and reduction in global distress, depression, and anxiety in parents following family-centered problem solving and online parent interventions respectively. However, the effects on families of prolonged recovery from concussion in children have not been systematically studied and interventions have not been tested in such families.

ACCESS TO CARE FOR INDIVIDUALS
WITH PROLONGED RECOVERY

It is important for individuals with a concussion to receive care from providers knowledgeable about concussions, and a number of state concussion laws require that high school athletes with a concussion be cleared to return to play by providers knowledgeable in concussion diagnosis and management. Individuals experiencing a prolonged recovery may have a particular need for knowledgeable and coordinated management of their symptoms. During the past several years, there has been a proliferation of clinics around the United States specializing in the management of youth with sports-related concussion (Pennington, 2013). However, access to this sort of specialized concussion care may be limited for youth who lack sufficient health insurance or financial resources as well as for those living in areas where such specialized care is not readily available. The latter may include individuals living in rural areas of the United States and, potentially, military personnel and their dependents who are stationed in other countries.

Telemedicine (i.e., the use of technology to provide medical consultation over a distance) may be a way to provide access to specialized concussion care for some individuals who would otherwise be unable to access such services. The military and Department of Veterans Affairs (VA) Veterans Health Administration have implemented the use of technologies (e.g., Web-based applications, interactive video teleconferencing, electronic health records) to assist in the identification, acute and long-term management, and rehabilitation of individuals with TBI in military and VA settings (Girard, 2007). Telemedicine has been found to be effective in the examination and treatment of stroke victims by permitting evaluation of the patient by a stroke specialist at a remote location, who then directs treatment of the patient by local providers (Schwamm et al., 2009). The Mayo Clinic in Arizona, which has telemedicine programs for stroke, epilepsy, and neurology (Mayo Clinic, 2011), implemented a "teleconcussion" pilot program in 2011 to help provide concussion expertise to patients and their providers in rural areas of Arizona (Vargas et al., 2012). Research is needed to validate the safety and efficacy of telemedicine for concussion identification and management.

FINDINGS

The committee offers the following findings concerning the treatment and management of prolonged symptoms and PCS:

- Typically youth athletes recover from a concussion within 2 weeks of the injury, but in 10 to 20 percent of cases the symptoms of concussion persist for a number of weeks, months, or even years.
- Short-term predictors of prolonged recovery and PCS vary across studies but appear to include older age (adolescent versus child), high initial symptom load, initial presenting symptoms of amnesia and loss of consciousness, and some evidence to support premorbid conditions as contributing to symptom persistence (e.g., previous concussion, learning difficulties, psychiatric difficulties).
- There is a paucity of prospective studies on the course of recovery for youth from sports concussion, and none of these include pre–high school athletes.
- There are no randomized clinical trials testing the efficacy of psychosocial or psychopharmacological treatments for children and adolescents with post-concussive symptoms and prolonged recovery.
- There currently are no data to evaluate the relationship between concussion history and risk of suicide in young athletes because existing post-concussion symptoms inventories do not assess suicidal ideation.

REFERENCES

Al Sayegh, A., D. Sandford, and A. J. Carson. 2010. Psychological approaches to treatment of postconcussion syndrome: A systematic review. *Journal of Neurology, Neurosurgery, and Psychiatry* 81(10):1128-1134.

APA (American Psychiatric Association). 2013. *Diagnostic and Statistical Manual of Mental Disorders*, fifth edition. Arlington, VA: American Psychiatric Association.

Archbold, K. H., B. Giordani, D. L. Ruzicka, and R. D. Chervin. 2004. Cognitive executive dysfunction in children with mild sleep-disordered breathing. *Biological Research for Nursing* 5(3):168-176.

Ayr, L. K., K. O. Yeates, H. G. Taylor, and M. Browne. 2009. Dimensions of postconcussive symptoms in children with mild traumatic brain injuries. *Journal of the International Neuropsychological Society* 15(1):19-30.

Bailey, C. M., H. L. Samples, D. K. Broshek, J. R. Freeman, and J. T. Barth. 2010. The relationship between psychological distress and baseline sports-related concussion testing. *Clinical Journal of Sport Medicine* 20:272-277.

Bendz, L. M., and A. C. Scates. 2010. Melatonin treatment for insomnia in pediatric patients with attention-deficit/hyperactivity disorder. *Annals of Pharmacotherapy* 44(1):185-191.

Birmaher, B., D. Brent; AACAP Work Group on Quality Issues, W. Bernet, O. Bukstein, H. Walter, R. S. Benson, A. Chrisman, T. Farchione, L. Greenhill, J. Hamilton, H. Keable, J. Kinlan, U. Schoettle, S. Stock, K. K. Ptakowski, and J. Medicus. 2007. Practice parameter for the assessment and treatment of children and adolescents with depressive disorders. *Journal of the American Academy of Child and Adolescent Psychiatry* 46(11):1503-1526.

Bloom, G. A., A. S. Horton, P. McCrory, and K. M. Johnston. 2004. Sport psychology and concussion: New impacts to explore. *British Journal of Sports Medicine* 38(5):519-521.

Blume, H. K., M. S. Vavilala, K. M. Jaffe, T. D. Koepsell, J. Wang, N. Temkin, D. Durbin, A. Dorsch, and F. P. Rivara. 2012. Headache after pediatric traumatic brain injury: A cohort study. *Pediatrics* 129(1):e31-e39.

Blunden, S., K. Lushington, and D. Kennedy. 2001. Cognitive and behavioural performance in children with sleep-related obstructive breathing disorders. *Sleep Medicine Reviews* 5(6):447-461.

Carro, E., J. L. Trejo, S. Busiguina, and I. Torres-Aleman. 2001. Circulating insulin-like Growth Factor I mediates the protective effects of physical exercise against brain insults of different etiology and anatomy. *Journal of Neuroscience* 21(15):5678-5684.

Chen, J. K., K. M. Johnston, M. Petrides, and A. Ptito. 2008. Neural substrates of symptoms of depression following concussion in male athletes with persisting postconcussion symptoms. *Archives of General Psychiatry* 65(1):81-89.

Chrisman, S. P., F. P. Rivara, M. A. Schiff, C. Zhou, and R. D. Comstock. 2013. Risk factors for concussive symptoms 1 week or longer in high school athletes. *Brain Injury* 27(1):1-9.

Clarke, G., and A. G. Harvey. 2012. The complex role of sleep in adolescent depression. *Child and Adolescent Psychiatric Clinics of North America* 21(2):385-400.

Collins, M. W., M. R. Lovell, G. L. Iverson, R. C. Cantu, J. C. Maroon, and M. Field. 2002. Cumulative effects of concussion in high school athletes. *Neurosurgery* 51(5):1175-1179; discussion 1180-1181.

Collins, M. W., M. Field, M. R. Lovell, G. Iverson, K. M. Johnston, J. Maroona, and F. H. Fu. 2003. Relationship between postconcussion headache and neuropsychological test performance in high school athletes. *American Journal of Sports Medicine* 31(2):168-173.

Cortesi, F., F. Giannotti, T. Sebastiani, S. Panunzi, and D. Valente. 2012. Controlled-release melatonin, singly and combined with cognitive behavioural therapy, for persistent insomnia in children with autism spectrum disorders: A randomized placebo-controlled trial. *Journal of Sleep Research* 21(6):700-709.

Cotman, C. W., and N. C. Berchtold. 2002. Exercise: A behavioral intervention to enhance brain health and plasticity. *Trends in Neurosciences* 25(6):295-301.

Covassin, T., R. Elbin, and Y. Nakayama. 2010. Examination of recovery time from sport-related concussion in high school athletes. *Physician and Sportsmedicine* 4(38):1-6.

Ding, Q., S. Vaynman, P. Souda, J. P. Whitelegge, and F. Gomez-Pinilla. 2006. Exercise affects energy metabolism and neural plasticity-related proteins in the hippocampus as revealed by proteomic analysis. *European Journal of Neuroscience* 24(5):1265-1276.

Ding, Y. H., X. D. Luan, J. Li, J. A. Rafols, M. Guthinkonda, F. G. Diaz, and Y. Ding. 2004. Exercise-induced overexpression of angiogenic factors and reduction of ischemia/reperfusion injury in stroke. *Current Neurovascular Research* 1(5):411-420.

Eccleston, C., T. M. Palermo, A. C. de C. Williams, A. Lewandowski, S. Morley, E. Fisher, and E. Law. 2012. Psychological therapies for the management of chronic and recurrent pain in children and adolescents. *Cochrane Database of Systematic Reviews* 12:CD003968.

Eisenberg, M. A., J. Andrea, W. Meehan, and R. Mannix. 2013. Time interval between concussions and symptom duration. *Pediatrics* 132(1):8-17.

Field, M., M. W. Collins, M. R. Lovell, and J. Maroon. 2003. Does age play a role in recovery from sports-related concussion? A comparison of high school and collegiate athletes. *Journal of Pediatrics* 142(5):546-553.

Gagnon, I., C. Galli, D. Friedman, L. Grilli, and G. L. Iverson. 2009. Active rehabilitation for children who are slow to recover following sport-related concussion. *Brain Injury* 23(12):956-964.

Galland, B. C., D. E. Elder, and B. J. Taylor. 2012. Interventions with a sleep outcome for children with cerebral palsy or a post-traumatic brain injury: A systematic review. *Sleep Medicine Reviews* 16(6):561-573.

Girard, P. 2007. Military and VA telemedicine systems for patients with traumatic brain injury. *Journal of Rehabilitation Research & Development* 44(7):1017-1026.

Giza, C. C., J. S. Kutcher, S. Ashwal, J. Barth, T. S. D. Getchius, G. A. Gioia, G. S. Gronseth, K. Guskiewicz, S. Mandel, G. Manley, D. B. McKeag, D. J. Thurman, and R. Zafonte. 2013. *Evidence-Based Guideline Update: Evaluation and Management of Concussion in Sports.* Report of the Guideline Development Subcommittee of the American Academy of Neurology. American Academy of Neurology.

Gozal, D., and L. M. O'Brien. 2004. Snoring and obstructive sleep apnoea in children: Why should we treat? *Paediatric Respiratory Reviews* 5(Suppl A):S371-S376.

Gradisar, M., H. Dohnt, G. Gardner, S. Paine, K. Starkey, A. Menne, A. Slater, H. Wright, J. L. Hudson, E. Weaver, and S. Trenowden. 2011. A randomized controlled trial of cognitive-behavior therapy plus bright light therapy for adolescent delayed sleep phase disorder. *Sleep* 34(12):1671-1680.

Griesbach, G. S., D. A. Hovda, R. Molteni, A. Wu, and F. Gomez-Pinilla. 2004. Voluntary exercise following traumatic brain injury: Brain-derived neurotrophic factor upregulation and recovery of function. *Neuroscience* 125(1):129-139.

Guskiewicz, K. M., M. McCrea, S. W. Marshall, R. C. Cantu, C. Randolph, W. Barr, J. A. Onate, and J. P. Kelly. 2003. Cumulative effects associated with recurrent concussion in collegiate football players: The NCAA Concussion Study. *JAMA* 290(19):2549-2555.

Harmon, K. G., J. A. Drezner, M. Gammons, K. M. Guskiewicz, M. Halstead, S. A. Herring, J. S. Kutcher, A. Pana, M. Putukian, and W. O. Roberts. 2013. American Medical Society for Sports Medicine position statement: Concussion in sport. *British Journal of Sports Medicine* 47(1):15-26.

Hollway, J. A., and M. G. Aman. 2011. Pharmacological treatment of sleep disturbance in developmental disabilities: a review of the literature. *Research in Developmental Disabilities* 32(3):939-962.

Hutchison, M., L. M. Mainwaring, P. Comper, D. W. Richards, and S. M. Bisschop. 2009. Differential emotional responses of varsity athletes to concussion and musculoskeletal injuries. *Clinical Journal of Sport Medicine* 19(1):13-19.

Iverson, G. 2007. Predicting slow recovery from sport-related concussion: The new simple-complex distinction. *Clinical Journal of Sport Medicine* 17(1):31-37.

Johnston, K. M., G. A. Bloom, J. Ramsay, J. Kissick, D. Montgomery, D. Foley, J.-K. Chen, and A. Ptito. 2004. Current concepts in concussion rehabilitation. *Current Sports Medicine Reports* 3(6):316-323.

Kerr, Z. Y., S. W. Marshall, H. P. Harding, Jr., and K. M. Guskiewicz. 2012. Nine-year risk of depression diagnosis increases with increasing self-reported concussions in retired professional football players. *American Journal of Sports Medicine* 40(10):2206-2212.

Kontos, A. P., T. Covassin, R. J. Elbin, and T. Parker. 2012. Depression and neurocognitive performance after concussion among male and female high school and collegiate athletes. *Archives of Physical Medicine and Rehabilitation* 93(10):1751-1756.

Larun, L., L. V. Nordheim, E. Ekeland, K. B. Hagen, and F. Heian. 2006. Exercise in prevention and treatment of anxiety and depression among children and young people. *Cochrane Database of Systematic Reviews* 3:CD004691.

Lau, B. C., M. W. Collins, and M. R. Lovell. 2011a. Sensitivity and specificity of subacute computerized neurocognitive testing and symptom evaluation in predicting outcomes after sports-related concussion. *American Journal of Sports Medicine* 39(6):1209-1216.

Lau, B. C., A. P. Kontos, M. W. Collins, A. Mucha, and M. R. Lovell. 2011b. Which on-field signs/symptoms predict protracted recovery from sport-related concussion among high school football players? *American Journal of Sports Medicine* 39(11):2311-2318.

Lau, B. C., M. W. Collins, and M. R. Lovell. 2012. Cutoff scores in neurocognitive testing and symptom clusters that predict protracted recovery from concussions in high school athletes. *Neurosurgery* 70(2):371-379.

Leddy, J. J., K. Kozlowski, J. P. Donnelly, D. R. Pendergast, L. H. Epstein, and B. Willer. 2010. A preliminary study of subsymptom threshold exercise training for refractory post-concussion syndrome. *Clinical Journal of Sport Medicine* 20(1):21-27.

Leddy, J., H. Sandhu, V. Sodi, J. Baker, and B. Willer. 2012. Rehabilitation of concussion and post-concussion syndrome. *Sports Health: A Multidisciplinary Approach* 4(2):147-154.

Leddy, J. J., J. L. Cox, J. G. Baker, D. S. Wack, D. R. Pendergast, R. Zivadinov, and B. Willer. 2013. Exercise treatment for postconcussion syndrome: A pilot study of changes in functional magnetic resonance imaging activation, physiology, and symptoms. *Journal of Head Trauma and Rehabilitation* 28(4):241-249.

Makdissi, M., D. Darby, P. Maruff, A. Ugoni, P. Brukner, and P. R. McCrory. 2010. Natural history of concussion in sport: Markers of severity and implications for management. *American Journal of Sports Medicine* 38(3):464-471.

Makdissi, M., R. C. Cantu, K. M. Johnston, P. McCrory, and W. H. Meeuwisse. 2013. The difficult concussion patient: What is the best approach to investigation and management of persistent (>10 days) postconcussive symptoms? *British Journal of Sports Medicine* 47(5):308-313.

Maller, J. J., R. H. Thomson, P. M. Lewis, S. E. Rose, K. Pannek, and P. B. Fitzgerald. 2010. Traumatic brain injury, major depression, and diffusion tensor imaging: Making connections. *Brain Research Reviews* 64(1):213-240.

Management of Concussion/mTBI Working Group. 2009. *VA/DoD Clinical Practice Guideline for the Management of Concussion/Mild Traumatic Brain Injury (mTBI).* http://www.healthquality.va.gov/mtbi/concussion_mtbi_full_1_0.pdf (accessed October 3, 2013).

Mayo Clinic. 2011. Telemedicine technology links rural Arizona to concussion care at Mayo Clinic. Press Release. http://www.mayoclinic.org/news2011-sct/6427.html (accessed August 6, 2013).

McBeath, J. G., and A. Nanda. 1994. Use of dihydroergotamine in patients with postconcussion syndrome. *Headache* 34(3):148-151.

McClincy, M. P., M. R. Lovell, J. Pardini, M. W. Collins, and M. K. Spore. 2006. Recovery from sports concussion in high school and collegiate athletes. *Brain Injury* 20(1):33-39.

McCrea, M., K. Guskiewicz, C. Randolph, W. B. Barr, T. A. Hammeke, S. W. Marshall, and J. P. Kelly. 2009. Effects of a symptom-free waiting period on clinical outcome and risk of reinjury after sport-related concussion. *Neurosurgery* 65(5):876-882; discussion 882-883.

McCrea, M., K. Guskiewicz, C. Randolph, W. B. Barr, T. A. Hammeke, S. W. Marshall, M. R. Powell, K. Woo Ahn, Y. Wang, and J. P. Kelly. 2013. Incidence, clinical course, and predictors of prolonged recovery time following sport-related concussion in high school and college athletes. *Journal of the International Neuropsychological Society* 19(1):22-33.

McCrory, P., W. H. Meeuwisse, M. Aubry, B. Cantu, J. Dvořák, R. J. Echemendia, L. Engebretsen, K. Johnston, J. S. Kutcher, M. Raftery, A. Sills, B. W. Benson, G. A. Davis, R. G. Ellenbogen, K. Guskiewicz, S. A. Herring, G. L. Iverson, B. D. Jordan, J. Kissick, M. McCrea, A. S. McIntosh, D. Maddocks, M. Makdissi, L. Purcell, M. Putukian, K. Schneider, C. H. Tator, and M. Turner. 2013. Consensus statement on concussion in sport: The 4th International Conference on Concussion in Sport held in Zurich, November 2012. *British Journal of Sports Medicine* 47(5):250-258.

Mihalik, J. P., J. Register-Mihalik, Z. Y. Kerr, S. W. Marshall, M. C. McCrea, and K. M. Guskiewicz. 2013. Recovery of posttraumatic migraine characteristics in patients after mild traumatic brain injury. *Amercian Journal of Sports Medicine* 41(7):1490-1496.

Milroy, G., L. Dorris, and T. M. McMillan. 2008. Brief report: Sleep disturbances following mild traumatic brain injury in childhood. *Journal of Pediatric Psychology* 33(3):242-247.

Mittenberg, W., G. Tremont, R. E. Zielinski, S. Fichera, and K. R. Rayls. 1996. Cognitive-behavioral prevention of postconcussion syndrome. *Archives of Clinical Neuropsychology* 11(2):139-145.

Nampiaparampil, D. E. 2008. Prevalence of chronic pain after traumatic brain injury: A systematic review. *JAMA* 300(6):711-719.

Neeper, S. A., F. Gomez-Pinilla, J. Choi, and C. Cotman. 1995. Exercise and brain neurotrophins. *Nature* 373(6510):109.

Packard, R. C. 2000. Treatment of chronic daily posttraumatic headache with divalproex sodium. *Headache* 40(9):736-739.

Paine, S., and M. Gradisar. 2011. A randomised controlled trial of cognitive-behaviour therapy for behavioural insomnia of childhood in school-aged children. *Behaviour Research and Therapy* 49(6-7):379-388.

Pangilinan, P. H., A. Giacoletti-Argento, R. Shellhaas, E. A. Hurvitz, and J. E. Hornyak. 2010. Neuropharmacology in pediatric brain injury: A review. *PM & R* 2(12):1127-1140.

Papetti, L., A. Spalice, F. Nicita, M. C. Paolino, R. Castaldo, P. Iannetti, M. P. Villa, and P. Parisi. 2010. Migraine treatment in developmental age: Guidelines update. *Journal of Headache and Pain* 11(3):267-276.

Pennington, B. 2013. A new way to care for young brains. *New York Times* (May 5). http://www.nytimes.com/2013/05/06/sports/concussion-fears-lead-to-growth-in-specialized-clinics-for-young-athletes.html?pagewanted=all&_r=0 (accessed August 5, 2013).

Peterson, R. L., M. W. Kirkwood, H. G. Taylor, T. Stancin, T. M. Brown, and S. L. Wade. 2013. Adolescents' internalizing problems following traumatic brain injury are related to parents' psychiatric symptoms. *Journal of Head Trauma Rehabilitation* 28(5):E1-E12.

Petraglia, A. L., J. C. Maroon, and J. E. Bailes. 2012. From the field of play to the field of combat: A review of the pharmacological management of concussion. *Neurosurgery* 70(6):1520-1533; discussion 1533.

Piao, C. S., B. A. Stoica, J. Wu, B. Sabirzhanov, Z. Zhao, R. Cabatbat, D. J. Loane, and A. I. Faden. 2013. Late exercise reduces neuroinflammation and cognitive dysfunction after traumatic brain injury. *Neurobiology of Disease* 54(June):252-263.

Ponsford, J., C. Willmott, A. Rothwell, P. Cameron, G. Ayton, R. Nelms, C. Curran, and K. Ng. 2001. Impact of early intervention on outcome after mild traumatic brain injury in children. *Pediatrics* 108(6):1297-1303.

Quach, J., H. Hiscock, O. C. Ukoumunne, and M. Wake. 2011. A brief sleep intervention improves outcomes in the school entry year: A randomized controlled trial. *Pediatrics* 128(4):692-701.

Rao, V., M. Mielke, X. Xu, G. S. Smith, U. D. McCann, A. Bergev, V. Doshi, D. L. Pham, D. Yousem, and S. Mori. 2012. Diffusion tensor imaging atlas-based analyses in major depression after mild traumatic brain injury. *Journal of Neuropsychiatry and Clinical Neuroscience* 24(3):309-315.

Reddy, C. C., M. Collins, M. Lovell, and A. P. Kontos. 2013. Efficacy of amantadine treatment on symptoms and neurocognitive performance among adolescents following sports-related concussion. *Journal of Head Trauma Rehabilitation* 28(4):260-265.

Rimer, J., K. Dwan, D. A. Lawlor, C. A. Greig, M. McMurdo, W. Morley, and G. E. Mead. 2012. Exercise for depression. *Cochrane Database of Systematic Reviews* 7:CD004366.

Rivara, J. M., K. M. Jaffe, N. L. Polissar, G. C. Fay, S. Liao, and K. M. Martin. 1996. Predictors of family functioning and change 3 years after traumatic brain injury in children. *Archives of Physical Medicine and Rehabilitation* 77(8):754-764.

Ruff, R. M. 2011. Mild traumatic brain injury and neural recovery: Rethinking the debate. *NeuroRehabilitation* 28(3):167-80.

Sadeh, A., R. Gruber, and A. Raviv. 2003. The effects of sleep restriction and extension on school-age children: What a difference an hour makes. *Child Development* 74(2):444-455.

Schatz, P., R. S. Moser, T. Covassin, and R. Karpf. 2011. Early indicators of enduring symptoms in high school athletes with multiple previous concussions. *Neurosurgery* 68(6):1562-1567; discussion 1567.

Schneider, K. J., G. L. Iverson, C. A. Emery, P. McCrory, S. A. Herring, and W. H. Meeuwisse. 2013. The effects of rest and treatment following sport-related concussion: A systematic review of the literature. *British Journal of Sports Medicine* 47(5):304-307.

Schwamm, L. H., R. G. Holloway, P. Amarenco, H. J. Audebert, T. Bakas, N. R. Chumbler, R. Handschu, E. C. Jauch, W. A. Knight, IV, S. R. Levine, M. Mayberg, B. C. Meyer, P. M. Meyers, E. Skalabrin, and L. R. Wechsler, on behalf of the American Heart Association Stroke Council and the Interdisciplinary Council on Peripheral Vascular Disease. 2009. A review of the evidence for the use of telemedicine within stroke systems of care: A scientific statement from the American Heart Association/American Stroke Association. *Stroke* 40(7):2616-2634.

Silverberg, N. D., B. J. Hallam, A. Rose, H. Underwood, K. Whitfield, A. E. Thornton, and M. L. Whittal. 2013. Cognitive-behavioral prevention of postconcussion syndrome in at-risk patients: A pilot randomized controlled trial. *Journal of Head Trauma Rehabilitation* 28(4):313-322.

Snedaker, K. 2013. *Concerns and Issues Faced by Families of Concussed Youth.* Presentation before the committee, Washington, DC, February 25.

Strawn, J. R., D. J. Sakolsky, and M. A. Rynn. 2012. Psychopharmacologic treatment of children and adolescents with anxiety disorders. *Child and Adolescent Psychiatric Clinics of North America* 21(3):527-539.

Tham, S. W., T. M. Palermo, M. S. Vavilala, J. Wang, K. M. Jaffe, T. D. Koepsell, A. Dorsch, N. Temkin, D. Durbin, and F. P. Rivara. 2012. The longitudinal course, risk factors, and impact of sleep disturbances in children with traumatic brain injury. *Journal of Neurotrauma* 29(1):154-61.

Vargas, B. B., D. D. Channer, D. W. Dodick, and B. M. Demaerschalk. 2012. Teleconcussion: An innovative approach to screening, diagnosis, and management of mild traumatic brain injury. *Telemedicine and e-Health* 18(10):803-806.

Vaughan, B., and C. J. Kratochvil. 2012. Pharmacotherapy of pediatric attention-deficit/hyperactivity disorder. *Child and Adolescent Psychiatric Clinics of North America* 21(4):941-955.

Wade, S. L., J. Carey, and C. R. Wolfe. 2006a. An online family intervention to reduce parental distress following pediatric brain injury. *Journal of Consulting and Clinical Psychology* 74(3):445-454.

Wade, S. L., L. Michaud, and T. M. Brown. 2006b. Putting the pieces together: Preliminary efficacy of a family problem-solving intervention for children with traumatic brain injury. *Journal of Head Trauma Rehabilitation* 21(1):57-67.

Walkup, J. T., A. M. Albano, J. Piacentini, B. Birmaher, S. N. Compton, J. T. Sherrill, G. S. Ginsburg, M. A. Rynn, J. McCracken, B. Waslick, S. Iyengar, J. S. March, and P. C. Kendall. 2008. Cognitive behavioral therapy, sertraline, or a combination in childhood anxiety. *New England Journal of Medicine* 359(26):2753-2766.

Weiss, H. D., B. J. Stern, and J. Goldberg. 1991. Post-traumatic migraine: Chronic migraine precipitated by minor head or neck trauma. *Headache* 31(7):451-456.

WHO (World Health Organization). 2010. *International Statistical Classification of Diseases and Related Health Problems*, 10th Revision. [Online version.] http://apps.who.int/classifications/icd10/browse/2010/en (accessed October 3, 2013).

Zemek, R. L., K. J. Farion, M. Sampson, and C. McGahern. 2013. Prognosticators of persistent symptoms following pediatric concussion: A systematic review. *JAMA Pediatrics* 167(3):259-265.

Zemper, E. D. 2003. Two-year prospective study of relative risk of a second cerebral concussion. *American Journal of Physical Medicine and Rehabilitation* 82(9):653-659.

5

Consequences of Repetitive Head Impacts and Multiple Concussions

In recent years there has been an increase in research on the cognitive and neuropathological consequences of repetitive head impacts and multiple concussions in athletes. Given the frequency of head impacts in contact sports, the public health implications of these consequences may be significant. This chapter addresses those elements of the committee's statement of task that concern the effects of "subconcussive" head impacts (i.e., head impacts that do not result in symptoms consistent with a diagnosis of concussion) and multiple concussions. The chapter reviews the clinical manifestations, neuroimaging features, risk factors, and animal studies related to repetitive head impacts and multiple concussions. It also discusses the possible long-term neuropathological consequences associated with repetitive head impacts and multiple concussions, including chronic traumatic encephalopathy (CTE), an emerging diagnostic entity associated with retired athletes with a history of head injury as well with as military personnel exposed to repeated brain injury from blast and other causes. The goals of this chapter are to provide a comprehensive review of the current literature, to clarify controversies, and to point out important directions for future research.

NEUROPSYCHOLOGICAL AND NEUROPHYSIOLOGICAL CONSEQUENCES

Studies of Repetitive Head Impacts

As with much of the clinical literature on the consequences of concussions in sports, the generalizability of many studies of the effects of repetitive head impacts is limited by methodological weaknesses. For example, helmet-based head impact recording devices are typically set to record only impact forces over a minimum threshold (e.g., 10 g of linear acceleration; see Duma et al., 2005) and, therefore, do not record all impacts to the head. Although recent advances in technical, statistical, and clinical knowledge have helped to improve research on repetitive head impacts, earlier findings have to be viewed in the context of history: Their importance lies more in their groundbreaking attempts to quantify relevant variables and not necessarily in their specific findings.

Findings from Soccer Studies

In soccer, athletes experience repetitive head impacts from using their heads to strike the ball for passing and shooting. Older research involving amateur and professional soccer players indicated an association between cumulative heading and neuropsychological impairments (see, for example, Matser et al., 1998, 1999, 2001; Sortland and Tysvaer, 1989; Tysvaer and Lochen, 1991). One study of 37 former professional soccer players found mild to severe deficits in the areas of attention, concentration, memory, and judgment in 81 percent of the players. The authors speculated that this finding could be indicative of permanent organic brain damage resulting from repeated traumas from heading the ball (Tysvaer and Lochen, 1991). In another study involving 53 active professional soccer players, impairments in memory, planning, and visuo-perceptual tasks were observed and compared with those in non-contact-sport athlete controls. Among the soccer players, performance on these tasks was inversely related to the frequency of heading the ball (Matser et al., 1998). Computed tomography scans of 33 former professional soccer players identified central brain atrophy in one-third of study participants, although scans were only visually inspected, and there were no baseline or control comparisons (Sortland and Tysvaer, 1989).

Several other studies, including more recent ones, involving youth soccer players have found no effect of heading on neurocognitive performance (Broglio and Guskiewicz, 2001; Guskiewicz et al., 2002; Kaminski et al., 2007, 2008; Kontos et al., 2011; Stephens et al., 2010; Straume-Naesheim et al., 2005). For example, Guskiewicz and colleagues (2002) found no differences in neurocognitive function or Scholastic Aptitude Test scores between collegiate soccer players (n=91) and groups of athletes from other contact and non-contact sports (n=96) or between the collegiate soccer players and non-athletic controls (n=53), suggesting that soccer players are not differentially affected by soccer playing (and, by extension, heading).

Furthermore, studies that have directly assessed changes in cognition related to heading a soccer ball have failed to establish any relationship between heading and neurocognitive changes. Following detailed observation of heading frequencies by 63 high school soccer players and the administration of Immediate Post-Concussion Assessment and Cognitive Testing (ImPACT), Kontos and colleagues (2011) found no differences in neurocognitive performance or symptoms among low-, moderate-, and high-exposure header groups. Similarly, Putukian and colleagues (2000) found no changes in neuropsychological test scores between pairs of collegiate soccer players who headed the ball in practice for 20 minutes compared with those who did not head in practice. Kaminski and colleagues conducted two studies with 71 (2007) and 393 (2008) female collegiate soccer players. Using heading counts as the independent variable and pre- and post-season balance and neuropsychological tests to determine neuropsychological changes, they found no significant relationships on any test measure.

Early research using magnetic resonance imaging (MRI) and cognitive tests found no significant cognitive impairments or differences on MRI scans among soccer players, boxers, and track and field athletes (Haglund and Eriksson, 1993). In a recent study using diffusion tensor imaging (DTI) scans on 12 German soccer players and 11 swimmers, several group differences in brain white matter were noted, including increased radial diffusivity and axial diffusivity in soccer players compared to swimmers (Koerte et al., 2012). Although the authors of the study suggest that heading in soccer may lead to neurophysiological changes in the brain, this study's generalizability is limited because of the small number of participants and because it did not include a baseline scan. Furthermore, it is not clear what the functional significance of such findings would be.

In summary, studies of the consequences of heading in soccer have obtained mixed results, with more recent studies showing no relationship between heading and neuropsychological impairment. The positive findings of some older studies may have been due in part to the more frequent use in the 1980s and 1990s of soccer balls that absorbed more water, increasing the weight of the ball by up to 20 percent and potentially making them more dangerous for heading (Smodlaka, 1984). Today, players use waterproof synthetic soccer balls that absorb less water (Kirkendall and Garrett, 2001). The DTI study (Koerte et al., 2012) appeared to show neurological differences in a very small sample. Due to small sample sizes and other methodological limitations, caution is required in interpretation of these studies' findings.

Findings from Football and Ice Hockey Studies

As is the case with soccer players, football and ice hockey players can incur repetitive head impacts (Brainard et al., 2012; Crisco et al., 2010, 2011, 2012). For example, a lineman in football who tackles another player with his head in successive plays experiences a series of repetitive head impacts. Hockey players may experience repetitive head impacts from collisions with the board and with other players.

McAllister and colleagues (2012) examined repetitive head impacts over a single season in collegiate football and ice hockey athletes and compared those athletes with a group of athletes who played a non-contact sport on a variety of measures. Contact athletes wore accelerometer-instrumented helmets and took pre- and post-season ImPACT tests. A subset from one of the three Division I universities also completed a paper-and-pencil neuropsychological battery and had preseason and postseason neuroimaging. There were no group differences on cognitive tasks over a sport season. The researchers also examined baseline neurocognitive tests scores across three sport seasons and found no differences on baseline assessments among the sport groups, suggesting that previous exposures to contact did not affect test scores negatively. However, the researchers did report that a higher percentage of the contact sport athletes performed worse than those in the non-contact group on a measure of new learning (California Verbal Learning Test), with no ImPACT composites showing significant change. Furthermore, the authors found that impact exposure above the 95th percentile in frequency during the last week of the season was related to poorer performance on the Trail Making test, a measure of visual attention and task switching, and that the peak linear acceleration for the season was related to slower ImPACT reaction times. A relationship among recent biomechanical exposures, brain white matter integrity, and lower scores was also found, although the absolute value of (significant) test score decline did not reach impairment level.

Other studies of the effects of repetitive head impacts in high school and collegiate football players have found no association with neurocognitive impairment or physiological changes (see, for example, Broglio et al., 2011; Gysland et al., 2012; Miller et al., 2007). However, these studies all have methodological weaknesses. Only McAllister and colleagues (2012) used non-contact controls and adjusted neurocognitive test scores for practice effects, baseline levels, regression to the mean, and relevant demographic factors, while also comparing seasonal exposure and recent exposures across biomechanical measurements of magnitude and frequency.

A few small studies of high school and collegiate football and hockey players have looked at DTI, neurocognitive test scores, and biomechanical data; these have found axonal changes but mixed neuropsychological findings (Bazarian et al., 2012; Breedlove et al., 2012; Talvage et al., 2010). Evidence for the effects of repetitive head impacts on diffuse axonal injury in humans comes largely from DTI studies that measure directionality (fractional anisotropy, or FA) and regularity (mean diffusivity, or MD) of white matter tracts. This technique showed pre-season to post-season changes in a small sample of high school athletes (n=10, 16 to 18 years old, hockey or football) relative to controls (n=5, 16 to 35 years old) following self-reported repetitive head impacts (Bazarian et al., 2012). While pre- and post-season FA and MD changes (calculated as the percentage of white matter voxels showing either a significant increase or a significant decrease) were largest in a concussed player with greater than 3 percent change, those athletes with repetitive head impacts had intermediary changes of more than 1 percent on average, while the controls had insignificant changes of less than 0.5 percent on average. These findings warrant further investigation in larger samples with same-aged comparison groups.

Traumatic brain injury may result in disruption of the blood-brain barrier (i.e., increased permeability of the brain vasculature) (Neuwelt et al., 2011). Marchi and colleagues used DTI and serum measurements of S100B (a protein secreted by cells in the central nervous system and used as a marker of blood-brain barrier disruption [Blyth et al., 2009, 2011; Marchi et al., 2004]) and S100B auto-antibodies, to evaluate whether head impacts below the threshold for a diagnosis of concussion can disrupt the blood-brain barrier. Sixty-seven college football players were enrolled. In a subset of players (n=15) for whom pre- and post-game blood samples were available, only those players with the most subconcussive head impacts based on self-report and post-game review of the game film had detectable serum levels of S100B and elevated levels of auto-antibodies against S100B. Serum S100B antibodies predicted lasting changes in mean brain white matter diffusivity in a subset of players (n=10) who had preseason and postseason and 6-month follow-up DTI scans. Post-season S100B auto-antibodies also correlated with impulse control and balance problems. Although the study sample is too small to make firm inferences, this research provides preliminary evidence that repetitive head impacts that do not result in a diagnosis of concussion may disrupt the blood-brain barrier. It is important to note that there are sources of serum S100B outside of the central nervous system (e.g., fat cells), although this does not preclude use of S100B as a biomarker of brain injury (Marchi et al., 2013).

Functional magnetic resonance imaging (fMRI) studies have begun to examine blood-oxygen-level dependent brain activity following repetitive head impacts. Talvage and colleagues (2010) prospectively followed 11 male high school football players ages 15 to 19 both preseason and postseason. A negative association was observed between the number of subconcussive repetitive impacts to the front of the head and activity in the prefrontal cortex, as indicated by blood-oxygen-level dependent signals on the fMRI during the performance of a working memory test. These players also exhibited neurocognitive deficits as measured by ImPACT scores on visual memory.

Together these studies suggest changes in cognitive function the brain following repetitive head impacts in football and hockey players. However, the types of cognitive impairment and brain changes that are observed vary by study, and the results are based on small sample sizes, which raises questions about the reliability of these studies.

Findings from Boxing Studies

Many youth continue to participate in boxing even though several medical groups have called for its discontinuation due to the incidence of brain injury (Purcell and LeBlanc, 2012). Although many youth and amateur boxers wear protective gear and follow rules that are different from those for professional boxers, a primary goal of boxing is to attack the head and face of the opponent, which often results in a concussion or more severe brain injury (Jordan, 1987). Indeed, the association of boxing and traumatic brain injury (TBI) is very well-recognized in the medical literature. The so-called punch-drunk syndrome was first recognized as early as 1928 (Wilberger and Maroon, 1989), and it is associated with personality disturbances, dysarthria, or Parkinson-like disturbances.

There is ample evidence supporting the association of boxing with chronic traumatic brain injury. Several researchers have found brain abnormalities in professional boxers (see, for example, Casson et al., 1984; Drew et al., 1986; Kaste et al., 1982; Morrison, 1986; Ross et al., 1983). Jordan and colleagues (1997) examined boxers who had a high exposure to head contact (defined as having had 12 or more professional bouts) to boxers with low exposure to head contact (defined by less than 12 professional bouts) on neurocognitive performance, symptoms, and genetic testing. The authors reported that athletes with a high exposure to head contact had lower cognitive function than did those with low head contact exposure.

The largest DTI studies to date on repetitive head impacts are those involving professional boxers (ages 20 to 52), with sample sizes ranging from 24 to 81. Across these studies, microstructural abnormalities were found as indicated by increased regional and whole brain diffusion and decreased FA in boxers relative to control subjects (Chappell et al., 2006; Zhang et al., 2003, 2006). These findings are further supported by a high-resolution MRI study of 100 boxers (85 with complete data, ages 19 to 42 years) showing a significant correlation between years of boxing and diffuse axonal injury (Orrison et al., 2009).

Together these studies suggest that boxing is associated with possible long-term cognitive decline and axonal injury. Although boxing is an extreme example of a contact sport, the neuropsychological and imaging findings from studies of boxers supplement those of athletes who play other contact sports such as football and hockey.

Studies of Multiple Concussions

As discussed in Chapter 2, there is some evidence from both animal studies and research involving humans that the brain is at increased risk while recovering from a concussion. Thus, a repeat injury while recovering from a prior concussion may occur with less force, take longer to resolve, and in rare cases lead to catastrophic results (e.g., second impact syndrome) (Bey and Ostick, 2009; Simma et al., 2013, Slobounov et al., 2007). Indeed, this is the purpose of the advice "When in doubt, sit them out" (McCrory et al., 2013). A related concern is the effect of a history of concussions on cognition and brain physiology. In a retrospective survey of 223 high school athletes, 20 percent reported a history of at least one concussion (Moser et al., 2005), suggesting that many youth sustain multiple concussions over the course of their athletic careers.

The committee reviewed 16 studies that attempted to answer various questions regarding the effects of multiple concussions. Four additional studies focused on professional and adult athletes and so were not included. Most of the 16 studies assessed the neurocognitive function and symptom load of "stable" athletes (those not currently concussed) and compared groups based on the reported histories of previous concussions. This cross-sectional approach has many limitations, as noted by Iverson and colleagues (2012). A primary difficulty is finding enough athletes with a history of three or more concussions to provide sufficient statistical power. Concussions are a relatively low-base-rate phenomenon, which means that obtaining a large enough sample of individuals who have sustained multiple concussions is particularly difficult.

High School–Age Athletes

Five studies of high school athletes compared symptom presentations, and three compared neurocognitive findings. Schatz and colleagues (2011) compared baseline symptoms of 251 high school athletes who had no reported concussions with 260 athletes who had had one concussion and 105 athletes who had had two or more. The athletes with a history of two or more concussions had significantly more cognitive problems, physical symptoms, and sleep problems at the time of pre-season baseline evaluation than those with no history of concussions. On the other hand, in a study of 867 male high school and college athletes with no (n=664), one (n=149), and two (n=54) previous concussions, Iverson and colleagues (2006) found no group differences in neuropsychological test performance or symptom reporting.

Collins and colleagues (2002) attempted to study the effect of previous concussions in high school athletes by characterizing the on-field signs and symptoms of a subsequent concussion. Sixty athletes with no concussion history were compared with 28 athletes who had had three or more concussions. Those with a history of three or more concussions were significantly more likely to suffer loss of consciousness, anterograde amnesia, and mental status changes lasting longer than 5 minutes.

Among studies that examined neuropsychological test scores, two had conflicting results (Iverson et al., 2006; Moser et al., 2005), and two had too few subjects to have confidence in the results (Elbin et al., 2012; Moser and Schatz, 2002). Moser and colleagues (2005) compared 82 athletes with no concussions to 56 with one concussion, 45 with two or more (although they had had no injuries for at least 6 months), and 40 recently concussed athletes. Athletes were compared on neuropsychological test scores (Repeatable Battery for the Assessment of Neuropsychological Status, Trail Making). While there was a significant difference between groups, the only post hoc result reported was that those with two or more concussions were not different from the recently concussed. Inspection of the data indicates that scores of the recently concussed athletes were lower than those of the no- and one-concussion groups. In contrast, Iverson and colleagues (2006) compared baseline ImPACT scores for 664 athletes with no history of concussion, 149 with a history of one previous concussion, and 54 with a history of two. After controlling for education level, no significant differences were found between the groups.

Overall the findings from studies of the effects of multiple concussions on high school athletes are mixed. In addition to the number of concussions, the interval between concussions may be an important recovery-related factor to consider.

College-Age Athletes

Ten studies of college-age athletes were reviewed. Four studies used symptom presentation as the dependent variable (Collins et al., 1999; Covassin et al., 2008; Guskiewicz et al., 2003; Iverson et al., 2012). Collins and colleagues (1999) found increased symptoms among those athletes with more concussions at baseline, while Guskiewicz assessed the time to symptom resolution of a current concussion based on the number of previous concussions. Neither Covassin and colleagues (2008) nor Iverson and colleagues (2012) found a relationship between symptom levels at baseline testing and the number of previous concussions. However, among those studies that looked at neuropsychological test scores, four found significant differences between previously concussed and non-concussed athletes (Collins et al., 1999; Covassin et al., 2008, 2010; De Beaumont et al., 2009), while four failed to find differences (Broglio et al., 2006; Bruce and Echemendia, 2009; Guskiewicz et al., 2002; Iverson et al., 2012). Three studies had too few cases to be considered (De Beaumont et al., 2007; Elbin et al., 2012; Killam et al., 2005).

In 1999, Collins and colleagues compared baseline symptom totals among 179 athletes with no concussion history, 129 with one, and 78 with a history of two or more. Significant differences were found for symptoms. The researchers also noted that baseline symptom scores increased with the frequency of previous concussions. In a large sample of 184 college football players who suffered concussions, Guskiewicz and colleagues (2003) found that 30 percent of the athletes with more than three concussions took longer than 1 week for symptoms to resolve, compared to only 15 percent of those with one concussion taking more than a week to resolve.

Collins and colleagues (1999) also compared baseline neuropsychological test scores. Significant differences were found on two tests of processing speed. However, the average neuropsychological test scores for the group with two or more concussions were within normal limits. In 2002, Guskiewicz and colleagues compared collegiate soccer players with histories of concussion to soccer players, other athletes, and non-athletes with no histories of concussion. He found no significant differences at baseline on any of a battery of neuropsychological tests. Broglio and colleagues (2006) compared baseline test scores of 163 athletes with no history of concussions to 43 athletes with one previous concussion, 18 with two, and 11 with three. The researchers administered both the Concussion Resolution Index (CRI), an Internet-based neurocognitive test that assesses "simple" and "complex reaction time and process speed, and ImPACT and found no differences in any scores. The small number of athletes with two or more concussions limited the study.

Covassin and colleagues (2010) found no differences on any ImPACT composite test between athletes with no previous concussions and those with one previous concussion. However, both the two-concussion (n=50) and three-plus concussion (n=48) groups scored significantly lower on the verbal memory test than did the no-concussion group (n=50); furthermore, visual memory scores were significantly lower for those with a history of three or more concussions (n=48) than those with no concussion history. The authors concluded that they had demonstrated a partial dose-response relationship for those tests.

In a prospective study Guskiewicz and colleagues (2003) followed a large sample of collegiate football players over 3 years; of those athletes, 184 experienced concussions during the study. The researchers reported that athletes with a history of three or more previous concussions had three times the risk of getting a subsequent concussion than those with no previous history.

In a study of the effects of concussion history on recovery after a subsequent concussion, Covassin and colleagues (2008) compared post-injury neurocognitive test scores 1 day out and 5 days out from the injury between 56 athletes with no previous concussion and 21 with a history of two or more concussions. While they found significant differences in all four composite scores at day 1 and in two composite scores at day 5 (verbal memory and reaction time), they did not control for baseline scores or compare the number of significantly changed scores (CRI) between groups. There were no symptom level differences at any point.

Methodological differences make comparisons among these studies difficult. Differences in how concussion history is measured (e.g., two and more, three and more, etc.) may obscure an important threshold. Variable controls, small sample sizes, and cross-sectional designs make generalizations difficult. Group-level studies are mixed in terms of results, and better methodologies are needed to identify the timing and cumulative effects of multiple concussions. Longitudinal studies and studies highlighting individual differences are lacking. Collaborative studies may be needed to accumulate larger samples of multiply concussed athletes.

MULTIPLE CONCUSSIONS AND DEPRESSION AND SUICIDE

Surveys of retired professional athletes provide some evidence that a history of multiple concussions increases risk for depression (Didehbani et al., 2013; Guskiewicz et al., 2007; Kerr et al., 2012). In a survey of more than 2,500 retired professional football players, 269 of the respondents (11.1 percent) reported having had a prior or current diagnosis of clinical depression. After controlling for parameters such as age, number of years since retirement, number of years played, physical condition, and diagnosed comorbidities such as osteoarthritis, coronary heart disease, stroke, cancer, and diabetes (but not substance abuse or intervening psychosocial issues), the authors found an increasing linear relationship between history of concussion and diagnosis of lifetime depression ($p < 0.005$). Compared with retired players with no history of concussion, retired players reporting three or more previous concussions (24.4 percent) were three times more likely to have been diagnosed with depression; those with a history of one or two previous concussions (36.3 percent) were 1.5 times more likely to have been diagnosed with depression (Guskiewicz et al., 2007). In another study of 30 retired professional football players with a history of concussion versus 29 age- and IQ-matched controls without a history of concussion, a significant correlation was observed between number of lifetime concussions and current cognitive symptoms of depression as measured by the Beck Depression Inventory II. These findings suggest that the number of concussions an individual has sustained may be related to later depressive symptomology (Didehbani et al., 2013). Imaging research is beginning to explore the relationship between depression symptoms and brain white matter abnormalities in retired athletes (Hart et al., 2013; Strain et al., 2013).

Athletes who retire as a result of suffering multiple concussions may experience distress and reduced quality of life, similar to outcomes reported following other serious athletic injuries (Caron et al., 2013; Kuehl et al., 2010; Mihovilovic, 1968). Social support has been identified as important to psychological recovery following more severe brain injuries (Gan et al., 2006) as well as within the sport injury and rehabilitation process (Bianco, 2001; Clement and Shannon, 2011; Wiese-Bjornstal et al., 1998). Individuals who have sustained concussions are also likely to benefit from social support. However, little is known about the role of social support in managing athletes' concussion symptoms and related psychosocial outcomes. The effect of support may be complicated in situations where norms encourage athletes to play through their injuries and when athletes fear being stigmatized by peers as lacking toughness (Safai, 2003; Young et al., 1994). Qualitative interviews with five retired National Hockey League players who had retired due to symptoms following multiple concussions revealed that they were significantly affected by their injuries in their postathletic careers and in their personal relationships. They continued to feel debilitated by post-concussive symptoms and experienced symptoms of anxiety and depression. Three of the participants reported thoughts of suicide in the months immediately following their retirement. Though it is difficult to distinguish whether the experiences of these former athletes were a result of multiple concussions or the end of their careers in professional ice hockey, these findings indicate a need for professional support for athletes when they are recovering from concussions and during the transition to their post-athletic careers (Caron et al., 2013).

Recently, after several highly publicized suicides by professional athletes who showed evidence of CTE, there has been growing interest in understanding the relationship between multiple concussions and suicide (Omalu et al., 2006; Reider, 2012). Though there is some indication of a relationship between number of previous concussions and risk of developing depression, very little research has evaluated the relationship between concussions and suicidal thoughts and behaviors. There are certainly theoretical reasons why individuals who have sustained concussions might be predisposed to suicidal ideation and behavior. For example, there is growing evidence that individuals who attempt suicide, particularly those who engage in high lethality attempts, show deficits in attention, working memory, and risk assessment, which overlap with the neurocognitive residua of concussions, both in the short term and, for those with longer-lasting post-concussive symptoms, in the long term as well (Bridge et al., 2012; Jollant et al., 2005; Keilp et al., 2001, 2013). Thus, the deficits associated with a concussion may lower the threshold for a person with suicidal thoughts to act on them. In addition, some of the associated symptoms of concussion, namely pain, depressive symptoms, and sleep impairment, are common antecedents of suicidal behavior (Goldstein et al., 2008; Wong et al., 2011).

There is a growing literature on the relationship between more severe TBI and suicidal behavior. Oquendo and colleagues (2004) examined a clinical sample of depressed patients and found that while a past history of TBI was a risk factor for suicidal behavior, this increased risk for suicidal behavior was explained by the higher rates of substance abuse, cluster B personality disorder, and higher self-reported aggression and hostility in those with TBI. Because this was a cross-sectional study, it was not possible to determine if these characteristics antedated—and perhaps contributed to—the TBI or if they were sequelae of the TBI. Mainio and colleagues (2007) found that among suicide victims, those with TBI were more likely to have been hospitalized for a psychiatric disorder and to have a substance abuse disorder. In a review paper Simpson and Tate (2007) found that pre-morbid psychiatric disorder and substance abuse, a previous suicide attempt, and severe hopelessness were all related to patients with TBI making a suicide attempt. Similar correlates of suicidal ideation were found in community-dwelling adults with a history of TBI (Tsaudousidies et al., 2011), namely, a current psychiatric diagnosis of depression, anxiety, or posttraumatic stress disorder (PTSD) and a history of pre-morbid substance misuse. In this sample there was no relationship between injury severity and suicidal ideation, with 32 percent of those with moderate to severe TBI and 25 percent of those with mild TBI (mTBI) reporting suicidal ideation. Conversely, among patients undergoing treatment for substance abuse, those with a history of TBI were more likely to have had parental loss and childhood conduct disorders and, as an adult, to have made a suicide attempt (48 percent versus 37 percent) (Felde et al., 2006).

In military populations, those under care in the Department of Veterans Affairs (VA) system with a history of TBI were 1.55 times more likely to die by suicide than were those without a history of TBI (Brenner et al., 2011). Greater injury severity was associated with a greater risk of suicide. Among deployed military personnel with mTBI, increased suicidality was associated with depression and with its interaction with the presence of PTSD (Bryan et al., 2013). Similarly, in veterans with TBI, PTSD is a significant risk factor for suicide attempts (Brenner et al., 2011). A study of military personnel (n=161) provides preliminary evidence of a dose-response relationship between the number of TBIs (none, single, multiple), including concussions, an individual has sustained during his or her lifetime and suicidal thoughts or behavior (Bryan and Clemans, 2013). These results persisted even after controlling for the effects of depression, PTSD, and TBI symptom severity. Further research is needed to confirm these findings.

In summary, the long-term effects of repeated concussions have been linked to risk for depression in retired professional football players, although suicidal ideation and behavior have not been reported in these samples (Didehbani et al., 2013; Guskiewicz et al., 2007). In both military and non-military samples, while there appears to be an increased risk for suicidal behavior and suicide associated with TBI, the increased risk has been reported to occur with injuries of greater severity than concussion in most studies (Brenner et al. 2011; Tsaudousidies et al., 2011). In military samples, depression and PTSD are strong contributors to suicidal risk in those with TBI (Brenner et al., 2011; Bryan et al., 2013), and one recent study found that TBI makes a unique contribution to the risk for suicidal ideation or behavior even after controlling for depression and PTSD (Bryan and Clemans, 2013). Prospective studies that examine changes in depression and suicidal ideation behavior pre- and post-concussion will be required to address whether there are increased risks for suicidal behavior in individuals who have suffered a sports-related concussion. Only one intervention study for suicide prevention in individuals with TBI has been reported. In a pilot study Simpson and colleagues randomly assigned 17 patients with TBI and moderate to severe hopelessness or suicidal ideation, or both, to cognitive psychotherapy or usual care, and they found significant decreases in hopelessness in the treatment group versus the usual care group (Simpson et al., 2011). Clearly more work needs to be done on identifying individuals with concussion who are at risk for suicide as well as in developing effective interventions to reduce suicidal risk.

EXPERIMENTAL MODELS

Behavioral and Cognitive Consequences

Several experimental models of repeat TBI have demonstrated changes in behavioral outcome in the absence of overt pathology (DeFord et al., 2002; Prins et al., 2010; Shitaka et al., 2011). The Morris water maze (MWM) task has been traditionally used to quantify memory and learning impairments after moderate TBI and has been used to detect acute deficits after mTBI. In two models of repeat weight drop injury and controlled cortical impact (CCI) injury in the adult mouse, repeat TBI produced significant latency deficits in the MWM 7 days post injury in the absence of histopathology as measured (Creeley et al., 2004; DeFord et al., 2002; Shitaka et al., 2011). Among the studies addressing the cognitive consequences of repeat TBI in the younger brain, MWM deficits at 2 weeks post injury were not detected in 11-day-old rats that received one to three closed-skull CCI injuries (Huh et al., 2007). Because deficits detected by the MWM task following mTBI can be subtle and short-lived, other behavioral assessments have been used to quantify cognitive dysfunction. In a juvenile repeat closed-head CCI injury model, the novel object recognition (NOR) task was used to evaluate transient memory impairments, in the absence of overt cell death, in rats (Prins et al., 2010). Thirty-five-day-old rats were given sham, single, or two injuries (over a 24-hour interval) and were tested in the NOR task 24 hours after the last injury. All groups were able to recognize the novel object when the interval between familiar objects and novel object was 1 hour. Increasing the interval to 24 hours made the task more difficult and resulted in both injured groups showing significant impairments that were alleviated after 3 days of recovery only in the once-injured group (Prins et al., 2010). Findings from this study demonstrate the value of using other testing paradigms to characterize the nature of behavioral and cognitive deficits after mTBI and repeat mTBI. Collectively, experimental models have been able to mimic the acute memory deficits often clinically reported in the absence of gross pathology in both the adult and younger age groups. Future studies need to focus on age and gender differences following multiple concussions.

Acute Cellular Pathology

Experimental models have also been able to show axonal pathology following repeat TBI. Huh and colleagues (2007) used a modified convex silicone 5-millimeter tip to deliver an impact to 11-day-old rats held within a stereotaxic frame. The effects of a single impact were compared to those of sham impacts and of two or three injuries delivered at 5-minute intervals. Histological samples were collected at 1, 3, or 7 days post injury, and cognitive function was assessed 14 days post injury with the MWM. While single injury did not result in gross damage at 7 days, multiple (two or three) impacts caused ventricular enlargement and white matter atrophy. Both reactive astrocytosis throughout the cortical layers and axonal swellings increased with repeat TBI. There were no latency differences between the sham group and any of the injury groups. While the majority of experimental repeat TBI models are rodents, one research group has developed a novel rotational piglet injury model (Raghupathi and Margulies, 2002) that has been used to address axonal injury and cognition after repetitive injury. Piglets (3-5 days old) were given one injury or two injuries 15 minutes apart and were histologically assessed at 6 hours post injury. There were no physiological responses to the injury, with the exception of a mild decrease in blood pressure. While the density of the injured axons did not differ between once- and twice-injured groups, the number of axonal swellings per axon did increase in the twice-injured brains (Raghupathi et al., 2004). In the next study, piglets were a given single rotational injury, two injuries at a 1-day interval, or two injuries at a 1-week interval. Animals given repeat TBI at the 1-day interval showed 43 percent mortality and poorer cognitive composite scores. Those with repeat TBI at the 1-week interval showed greater βAPP staining. No differences were observed between groups on open field testing, T-maze testing, or glass barrier task (Friess et al., 2009).

More recently the CCI injury has been used in a juvenile rat to mimic some of the common pathophysiological processes described after mTBI and concussions, including mild or transient memory impairment, white matter and axonal dysfunction, and the absence of overt cell death (Prins et al., 2010). Adolescent (35-day-old) mice were given either a sham injury, a single injury, or two injuries 24 hours apart, and axonal damage and astrocytic reactivity were histologically assessed 24 hours post injury. The βAPP immunohistochemical labeling was positive in the ipsilateral white matter and was significantly greater in animals exposed to repeat TBI than in the single-injury or sham-injury animals. GFAP labeling revealed slight increases in the ipsilateral gray-white matter junction in single-injury animals. In contrast, the animals with repeat injuries showed a bilateral increase in GFAP with clear morphological changes in the astrocytes. The study is currently the only research addressing the additive effects of repeat TBI in the "adolescent" brain. Experimental models of repeat TBI that report a lack of gross histological pathology have also shown evidence of axonal damage and astrocytic reactivity in both the adult and young developing brain.

Acute Metabolic Dysfunction

As discussed in Chapter 2, one sort of metabolic dysfunction that is known to follow a TBI is a change in the cerebral metabolic rate of glucose consumption (CMRglc). Shortly after an injury the brain enters a prolonged period of glucose metabolic depression. This decrease in CMRglc has been observed in various types of experimental injury models (Andersen and Marmarou, 1992; Chen et al., 2004; Kawamata et al., 1992; Prins and Hovda, 2009; Richards et al., 2001; Sutton et al., 1994; Yoshino et al., 1991, 1992) and in human TBI (Bergsneider et al., 1997; O'Connell et al., 2005). The magnitude and duration of CMRglc depression increases with the severity of the injury and correlates with behavioral dysfunction (Hovda et al., 1994; Moore et al., 2000; Queen et al., 1997). This relationship between CMRglc and injury severity has also been observed in human TBI patients (Hattori et al., 2003). TBIs that do not cause overt cell death or gross pathology can still produce dysfunction. Instances of mTBI, which may be associated with axonal damage or dysfunction as detected from DTI, also show measurable decreases in CMRglc (Gross et al., 1996; Humayun et al., 1989).

Changes in cerebral metabolism have also been examined following repeat TBI at different intervals in adults and in juveniles. Although most of the studies compare single and repeat injury to sham, few studies have incorporated a design in which the interval between injuries was varied. Vagnozzi and colleagues (2007) used a varied interval injury design in adult rats to examine the effects of multiple mild injuries on mitochondrial function and oxidative damage. A weight drop injury was delivered between 1 and 5 days after the primary injury. The greatest cumulative effects on adenosine triphosphate, N-Acetylaspartic acid (NAA), redox, and oxidative damage were all seen with the 3-day injury interval. This research is the first to examine the temporal window of cerebral vulnerability after a mild primary TBI. A more recent study conducted in adolescent rats showed decreases in brain glucose metabolism after a single concussion, with CMRglc recovering in 3 days. The duration of the change in brain glucose metabolism was prolonged if the second concussion was delivered within the first 24 hours, but the effects were not cumulative if the second blow was delivered after the rat had recovered from the first concussion (Prins et al., 2013). These results demonstrate that the window of vulnerability for the adult and adolescent brain may be related to post-concussive metabolic derangements, which could be used as a biomarker. Given that the duration of metabolic depression varies with age (Prins and Hovda, 2001; Thomas et al., 2000; Yoshino et al., 1991), it is likely that the metabolic window of vulnerability will also vary with cerebral maturation. These studies emphasize the need for establishing age-appropriate biomarkers for cerebral vulnerability to help inform return-to-play guidelines.

The human findings concerning the effects of repetitive head impact on brain physiology are supported by controlled animal studies which show increased vulnerability to axonal damage and cognitive impairment with repeated mild head injury (Barkhoudarian et al., 2011; Laurer et al., 2001) that are amplified when injuries occur within a day apart (Prins et al., 2010). Moreover, animal studies show that the pathologies differ in myelinated versus unmyelinated fibers (Reeves et al., 2005), which may suggest that myelin provides some protection against concussive injury so that the immature brain with less myelin may be more vulnerable to brain trauma (Shrey et al., 2011). Although this research involved rodents, epidemiological evidence is consistent with children having poorer outcomes than adolescents or adults following mTBI. There is not yet evidence from imaging studies of greater or more sustained diffuse axonal injury in children relative to older individuals.

BIOMARKERS AND RISK FACTORS

TBI biomarkers have been well researched, with hundreds of published articles. However, there are significantly fewer articles on neurochemical or serum markers for mTBI or concussions and even fewer on issues related to children. There are currently no serum biomarkers that have been shown to be related to the risk of subsequent concussions following the first concussion.

Magnetic resonance spectroscopy (MRS) has been used to examine the effects of multiple concussions on brain metabolites. This research shows that changes in NAA, a marker of neuronal injury, take longer to resolve following a second concussion in nonprofessional athletes—an average of 45 days (n=13) versus an average of only 30 days following a first concussion (n=10) (Vagnozzi et al., 2008). Parallel MRS and cerebral glucose metabolism studies in rodents appear to be consistent with these findings in suggesting that the number of concussions and the interval between concussions both play a role in recovery (Longhi et al., 2005; Prins et al., 2013; Tavazzi et al., 2007; Vagnozzi et al., 2005, 2008). Nonetheless, larger studies may be needed to verify the effects of a second concussive event during this recovery curve.

There has been only one study to date that has addressed the issue of vulnerability of the developing brain after repeat concussions, and this was in an animal model. In this study cerebral glucose metabolism (i.e., CMRglc) was measured in 35-day-old (adolescent) rats that had been exposed to repeat concussive injuries (Prins et al., 2013). The closed-head, mild concussive injury model used in the experiment has been shown to generate mild axonal injury without overt pathology and to produce measurable cognitive dysfunction (Prins et al., 2010). Following a single closed-head mild injury, CMRglc was decreased at 24 hours and had recovered by 3 days post injury. When a second injury was introduced during the metabolic depression, both the magnitude and the duration of CMRglc depression were exacerbated. However, when the second injury was delivered after the metabolic depression had receded, CMRglc did not change significantly. These results demonstrate that the window of vulnerability for the adolescent brain may be related to post-concussive metabolic derangements, which could be used as a biomarker. Given that the duration of metabolic depression varies with age (Prins and Hovda, 2001; Thomas et al., 2000; Yoshino et al., 1991), it is likely that the metabolic window of vulnerability will also vary with cerebral maturation. These studies emphasize the need for establishing age-appropriate biomarkers for cerebral vulnerability in the development of return-to-play guidelines.

Beckwith and colleagues (2013) documented the time-course of diagnosis of a subset of concussions from a large dataset of football players at six Division I universities and related the time-course of diagnosis to biomechanical parameters. Of 105 concussions documented during a 6-year period involving more than 1,200 athletes, 45 concussions were diagnosed within the same day of injury, and athletes were removed immediately from the competition. The 60 concussions diagnosed sometime after the contest (with the athletes not removed from competition) were found to have a different pattern of accelerometer readings (Beckwith et al., 2013). Compared to the immediate diagnosis group, this delayed-diagnosis group sustained more impacts on the day of injury (33 compared to 17 impacts above 15 g) and also during the week before injury (70 impacts compared to 50 impacts). The study concluded that concussions diagnosed immediately were related to hits with a greater force, while those diagnosed later were preceded by a higher number of impacts.

LONG-TERM NEURODEGENERATIVE CONSEQUENCES

In general there is a paucity of literature on the long-term neuropathological consequences of repeated or chronic traumatic brain injury in athletes. However, the recent interest in the effects of repeat head injury on professional athletes, many of whom began playing sports in their youth, has prompted a series of studies aimed at identifying the neuroanatomical and neuropathological substrates that underlie the behavioral outcomes in these athletes. Notwithstanding these efforts, little is known about how TBI, either in acute or chronic form, affects the developing brain at the critical periods when circuit formation and synaptic connectivity are active.

Dementia Pugilistica

Much of the current understanding of the neuropathology of chronic traumatic brain injury in athletes comes from classical studies of professional boxers who experienced repeated impacts to the head throughout their careers (Corsellis et al., 1973). The committee recognizes that the nature of brain injury in boxers is quite different from—and its extent much more severe than—that experienced in other contact sports, so that the long-term neuropathological consequences in boxers may be quite different from those in athletes in other contact sports. However, it is possible that the available data on neurodegenerative features in boxers may provide insights for understanding less severe injury conditions.

Dementia pugilistica, also known as "punch-drunk syndrome," is a chronic progressive traumatic encephalopathy that has been detected in some professional boxers (Corsellis, 1989; Roberts et al., 1990; Tokuda et al., 1991). It exhibits distinct neuropathological features such as cerebral atrophy, thinning of the corpus callosum, enlarged ventricles, and large cavum septi pellucidi with multiple fenestrations, which presumably are caused by tearing of the septa. Microscopically, dementia pugilistica shares certain histological features with Alzheimer's disease, including tau-positive neurofibrillary tangles (NFTs) and diffuse Aβ amyloid plaques, although the distribution of NFTs and plaques in dementia pugilistica shows a greater abundance in the brainstem and the superficial layers of the neocortex. In addition, NFTs in boxers are often clustered as multifocal patches in the dorsolateral frontal cortex, temporal cortex, and orbital gyri, and they show unique perivascular distributions. The tau-positive protein aggregates have also been identified in glial cells and in neurites in the subcortical white matter (McKee et al., 2009; Saing et al., 2012).

As is seen in Alzheimer's disease, the presence of apolipoprotein E (APOE) e4 allele in boxers is associated with an increased risk of cognitive impairment. In particular, high-exposure boxers (those with 12 or more professional bouts) with an APOE e4 allele have been shown to have significantly greater (i.e., worse) chronic traumatic brain injury scores (mean, 3.9; standard deviation [SD], 2.3) than high-exposure boxers without APOE e4 (mean, 1.8; SD, 1.2) (p=0.04) (Jordan et al., 1997). These results were extended by several other studies which showed that, in moderate and severe TBI, APOE e4 allele carriers tend to perform worse on neuropsychological tasks that are presumed to be related to temporal lobe, frontal lobe, and white matter integrity (Ariza et al., 2006), and experience poorer clinical outcomes (Chiang et al., 2003; Friedman et al., 1999). While the underlying mechanisms that account for the increased risks and poor outcome in APOE e4 allele carriers after TBI remain unclear, studies on animal models show that transgenic mice expressing APOE e4 have increased propensity for Aβ amyloid deposits following traumatic brain injury (Hartman et al., 2002; Nicoll et al., 1995).

Chronic Traumatic Encephalopathy

The identification of tau-positive NFTs in boxers with dementia pugilistica raises the question of whether this is an early and a consistent diagnostic feature in repeated traumatic brain injury. In a study focusing on the neuropathological features in a 23-year-old boxer, Geddes and colleagues showed that NFTs, but not amyloid plaques, indeed could be identified in the orbitofrontal and temporal cortex (Geddes et al., 1996). This finding was verified in a follow-up study, in which argyrophilic, tau-positive NFTs, and neuropil threads were consistently identified in two boxers, two patients with repeated head injury due to seizures, and one amateur football player, all of whom died at young ages (Geddes et al., 1999). Although the mechanisms for the abnormal tau-positive NFTs remain unclear, it is postulated that repeated traumatic brain injury may cause mechanical injury in axons, leading to hyperphosphorylation and the formation of abnormal tau protein aggregates. NFTs in these cases tend to be more accentuated in the perivascular regions for reasons that are poorly understood.

CTE is a form of brain neurodegeneration that is thought to result from the sort of repeated head injuries that occur in many contact sports (Gavett et al., 2011). Clinical features of CTE include the progressive decline of memory and cognition, depression, suicidal behavior, poor impulse control, aggressiveness, Parkinsonism, and dementia (Stern et al., 2011). The term chronic traumatic encephalopathy first emerged in two case reports that described neuropathologic changes in two National Football League (NFL) players who suffered from a wide range of neuropsychological disorders after long careers playing football in high school and college and professionally (Omalu et al., 2005, 2006). Gross neuropathological examinations in these two index cases showed no evidence of brain atrophy or fenestrations in the septum pellucidum. Microscopically, the consistent findings were the presence of tau-positive NFTs and neuropil threads, most prominently in frontal, parietal, and temporal neocortex. The results from these two studies were similar to those reported by Geddes and colleagues (1996, 1999), and they strongly suggest that tau-positive NFTs are indeed a consistent and early feature in repeated traumatic brain injury. This notion has been extended by a series of studies that have also identified tau-positive NFTs as a consistent diagnostic neuropathology feature in athletes in professional American football (Goldstein et al., 2012; McKee et al., 2009, 2013; Omalu et al., 2010).

There are a few limitations to this research that should be noted. Most of the studies on CTE have been case reports that lacked proper controls, rendering the results difficult to interpret. Furthermore, unlike neurodegenerative diseases such as Alzheimer's disease and frontotemporal dementia, the diagnostic criteria for CTE are based on a relatively small sample size and have not been universally accepted in the field. Clinical history and comorbid factors, such as complications from other medical conditions and exposures (e.g., substance use) may make it difficult to determine whether the features of CTE are a result of head impacts or of other factors, which complicates the development of diagnostic criteria for CTE.

An important question is whether CTE represents a single "disease entity" that can be graded based on the severity and distribution of tau pathology (McKee et al., 2013), or is part of a spectrum of disease manifestations that happen to share a common finding of tau pathology.

One emerging finding is the high prevalence of patients diagnosed with CTE who also show clinical and neuropathological features of motor neuron disease, such as amyotrophic lateral sclerosis (ALS). These results raise the possibility that the mechanical impacts in repeated head injury trigger a pathological process similar to that reported in frontotemporal lobar degeneration (FTLD), which shares similar signatures of abnormal protein aggregates involving tau and TDP-43 (Mackenzie et al., 2010; McKee et al., 2010). Recent evidence indicates that abnormal tau protein aggregates can propagate from cell to cell in experimental models of neurodegeneration (de Calignon et al., 2012; Kfoury et al., 2012; Liu et al., 2012). In addition, it is possible that cases diagnosed with CTE represent a selected group of individuals who have a higher propensity to develop a spectrum of neurodegenerative disorders that are phenotypically similar to FTLD.

There is limited evidence that APOE e4 is a risk factor for CTE. In an analysis of 10 CTE cases verified by autopsy and where APOE status was known, APOE e4 was overrepresented in those with CTE versus its prevalence in the general population (McKee et al., 2009). A few studies of athletes found an association between APOE e4 and poorer clinical outcomes such as more severe concussion symptoms (Teasdale et al., 2005; Terrell et al., 2008) and lower neurocognitive performance (Kutner et al., 2000), but they do not provide any indication of the role of APOE e4 in the development of CTE.

Other Long-Term Consequences

Several studies indicate that head injury is a risk factor for the development of Alzheimer's disease and other dementias (Bazarian et al., 2009; Fleminger et al., 2003; Guskiewicz et al., 2005; Mortimer et al., 1985, 1991; Plassman et al., 2000; Reitz et al., 2011; Schofield et al., 1997). Plassman and colleagues showed that both moderate and severe head injuries sustained during early adulthood are associated with increased risk of Alzheimer's disease, whereas the relationship between mild head injury and Alzheimer's disease was inconclusive (Plassman et al., 2000). A meta-analysis of 75 published studies found that dementia of the Alzheimer's type was associated with moderate and severe TBI but not with mTBI unless there was loss of consciousness (Bazarian et al., 2009).

Within the past year a study of retired NFL players ages 45 to 73 years (n=5) with histories of mood and cognitive symptoms was published that used positron emission tomography (PET) following intravenous injection with FDDNP[1] (FDDNP-PET) to index both tau tangle and amyloid plaque deposition in vivo (Small et al., 2013). This technique was first described by Shoghi-Jadid and colleagues (2002) who observed higher FDDNP signals in brain regions where tau tangles accumulate in Alzheimer's disease and in later research was used to differentiate Alzheimer's from mild cognitive impairment as well as to predict later cognitive decline (Small et al., 2006, 2012). In the current study, FDDNP-PET signals in subcortical and cortical regions in retired athletes were similar to controls (n=5) of comparable age, education level, body mass index, and family histories of Alzheimer's disease, but greater depressive symptoms were seen in the retired athletes as measured by the Hamilton Rating Scale for Depression. The results

---

[1]FDDNP refers to 2-(1-{6-[(2-[F-18]fluorethyl)(methyl)amino]-2-napthyl}ethylidene)malononitrile, a chemical marker injected prior to brain imaging to help identify accumulation of abnormal protein deposits.

indicated higher FDDNP signals in athletes compared with controls in regions such as the amygdala that have been shown to produce tau deposits following trauma. Unfortunately, a small sample and lack of postmortem tissue to confirm the findings limit the implications of this study. The trend for higher FDDNP signals in the two oldest athletes (64 and 73 years) is consistent with previous reports of elevated FDDNP binding in geriatric depression (Kumar et al., 2011).

Some research indicates that TBI may be associated with higher incidence of ALS. For instance, two case-control studies found an increased risk of ALS among veterans of the armed forces who had experienced head injuries during the last 15 years (Schmidt et al., 2010) and among soccer players with multiple head injuries (Chen et al., 2007). The association of ALS with both severe and repeated traumatic brain injury is supported by another case-control study from a population-based registry (Pupillo et al., 2012). However, a systematic review of studies found insufficient evidence to support an association between TBI and ALS (Bazarian et al., 2009).

The presence of abnormal TDP-43 protein aggregates in certain CTE cases suggests similar proteinopathy might increase the propensity of ALS in individuals with CTE (McKee et al., 2010), although the exact nature of the relationship between these disease entities requires further research. Similar to the case with ALS, TBI and repeat TBI are associated with an increased risk for the development of Parkinson's disease (Bazarian et al., 2009; Goldman et al., 2006), but because α-synuclein pathology is not a common feature in CTE, the mechanisms that connect Parkinson's disease and CTE will require future larger-scale studies to confirm. Equally important will be the ability to accurately determine if the underlying neuropathology leading to Parkinson's disease in CTE patients is caused by the α-synucleinopathy seen in sporadic Parkinson's disease or the tauopathy seen in individuals with FTLD with atypical Parkinsonism.

Experimental Models of the Long-Term Consequences of Repeat TBI

It is important to note that, at present, all experimental models of repeat TBI addressing long-term neurodegenerative consequences involve injuries sustained in adulthood. Models of repeat injury have been developed for use in transgenic mice to determine whether repeat TBI increases susceptibility for Alzheimer's disease. Under pentobarbital anesthesia, 8- to 10-week-old mice were placed in a stereotaxic frame, and a 6-mm silicone tip was used to deliver a CCI injury to the exposed skull (Laurer et al., 2001). Mice given either a single injury or two injuries 24 hours apart were given motor, cognitive, and histological assessments. While no significant neuroscore or cognitive deficits were seen, the repeat TBI group showed impairments in the rotorod task. The repeat TBI group also showed significantly greater blood brain–barrier breakdown and axonal injury than the single-injury group. No βAPP or tau deposits were observed in any group at 56 days post injury. The same injury paradigm was applied to transgenic mice that expressed human Aβ precursor protein (Uryu et al., 2002). While the injured groups showed no motor deficits, the repeat group showed latency deficits in the MWM and increased cortical Aβ deposits at 16 weeks post injury. Treatment of these transgenic mice with vitamin E–enriched food for 4 weeks prior to the two injuries given 24 hours apart decreased the levels of lipid peroxidation and the number of Aβ deposits and improved cognitive performances relative to standard-fed transgenic mice (Conte et al., 2004). CCI injury has also been delivered to transgenic mice expressing the human tau isoform (Yoshiyama et al., 2005). Among all the published repeat TBI models, this is the only study that delivered impacts to both hemispheres. A 9-mm silicone tip delivered four injuries to the exposed skull with two injuries per hemisphere at 20-minute intervals. This series of four injuries was repeated once a week for 4 consecutive weeks. Neurobehavioral tests conducted at 6 months post injury showed no difference between wild-type and transgenic repeat TBI groups. The study reported that one transgenic mouse showed extensive neurofibrillary tangles and had significant behavioral deficits.

The effects of TBI on the development of Aβ and tau pathology have also been recapitulated in triple-transgenic Alzheimer's disease mice harboring mutant genes for Aβ, presenilin-1, and tau (P301L) (Oddo et al., 2003). Similar to the results from other studies, CCI in the triple-transgenic Alzheimer's disease mice also results in intra-axonal Aβ accumulation and phospho-tau immunoreactivity at 24 hours and up to 7 days after injury (Tran et al., 2011). Treatment with compound E, a γ-secretase inhibitor, successfully blocks the posttraumatic Aβ accumulation but not the tau protein pathology. Results from the Aβ and tau transgenic mice studies provide some of the first evidence that repeat TBI can increase accumulation of these proteins and increase the risk of neurocognitive complications.

In addition to the implications of Aβ and tau in the pathogenesis of TBI, there is emerging evidence that reactive astrogliosis and microgliosis may contribute to neuronal injury following TBI. Indeed, microarray analyses of gene expression profiles in wild-type adult mouse brains at multiple time points following TBI show dysregulations of multiple gene ontology categories, including trophic factors, transcription factors, inflammation-related factors, and many glial markers (Kobori et al., 2002). One of the astroglial genes, S100A4—which is markedly up-regulated in, and released by, white matter astroglia—has been shown to protect neurons from apoptosis during TBI (Dmytriyeva et al., 2012; Kozlova and Lukanidin, 2002). Genetic deletion of S100A4 exacerbates neuronal loss after TBI because of increases in oxidative cell damage and down-regulation of neuroprotective protein metallothioneins. These results raise the intriguing possibility that, in addition to the potential influences from neurodegeneration-related genes, there are many critical molecular and cellular responses that can contribute to the pathogenesis of neuronal injury following TBI. Many of these factors could serve as potential therapeutic targets to mitigate both the short-term and the long-term consequences of TBI.

FINDINGS

The committee offers the following findings on the consequences of repetitive head impacts and multiple concussions:

- Studies of repetitive head impacts (sometimes called "subconcussive" impacts) have had mixed findings, with some showing an association between such impacts and functional impairments, and others not. Preliminary imaging research suggests that there are changes in brain white matter following repetitive head impacts. This finding is supported by the animal literature.
- Although studies of the effects of multiple concussions on cognitive function and symptom presentation have had mixed results, more studies report unfavorable changes than do not. The most commonly observed neurocognitive impairments have been in the areas of memory and processing speed. In some studies, symptom load (i.e., the number and severity of concussion symptoms) has been found to be increased in athletes with a history of two or more concussions.
- Athletes with a history of concussion may have more severe subsequent concussions and may take longer to recover. Preliminary evidence suggests that, in addition to the number of concussions an individual has sustained, the time interval between concussions may be an important factor in the risk for and the severity of subsequent concussions.
- Surveys of retired professional athletes provide some evidence of a positive association between the number of concussions an individual has sustained and risk for depression. There has thus far been very little research on the relationship between multiple concussions and suicidal thoughts and behaviors.
- Whether repetitive head impacts and multiple concussions sustained in youth lead to long-term neurodegenerative diseases, such as CTE and Alzheimer's disease, remains unclear. Additional research is needed to determine whether CTE represents a unique disease entity and, if so, to develop diagnostic criteria for it. There is preliminary evidence that the genetic variant APOE e4 is associated with neuropathological features of CTE in individuals with a history of head injury.

REFERENCES

Andersen, B. J., and A. Marmarou. 1992. Post-traumatic selective stimulation of glycolysis. *Brain Research* 585(1-2):184-189.

Ariza, M., R. Pueyo, M. Matarin Mdel, C. Junque, M. Mataro, I. Clemente, P. Moral, M. A. Poca, A. Garnacho, and J. Sahuquillo. 2006. Influence of APOE polymorphism on cognitive and behavioural outcome in moderate and severe traumatic brain injury. *Journal of Neurology, Neurosurgery, and Psychiatry* 77(10):1191-1193.

Barkhoudarian, G., D. A. Hovda, and C. C. Giza. 2011. The molecular pathophysiology of concussive brain injury. *Clinics in Sports Medicine* 30(1):33-48.

Bazarian, J. J., I. Cernak, L. Noble-Haeusslein, S. Potolicchio, and N. Temkin. 2009. Long-term neurologic outcomes after traumatic brain injury. *Journal of Head Trauma Rehabilitation* 24(6):439-451.

Bazarian, J. J., T. Zhu, B. Blyth, A. Borrino, and J. H. Zhong. 2012. Subject-specific changes in brain white matter on diffusion tensor imaging after sports-related concussion. *Magnetic Resonance Imaging* 30(2):171-180.

Beckwith, J. G., R. M. Greenwald, J. J. Chu, J. J. Crisco, S. Rowson, S. M. Duma, S. P. Broglio, T. W. McAllister, K. M. Guskiewicz, J. P. Mihalik, S. Anderson, B. Schnebel, P. G. Brolinson, and M. W. Collins. 2013. Timing of concussion diagnosis is related to head impact exposure prior to injury. *Medicine and Science in Sports and Exercise* 45(4):747-754.

Bergsneider, M., D. A. Hovda, E. Shalmon, D. F. Kelly, P. M. Vespa, N. A. Martin, M. E. Phelps, D. L. McArthur, M. J. Caron, J. F. Kraus, and D. P. Becker. 1997. Cerebral hyperglycolosis following severe traumatic brain injury in humans: A positron emission tomography study. *Journal of Neurosurgery* 86(2):241-251.

Bey, T., and B. Ostick. 2009. Second impact syndrome. *Western Journal of Emergency Medicine* 10(1):6-10.

Bianco, T. 2001. Social suport and recovery from sport injury: Elite skiers share their experiences. *Research Quarterly for Exercise and Sport* 72(4):376-388.

Blyth, B. J., A. Farhavar, C. Gee, B. Hawthorn, H. He, A. Nayak, V. Stocklein, and J. J. Bazarian. 2009. Validation of serum markers for blood-brain barrier disruption in traumatic brain injury. *Journal of Neurotrauma* 26(9):1497-1507.

Blyth, B. J., A. Farahvar, H. He, A. Nayak, C. Yang, G. Shaw, and J. J. Bazarian. 2011. Elevated serum ubiquitin carboxy-terminal hydrolase L1 is associated with abnormal blood-brain barrier function after traumatic brain injury. *Journal of Neurotrauma* 28(12):2453-2462.

Brainard, L. L., J. G. Beckwith, J. J. Chu, J. J. Crisco, T. W. McAllister, A. C. Duhaime, A. C. Maerlender, and R. M. Greenwald. 2012. Gender differences in head impacts sustained by collegiate ice hockey players. *Medicine and Science in Sports and Exercise* 44(2):297-304.

Breedlove, E. L., M. Robinson, T. M. Talavage, K. E. Morigaki, U. Yoruk, K. O'Keefe, J. King, L. J. Leverenz, J. W. Gilger, and E. A. Nauman. 2012. Biomechanical correlates of symptomatic and asymptomatic neurophysiological impairment in high school football. *Journal of Biomechanics* 45(7):1265-1272.

Brenner, L. A., R. V. Ignacio, and F. C. Blow. 2011. Suicide and traumatic brain injury among individuals seeking Veterans Health Administration services. *Journal of Head Trauma and Rehabilitation* 26(4):257-264.

Bridge, J. A., S. M. McBee-Strayer, E. A. Cannon, A. H. Sheftall, B. Reynolds, J. V. Campo, K. A. Pajer, R. P. Barbe, and D. A. Brent. 2012. Impaired decision making in adolescent suicide attempters. *Journal of the American Academy of Child and Adolescent Psychiatry* 51(4):394-403.

Broglio, S., and K. Guskiewicz. 2001. Soccer heading: Are there risks involved? *Athletic Therapy Today* 6(1):28-32.

Broglio, S. P., M. S. Ferrara, S. G. Piland, R. B. Anderson, and A. Collie. 2006. Concussion history is not a predictor of computerised neurocognitive performance. *British Journal of Sports Medicine* 40(9):802-805.

Broglio, S. P., J. T. Eckner, T. Surma, and J. S. Kutcher. 2011. Post-concussion cognitive declines and symptomatology are not related to concussion biomechanics in high school football players. *Journal of Neurotrauma* 28(10):2061-2068.

Bruce, J. M., and R. J. Echemendia. 2009. History of multiple self-reported concussions is not associated with reduced cognitive abilities. *Neurosurgery* 64(1):100-106.

Bryan, C. J., and T. A. Clemans. 2013. Repetitive traumatic brain injury, psychological symptoms, and suicide risk in a clinical sample of deployed military personnel. *JAMA Psychiatry* 70(7):686-691.

Bryan, C. J., T. Clemans, A. M. Hernandez, and M. D. Rudd. 2013. Loss of consciousness, depression, PTSD, and suicide risk among deployed military personnel with mild TBI. *Journal of Head Trauma and Rehabilitation* 28(1):13-20.

Caron, J. G., G. A. Bloom, K. M. Johnston, and C. M. Sabiston. 2013. Effects of multiple concussions on retired National Hockey League players. *Journal of Sport and Exercise Psychology* 35(2):168-179.

Casson, I., O. Seigel, R. Sham, E. Campbell, M. Tarlau, and A. Didomenico. 1984. Brain damage in modern boxers. *JAMA* 251(20):2663-2667.

Chappell, M. H., A. M. Ulug, L. Zhang, M. H. Heitger, B. D. Jordan, R. D. Zimmerman, and R. Watts. 2006. Distribution of microstructural damage in the brains of professional boxers: A diffusion MRI study. *Journal of Magnetic Resonance Imaging* 24(3):537-542

Chen, H., M. Richard, D. P. Sandler, D. M. Umbach, and F. Kamel. 2007. Head injury and amyotrophic lateral sclerosis. *American Journal of Epidemiology* 166(7):810-816.

Chen, J. R., Y. J. Wang, and G. F. Tseng. 2004. The effects of decompression and exogenous NGF on compressed cerebral cortex. *Journal of Neurotrauma* 21(11):1640-1651.

Chiang, M. F., J. G. Chang, and C. J. Hu. 2003. Association between apolipoprotein E genotype and outcome after brain injury. *Acta Neurochirurgica* 145(8):649-653.

Clement, D., and V. R. Shannon. 2011. Injured athletes' perceptions about social support. *Journal of Sport Rehabilitation* 20(4):457-470.

Collins, M. W., S. H. Grindel, M. R. Lovell, D. E. Dede, D. J. Moser, B. R. Phalin, S. Nogle, M. Wasik, D. Cordry, K. M. Daugherty, S. F. Sears, G. Nicolette, P. Indelicato, and D. B. McKeag. 1999. Relationship between concussion and neuropsychological performance in college football players. *JAMA* 282(10):964-970.

Collins, M. W., M. Lovell, G. Iverson, R. Cantu, J. Maroon, and M. Field. 2002. Cumulative effects of concussion in high school athletes. *Neurosurgery* 51(5):1175-1179.

Conte, V., K. Uryu, S. Fujimoto, Y. Yao, J. Rocach, L. Longhi, J. Q. Trojanowski, V. M. Lee, T. K. McIntosh, and D. Pratico. 2004. Vitamin E reduced amyloidosis and improves cognitive function in Tg2576 mice following repetitive concussive brain injury. *Journal of Neurochemistry* 90(3):758-764.

Corsellis, J. A. 1989. Boxing and the brain. *British Medical Journal* 298(6666):105-109.

Corsellis, J. A., C. J. Bruton, and D. Freeman-Browne. 1973. The aftermath of boxing. *Psychological Medicine* 3(3):270-303.

Covassin, T., D. Stearne, and R. Elbin. 2008. Concussion history and postconcussion neurocognitive performance and symptoms in collegiate athletes. *Journal of Athletic Training* 43(2):119-124.

Covassin, T., R. Elbin, A. Kontos, and E. Larson. 2010. Investigating baseline neurocognitive performance between male and female athletes with a history of multiple concussion. *Journal of Neurology, Neurosurgery, and Psychiatry* 81(6):597-601.

Creeley, C. E., D. F. Wozniak, P. V. Bayly, J. W. Olney, and L. M. Lewis. 2004. Multiple episodes of mild traumatic brain injury result in impaired cognitive performance in mice. *Academic Emergency Medicine* 11(8):809-819.

Crisco, J. J., R. Fiore, J. G. Beckwith, J. J. Chu, P. G. Brolinson, S. Duma, T. W. McAllister, A. C. Duhaime, and R.M. Greenwald. 2010. Frequency and location of head impact exposures in individual collegiate football players. *Journal of Athletic Training* 45(6):549-559.

Crisco, J. J., B. J. Wilcox, J. G. Beckwith, J. J. Chu, A. C. Duhaime, S. Rowson, S. M. Duma, A. C. Maerlender, T. W. McAllister, and R. M. Greenwald. 2011. Head impact exposure in collegiate football players. *Journal of Biomechanics* 44(15):2673-2678.

Crisco, J. J., B. J. Wilcox, J. T. Machan, T. W. McAllister, A. C. Duhaime, S. M. Duma, S. Rowson, J. G. Beckwith, J. J. Chu, and R. M. Greenwald. 2012. Magnitude of head impact exposures in individual collegiate football players. *Journal of Applied Biomechanics* 28(2):174-183

De Beaumont, L., B. Brisson, M. Lassonde, and P. Jolicoeur. 2007. Long-term electrophysiological changes in athletes with a history of multiple concussions. *Brain Injury* 21(6): 189-201.

De Beaumont, L., H. Theoret, D. Mongeon, J. Messier, S. Leclerc, S. Tremblay, D. Ellemberg, and M. Lassonde. 2009. Brain function decline in healthy retired athletes who sustained their last sports concussion in early adulthood. *Brain* 132(Part 3):695-708.

de Calignon, A., M. Polydoro, M. Suarez-Calvet, C. William, D. H. Adamowicz, K. J. Kopeikina, R. Pitstick, N. Sahara, K. H. Ashe, G. A. Carlson, T. L. Spires-Jones, and B. T. Hyman. 2012. Propagation of tau pathology in a model of early Alzheimer's disease. *Neuron* 73(4):685-697.

DeFord, S. M., M. S. Wilson, A. C. Rice, T. Clausen, L. K. Rice, A. Barabnova, R. Bullock, and R. J. Hamm. 2002. Repeated mild brain injuries result in cognitive impairment in B6C3F1 mice. *Journal of Neurotrauma* 19(4):427-438.

Didehbani, N., C. Munro Cullum, S. Mansinghani, H. Conover, and J. Hart. 2013. Depressive symptoms and concussions in aging retired NFL players. *Archives of Clinical Neuropsychology* 28(5):418-424.

Dmytriyeva, O., S. Pankratova, S. Owczarek, K. Sonn, V. Soroka, C. M. Ridley, A. Marsolais, M. Lopez-Hovos, N. Ambartsumian, E. Lukanidin, E. Bock, V. Berezin, and D. Kirvushko. 2012. The metastasis-promoting S100A4 protein confers neuroprotection in brain injury. *Nature Communications* 3:1197.

Drew, R., D. Tempier, B. Schuyler, T. Newell, and W. Cannon. 1986. Neuropsychological deficits in active licensed professional boxers. *Journal of Clinical Psychology* 42(3):520-525.

Duma, S. M., S. J. Manoogian, W. R. Bussone, P. G. Brolinson, M. W. Goforth, J. J. Donnenwerth, R. M. Greenwald, J. J. Chu, and J. J. Crisco. 2005. Analysis of real-time head accelerations in collegiate football players. *Clinical Journal of Sport Medicine* 15(1):3-8.

Elbin, R. J., T. Covassin, J. Hakun, A. P. Kontos, K. Berger, K. Pfeiffer, and S. Ravizza. 2012. Do brain activation changes persist in athletes with a history of multiple concussions who are asymptomatic? *Brain Injury* 26(10):1217-1225.

Felde, A. B., J. Westermeyer, and P. Thuras. 2006. Co-morbid traumatic brain injury and substance abuse disorders: Childhood predictors and adult correlates. *Brain Injury* 20(1):41-49.

Fleminger, S., D. Oliver, S. Lovestone, S. Rabe-Hesketh, and A. Giora. 2003. Head injury as a risk factor for Alzheimer's disease: The evidence 10 years on; a partial replication. *Journal of Neurology, Neurosurgery, and Psychiatry* 74(7):857-862.

Friedman, G., P. Froom, L. Sazbon, I. Grinblatt, M. Shochina, J. Tsenter, S. Babaey, B. Yehuda, and Z. Groswasser. 1999. Apolipoprotein E-epsilon4 genotype predicts a poor outcome in survivors of traumatic brain injury. *Neurology* 52(2):244-248.

230

Friess, S. H., R. N. Ichord, J. Ralston, K. Ryall, M. A. Helfaer, C. Smith, and S. S. Margulies. 2009. Repeated traumatic brain injury affects composite cognitive function in piglets. *Journal of Neurotrauma* 26(7):1111-1121.

Gan, C., K. A. Campbell, M. Gemeinhardt, and G. T. McFadden. 2006. Predictors of family system functioning after brain injury. *Brain Injury* 20(6):587-600.

Gavett, B. E., R. A. Stern, and A. C. McKee. 2011. Chronic traumatic encephalopathy: A potential late effect of sport-related concussive and subconcussive head trauma. *Clinics in Sports Medicine* 30(1):179-188.

Geddes, J. F., G. H. Vowles, S. F. Robinson, and J. C. Sutcliffe. 1996. Neurofibrillary tangles, but not Alzheimer-type pathology, in a young boxer. *Neuropathology and Applied Neurobiology* 22(1):12-16.

Geddes, J. F., G. H. Vowles, J. A. Nicoll, and T. Revesz. 1999. Neuronal cytoskeletal changes are an early consequence of repetitive head injury. *Acta Neuropathologica* 98(2):171-178.

Goldman, S. M., C. M. Tanner, D. Oakes, G. S. Bhudhikanok, A. Gupta, and J. W. Langston. 2006. Head injury and Parkinson's disease risk in twins. *Annals of Neurology* 60(1):65-72.

Goldstein, L. E., A. M. Fisher, C. A. Tagge, X. L. Zhang, L. Velisek, J. A. Sullivan, C. Upreti, J. M. Kracht, M. Ericsson, M. W. Wojnarowicz, C. J. Goletiani, G. M. Maglakelidze, N. Casey, J. A. Moncaster, O. Minaeva, R. D. Moir, C. J. Nowinski, R. A. Stern, R. C. Cantu, J. Geiling, J. K. Blusztajn, B. L. Wolozin, T. Ikezu, T. D. Stein, A. E. Budson, N. W. Kowall, D. Chargin, A. Sharon, S. Saman, G. F. Hall, W. C. Moss, R. O. Cleveland, R. E. Tanzi, P. K. Stanton, and A. C. McKee. 2012. Chronic traumatic encephalopathy in blast-exposed military veterans and a blast neurotrauma mouse model. *Science Translational Medicine* 4(134):134-160.

Goldstein, T. R., J. A. Bridge, and D. A. Brent. 2008. Sleep disturbance preceding completed suicide in adolescents. *Journal of Consulting and Clinical Psychology* 76(1):84-91.

Gross, H., A. Kling, G. Henry, C. Herndon, and H. Lavretsky. 1996. Local cerebral glucose metabolism in patients with long-term behavioral and cognitive deficits following mild traumatic brain injury. *Journal of Neuropsychiatry and Clinical Neurosciences* 8(3):324-334.

Guskiewicz, K. M., S. W. Marshall, S. P. Broglio, R. C. Cantu, and D. T. Kirkendall. 2002. No evidence of impaired neurocognitive performance in collegiate soccer players. *American Journal of Sports Medicine* 30(2):157-162.

Guskiewicz, K. M., M. McCrea, S. W. Marshall, R. C. Cantu, C. Randolph, W. Barr, J. A. Onate, and J. P. Kelly. 2003. Cumulative effects associated with recurrent concussion in collegiate football players: The NCAA Concussion Study. *JAMA* 290(19):2549-2555.

Guskiewicz, K. M., S. W. Marshall, J. Bailes, M. McCrea, R. C. Cantu, C. Randolph, and B. D. Jordan. 2005. Association between recurrent concussion and late-life cognitive impairment in retired professional football players. *Neurosurgery* 57(4):719-726.

Guskiewicz, K. M., S. W. Marshall, J. Bailes, M. McCrea, H. P. Harding, A. Matthews, J. R. Mihalik, and R. C. Cantu. 2007. Recurrent concussion and risk of depression in retired professional football players. *Medicine and Science in Sports and Exercise* 39(6):903-909.

Gysland, S. M., J. P. Mihalik, J. K. Register-Mihalik, S. C. Trulock, E. W. Shields, and K. M. Guskiewicz. 2012. The relationship between subconcussive impacts and concussion history on clinical measures of neurologic function in collegiate football players. *Annals of Biomedical Engineering* 40(1):14-22.

Haglund, Y., and E. Eriksson. 1993. Does amatuer boxing lead to chronic brain damage? A review of recent investigations. *American Journal of Sports Medicine* 21(1):97-107.

Hart, J., M. A. Kraut, K. B. Womack, J. Strain, N. Didehbani, E. Bartz, H. Conover, S. Mansinghani, H. Lu, and C. M. Cullum. 2013. Neuroimaging of cognitive dysfunction and depression in aging retired National Football League players: A cross-sectional study. *JAMA* 70(3):326-335.

Hartman, R. E., H. Laurer, L. Longhi, K. R. Bales, S. M. Paul, T. K. McIntosh, and D. M. Holtzman. 2002. Apolipoprotein E4 influences amyloid deposition but not cell loss after traumatic brain injury in a mouse model of Alzheimer's disease. *Journal of Neuroscience* 22(23):10083-10087.

Hattori, N., S. C. Huang, H. M. Wu, E. Yeh, T. C. Glenn, P. M. Vespa, D. McArthur, M. E. Phelps, D. A. Hovda, and M. Bergsneider. 2003. Correlation of regional metabolic rates of glucose with Glasgow coma scale after traumatic brain injury. *Journal of Nuclear Medicine* 44(11):1709-1716.

Hovda, D. A., K. Fu, H. Badie, A. Samii, P. Pinanong, and D. P. Becker. 1994. Administration of an omega-conopeptide one hour following traumatic brain injury reduces 45calcium accumulation. *Acta Neurochirurgica* 60(Suppl):521-523.

Huh, J. W., A. G. Widing, and R. Raghupathi. 2007. Basic science; repetitive mild non-contusive brain trauma in immature rats exacerbates traumatic axonal injury and axonal calpain activation: A preliminary report. *Journal of Neurotrauma* 24(1):15-27.

Humayun, M. S., S. K. Presty, N. D. Lafrance, H. H. Holcomb, H. Loats, D. M. Long, H. N. Wagner, and B. Gordon. 1989. Local cerebral glucose abnormalities in mild closed head injured patients with cognitive impairments. *Nuclear Medicine Communications* 10(5):335-344.

Iverson, G. L., B. L. Brooks, M. R. Lovell, and M. W. Collins. 2006. No cumulative effects for one or two previous concussions. *British Journal of Sports Medicine* 40(1):72-75.

Iverson, G. L., R. J. Echemendia, A. K. Lamarre, B. L. Brooks, and M. B. Gaetz. 2012. Possible lingering effects of multiple past concussions. *Rehabilitation Research and Practice* 316575. doi: 10.1155/2012/316575. Epub February 26.

Jollant, F., F. Bellivier, M. Leboyer, B. Astruc, S. Torres, R. Verdier, D. Castelnau, A. Malafosse, and P. Courtet. 2005. Impaired decision making in suicide attempters. *American Journal of Psychiatry* 162(2):304-310.

Jordan, B. D. 1987. Neurologic aspects of boxing. *Archives of Neurology* 44(4):453-459.

Jordan, B. D., N. R. Relkin, L. D. Ravdin, A. R. Jacobs, A. Bennett, and S. Gandy. 1997. Apolipoprotein E epsilon4 associated with chronic traumatic brain injury in boxing. *JAMA* 278(2):136-140.

Kaminski, T. W., A. M. Wikstrom, G. M. Gutierrez, and J. J. Glutting. 2007. Purposeful heading during a season does not influence cognitive function or balance in female soccer players. *Journal of Clinical and Experimental Neuropsychology* 29(7):742-751.

Kaminski, T. W., E. S. Cousino, and J. J. Glutting. 2008. Examining the relationship between purposeful heading in soccer and computerized neuropsychological test performance. *Research Quarterly for Exercise and Sport* 79(2):235-244.

Kaste, M., T. Kuurne, J. Vilkki, K. Katevuo, K. Sainio, and M. Meurala. 1982. Is chronic brain damage in boxing a hazard of the past? *Lancet* 2(8309):1186-1188.

Kawamata, T., Y. Katayama, D. A. Hovda, A. Yoshino, D. P. Becker. 1992. Administration of excitatory amino acid antagonists via microdyalisis attenuates the increase in glucose utilization seen following concussive brain injury. *Journal of Cerebral Blood Flow and Metabolism* 12(1):12-24.

Keilp, J. G., H. A. Sackeim, B. S. Brodsky, M. A. Oquendo, K. M. Malone, and J. J. Mann. 2001. Neuropsychological dysfunction in depressed suicide attempters. *American Journal of Psychiatry* 158(5):735-741.

Keilp, J. G., M. Gorlyn, M. Russell, M. A. Oquendo, A. K. Burke, J. Harkavy-Friedman, and J. J. Mann. 2013. Neuropsychological function and suicidal behavior: attention control, memory, executive dysfunction in suicide attempt. *Psychological Medicine* 43(3):539-551.

Kerr, Z. Y., S. W. Marshall, and K. M. Guskiewicz. 2012. Reliability of concussion history in former professional football players. *Medicine and Science in Sports Exercise* 44(3):377-382.

Kfoury, N., B. B. Holmes, H. Jiang, D. M. Holtzman, and M. I. Diamond. 2012. Trans-cellular propagation of Tau aggregation by fibrillar species. *Journal of Biological Chemistry* 287(23):19940-19951.

Killam, C., R. L. Cautin, and A. C. Santucci. 2005. Assessing the enduring residual neuropsychological effects of head trauma in college athletes who participate in contact sports. *Archives of Clinical Neuropsychology* 20(5):599-611.

Kirkendall, D. T., and W. Garrett. 2001. Heading in soccer: Integral skill or grounds for cognitive dysfunction. *Journal of Athletic Training* 36(3):328-333.

Kobori, N., G. L. Clifton, and P. Dash. 2002. Altered expression of novel genes in the cerebral cortex following experimental brain injury. *Molecular Brain Research* 104(2):148-158.

Koerte, I. K., B. Ertl-Wagner, M. Reiser, R. Zafonte, and M. E. Shenton. 2012. White matter integrity in the brains of professional soccer players without a symptomatic concussion. *JAMA* 308(18):1859-1861.

Kontos, A. P., A. Dolese, R. J. Elbin, T. Covassin, and B. L. Warren. 2011. Relationship of soccer heading to computerized neurocognitive performance and symptoms among female and male youth soccer players. *Brian Injury* 25(12):1234-1241.

Kozlova, E. N., and E. Lukanidin. 2002. Mts1 protein expression in the central nervous system after injury. *Glia* 37(4):337-348.

Kuehl, M. D., A. R. Snyder, S. E. Erickson, and T. C. McLeod. 2010. Imact of prior concussions on health-related quality of life in collegiate athletes. *Clinical Journal of Sports Medicine* 20(2):86-91.

Kumar, A., V. Kepe, J. R. Barrio, P. Siddarth, V. Manoukian, V. Elderkin-Thompson, and G. W. Small. 2011. Protein binding in patients with late-life depression. *Archives of General Psychiatry* 68(11):1143-1150.

Kutner, K. C., D. M. Erlanger, J. Tsai, B. Jordan, and N. R. Relkin. 2000. Lower cognitive performance of older football players possessing apolipoprotein E episilon4. *Neurosurgery* 47(3):651-657.

Laurer, H., F. M. Bareyre, V. M. Lee, J. Q. Trojanowski, L. Longhi, R. Hoover, K. E. Saatman, R. Raghupathi, S. Hoshino, M. S. Grady, and T. K. McIntosh. 2001. Mild head injury increases the brain's vulnerability to a second traumatic impact. *Journal of Neurosurgery* 95(5):859-870.

Liu, L., V. Drouet, J. W. Wu, M. P. Witter, S. A. Small, C. Clelland, and K. Duff. 2012. Trans-synaptic spread of tau pathology in vivo. *PLoS One* 7(2):e31302.

Longhi, L., K. E. Saatman, S. Fujimoto, R. Raghupathi, D. F. Meaney, J. Davis, B. S. A. McMillan, V. Conte, H. L. Laurer, S. Stein, N. Stocchetti, and T. K. McIntosh. 2005. Temporal window of vulnerability to repetitive experimental concussive brain injury. *Neurosurgery* 56(2):364-374.

Mackenzie, I. R., M. Neumann, E. H. Bigio, N. J. Cairns, I. Alafuzoff, J. Kril, G. G. Kovacs, B. Ghetti, G. Halliday, I. E. Holm, P. G. Ince, W. Kamphorst, R. Revesz, A. J. Rozemuller, S. Kumar-Singh, H. Akiyama, A. Baborie, S. Spina, D. W. Dickson, J. Q. Trojanowski, and D. M. Mann. 2010. Nomenclature and nosology for neuropathologic subtypes of frontotemporal lobar degeneration: An update. *Acta Neuropathologica* 119(1):1-4.

Mainio, A., K. Viilo, H. Hakko, T. Sarkioja, and P. Rasanen. 2007. Traumatic brain injury, psychiatric disorders and suicide: A population-based study of suicide victims during the years 1988-2004 in Northern Finland. *Brain Injury* 21(8):851-855.

Marchi, N., M. Cavaglia, V. Fazio, S. Bhudia, K. Hallene, and D. Janigro. 2004. Peripheral markers of blood-brain barrier damage. *Clinica Chimica Acta* 342(1-2):1-12.

Marchi, N., J. J. Bazarian, V. Puvenna, M. Janigro, C. Ghosh, J. Zhong, T. Zhu, E. Blackman, D. Stewart, J. Ellis, R. Butler, and D. Janigro. 2013. Consequences of repeated blood-brain barrier disruption in football players. *PLoS One* 8(3):e56805.

Matser, E. J. T., A. Kessels, M. Lezak, B. D. Jordan, and J. Troost. 1999. Neuropsychological impairment in amateur soccer players. *JAMA* 282(10):971-973.

Matser, J. T., A. G. H. Kessels, B. D. Jordan, M. D. Lezak, and J. Troost. 1998. Chronic traumatic brain injuries in professional soccer players. *Neurology* 51(3):791-795.

Matser, J. T., A. G. Kessels, M. D. Lezak, and J. Troost. 2001. A dose-response relation of headers and concussions with cognitivie impairment in professional soccer players. *Journal of Clinical and Experimental Neuropsychology* 23(6):770-774.

McAllister, T. W., L. A. Flashman, A. Maerlender, R. M. Greenwald, J. G. Beckwith, T. D. Tosteson, J. J. Crisco, P. G. Brolinson, S. M. Duma, A. C. Duhaime, M. R. Grove, and J. H. Turco. 2012. Cognitive effects of one season of head impacts in a cohort of collegiate contact sport athletes. *Neurology* 78(22):1777-1784.

McCrory, P., W. H. Meeuwisse, M. Aubry, B. Cantu, J. Dvořák, R.J. Echemendia, L. Engebretsen, K. Johnston, J. S. Kutcher, M. Raftery, A. Sills, B. W. Benson, G. A. Davis, R. G. Ellenbogen, K. Guskiewicz, S. A. Herring, G. L. Iverson, B. D. Jordan, J. Kissick, M. McCrea, A .S. McIntosh, D. Maddocks, M. Makdissi, L. Purcell, M. Putukian, K. Schneider, C. H. Tator, and M. Turner. 2013. Consensus statement on concussion in sport: The 4th International Conference on Concussion in Sport held in Zurich, November 2012. *British Journal of Sports Medicine* 47(5):250-258.

McKee, A. C., R. C. Cantu, C. J. Nowinski, E. T. Hedley-Whyte, B. E. Gavett, A. E. Budson, V. E. Santini, H. S. Lee, C. A. Kubilus, and R. A. Stern. 2009. Chronic traumatic encephalopathy in athletes: Progressive tauopathy after repetitive head injury. *Journal of Neuropathology and Experimental Neurology* 68(7):709-735.

McKee, A. C., B. E. Gavett, R. A. Stern, C. J. Nowinski, R. C. Cantu, N. W. Kowall, D. P. Perl, E. T. Hedley-Whyte, B. Price, C. Sullivan, P. Morin, H. S. Lee, C. A. Kubilus, D. H. Daneshvar, M. Wulff, and A. E. Budson. 2010. TDP-43 proteinopathy and motor neuron disease in chronic traumatic encephalopathy. *Journal of Neuropathology and Experimental Neurology* 69(9):918-929.

McKee, A. C., T. D. Stein, C. J. Nowinski, R. A. Stern, D. H. Daneshvar, V. E. Alvarez, H. S. Lee, G. Hall, S. M. Wojtowicz, C. M. Baugh, D. O. Riley, C. A. Kubilus, K. A. Cormier, M. A. Jacobs, B. R. Martin, C. R. Abraham, T. Ikezu, R. R. Reichard, B. L. Wolozin, A. E. Budson, L. E. Goldstein, N. W. Kowall, and R. C. Cantu. 2013. The spectrum of disease in chronic traumatic encephalopathy. *Brain* 136(Part 1):43-64.

Mihovilovic, M. 1968. The status of former sportsmen. *International Review of Sport Sociology* 3:73-96.

Miller, J. R., G. J. Adamson, M. M. Pink, and J. C. Sweet. 2007. Comparison of preseason, midseason, and postseason neurocognitive scores in uninjured collegiate football players. *American Journal of Sports Medicine* 35(8):1284-1288.

Moore, A. H., C. L. Osteen, A. F. Chatzijoannou, D. A. Hovda, and S. R. Cherry. 2000. Quantitative assessment of longitudinal metabolic changes in vivo after traumatic brain injury in the adult rat using FDG-microPET. *Journal of Cerebral Blood Flow and Metabolism* 20(10):1492-1501.

Morrison, R. G. 1986. Medical and public health aspects of boxing. *JAMA* 255(18):2475-2480.

Mortimer, J. A., L. R. French, J. T. Hutton, and L. M. Schuman. 1985. Head injury as a risk factor for Alzheimer's disease. *Neurology* 35(2):264-267.

Mortimer, J. A., C. M. van Duijn, V. Chandra, L. Fratiglioni, A. B. Graves, A. Heyman, A. F. Jorm, E. Kokmen, K. Kondo, and W. A. Rocca. 1991. Head trauma as a risk factor for Alzheimer's disease: A collaborative re-analysis of case-control studies. EURODEM Risk Factor Research Group. *International Journal of Epidemiology* 20(Suppl 2):S28-S35.

Moser, R. S. and P. Schatz. 2002. Enduring effects of concussion in youth athletes. *Archives of Clinical Neuropsychology* 17(1):91-100.

Moser, R. S., P. Schatz, and B. D. Jordan. 2005. Prolonged effects of concussion in high school athletes. *Neurosurgery* 57(2):300-306.

Neuwelt, E. A., B. Bauer, C. Fahlke, G. Fricker, C. Iadecola, D. Janigro, L. Laybaert, Z. Molnár, M. E. O'Donnell, J. T. Povlishock, N. R. Saunders, F. Sharp, D. Stanimirovic, R. J. Watts, and L. R. Drewes. 2011. Engaging neuroscience to advance translational research in brain barrier biology. *Nature Reviews: Neuroscience* 12(3):169-182.

Nicoll, J. A., G. W. Roberts, and D. I. Graham. 1995. Apolipoprotein E epsilon 4 allele is associated with deposition of amyloid beta-protein following head injury. *Nature Medicine* 1(2):135-137.

O'Connell, M. T., A. Seal, J. Nortje, P. G. Al-Rawi, J. P. Coles, T. D. Fryer, D. K. Menon, J. D. Pickard, and P. J. Hutchinson. 2005. Glucose metabolism in traumatic brain injury: A combined microdialysis and [18F]-2-fluoro-2-deoxy-d-glucose-positron emission tomography (FDG-PET) study. *Acta Neurochirurgica Supplement* 95:165-168.

Oddo, S., A. Caccamo, M. Kitazawa, B. P. Tseng, and F. M. LaFerla. 2003. Amyloid deposition precedes tangle formation in a triple transgenic model of Alzheimer's disease. *Neurobiology of Aging* 24(8):1063-1070.

Omalu, B. I., S. T. DeKosky, R. L. Minster, M. I. Kamboh, R. L. Hamilton, and C. H. Wecht. 2005. Chronic traumatic encephalopathy in a National Football League player. *Neurosurgery* 57(1):128-134.

Omalu, B. I., S. T. DeKosky, R. L. Hamilton, R. L. Minster, M. I. Kamboh, A. M. Shakir, and C. H. Wecht. 2006. Chronic traumatic encephalopathy in a National Football League player: Part II. *Neurosurgery* 59(5):1086-1092.

Omalu, B. I., R. L. Hamilton, M. I. Kamboh, S. T. DeKosky, and J. Bailes. 2010. Chronic traumatic encephalopathy (CTE) in a National Football League player: Case report and emerging medicolegal practice questions. *Journal of Forensic Nursing* 6(1):40-46.

Oquendo, M. A., J. H. Friedman, M. F. Grunebaum, A. Burke, J. M. Silver, and J. J. Mann. 2004. Suicidal behavior and mild traumatic brain injury in major depression. *Journal of Nervous and Mental Disease* 192(6):430-434.

Orrison, W. W., E. H. Hanson, T. Alamo, D. Watson, M. Sharma, T. G. Perkins, and R. D. Tandy. 2009. Traumatic brain injury: A review and high-field MRI findings in 100 unarmed combatants using a literature-based checklist approach. *Journal of Neurotrauma* 26(5):689-701.

Plassman, B. L., R. J. Havlik, D. C. Steffens, M. J. Helms, T. N. Newman, D. Drosdick, C. Phillips, B. A. Gau, K. A. Welsh–Bohmer, J. R. Burke, J. M. Guralnik, and J. C. Breitner. 2000. Documented head injury in early adulthood and risk of Alzheimer's disease and other dementias. *Neurology* 55(8):1158-1166.

Prins, M. L., and D. A. Hovda. 2001. Mapping cerebral glucose metabolism during spatial learning: Interactions of development and traumatic brain injury. *Journal of Neurotrauma* 18(1):31-46.

Prins, M. L., and D. A. Hovda. 2009. The effects of age and ketogenic diet on local cerebral metabolic rates of glucose after controlled cortical impact injury in rats. *Journal of Neurotrauma* 26(7):1083-1093.

Prins, M. L., A. Hales, M. Reger, C. C. Giza, and D. A. Hovda. 2010. Repeat traumatic brain injury in the juvenile rate is associated with increased axonal injury and cognitive impairments. *Developmental Neuroscience* 32(5-6):510-518.

Prins, M. L., D. Alexander, C. C. Giza, and D. A. Hovda. 2013. Repeated mild traumatic brain injury: Mechanisms of cerebral vulnerability. *Journal of Neurotrauma* 30(1):30-38.

Pupillo, E., P. Messina, G. Logroscino, S. Zoccolella, A. Chio, A. Calvo, M. Corbo, C. Lunetta, A. Micheli, A. Millul, E. Vitelli, and E. Beghi. 2012. Trauma and amyotrophic lateral sclerosis: A case-control study from a population-based registry. *European Journal of Neurology* 19(12):1509-1517.

Purcell, L. K., and C. M. Leblanc. 2012. Boxing participation by children and adolescents: A joint statement with the American Academy of Pediatrics. *Pediatrics and Child Health* 17(1):39-40.

Putukian, M., R. J. Echemendia, and S. Mackin. 2000. The acute neuropsychological effects of heading in soccer: A pilot study. *Clinical Journal of Sport Medicine* 10(2):104-109.

Queen, S. A., M. J. Chen, and D. M. Feeney. 1997. D-Amphetamine attenuates decreased cerebral glucose utilization after unilateral sensorimotor cortex contusion in rats. *Brain Research* 777(1-2):42-50.

Raghupathi, R., and S. S. Margulies. 2002. Traumatic axonal injury after closed head injury in the neonatal pig. *Journal of Neurotrauma* 19(7):843-853.

Raghupathi, R., M. F. Mehr, M. A. Helfaer, and S. S. Margulies. 2004. Traumatic axonal injury is exacerbated following repetititve closed head injury in the neonatal pig. *Journal of Neurotrauma* 21(3):307-316.

Reeves, T. M., L. L. Phillips, and J. T. Povlishock. 2005. Myelinated and unmyelinated axons of the corpus callosum differ in vulnerability and functional recovery following traumatic brain injury. *Experimental Neurology* 196(1):126-137.

Reider, B. 2012. Melancholy thoughts. *American Journal of Sports Medicine* 40(10):2197-2199.

Reitz, C., C. Brayne, and R. Mayeux. 2011. Epidemiology of Alzheimer disease. *Nature Reviews: Neurology* 7(3):137-152.

Richards, H. K., S. Simac, S. Piechnik, and J. D. Pickard. 2001. Uncoupling of cerebral blood flow and metabolism after cerebral contusion in the rat. *Journal of Cerebral Blood Flow and Metabolism* 21(7):779-781.

Roberts, G. W., D. Allsop, and C. Bruton. 1990. The occult aftermath of boxing. *Journal of Neurology, Neurosurgery, and Psychiatry* 53(5):373-378.

Ross, R. J., M. Cole, J. S. Thompson, and K. H. Kim.1983. Boxers: Computed tomography, EEG and neurologic evaluation. *JAMA* 249(2):211-213.

Safai, P. 2003. Healing the body in the "culture of risk": Examining the negotiation of treatment between sport medicine clinicians and injured athletes in Canadian intercollegiate sport. *Sociology of Sport Journal* 20(2):127-146.

Saing, T., M. Dick, P. T. Nelson, R. C. Kim, D. H. Cribbs, and E. Head. 2012. Frontal cortex neuropathology in dementia pugilistica. *Journal of Neurotrauma* 29(6):1054-1070.

Schatz, P., R. S. Moser, T. Covassin, and R. Karpf. 2011. Early indicators of enduring symptoms in high school athletes with multiple previous concussions. *Neurosurgery* 68(6):1562-1567.

Schmidt, S., L. C. Kwee, K. D. Allen, and E. Z. Oddone. 2010. Association of ALS with head injury, cigarette smoking and APOE genotypes. *Journal of Neurological Science* 291(1-2):22-29.

Schofield, P. W., M. Tang, K. Marder, K. Bell, G. Dooneief, M. Chun, M. Sano, Y. Stern, and R. Mayeux. 1997. Alzheimer's disease after remote head injury: An incidence study. *Journal of Neurology, Neurosurgery, and Psychiatry* 62(2):119-124.

Shitaka, Y., H. T. Tran, R. E. Bennett, L. Sanchez, M. A. Levy, K. Dikranian, and D. L. Brody. 2011. Repetitive closed-skull traumatic brain injury in mice causes persistent multifocal axonal injury and microglial reactivity. *Journal of Neuropathology and Experimental Neurology* 70(7):551-567.

Shoghi-Jadid, K., G. W. Small, E. D. Agdeppa, V. Kepe, L. M. Ercoli, P. Siddarth, S. Read, N. Satyamurthy, A. Petric, S. C. Huang, and J. R. Barrio. 2002. Localization of neurofibrillary tangles and beta-amyloid plaques in the brains of living patients with Alzheimer disease. *American Journal of Geriatric Psychiatry* 10(1):24-35.

Shrey, D. W., G. S. Griesbach, and C. C. Giza. 2011. The pathophysiology of concussions in youth. *Physical Medicine and Rehabilitation Clinics of North America* 22(4):577-602.

Simma, B., J. Lutschg, and J. M. Callahan. 2013. Mild head injury in pediatrics: Algorithms for management in the ED and in young athletes. *American Journal of Emergency Medicine* 31(7):1133-1138.

Simpson, G. K., and R. Tate. 2007. Review: Suicidality in people surviving a TBI: Prevalence, risk factors, and implications for clinical management. *Brain Injury* 21(13-14):1335-1351

Simpson, G. K., R. L. Tate, D. L. Whiting, and R. E. Cotter. 2011. Suicide prevention after traumatic brain injury: A randomized controlled trial of a program for the psychological treatment of hopelessness. *Journal of Head Trauma Rehabilitation* 26(4):290-300.

Slobounov, S., E. Slobounov, W. Sebastianelli, C. Cao, and K. Newell. 2007. Differential rate of recovery in athletes after first and second concussion episodes. *Neurosurgery* 61(2):338-344.

Small, G. W., V. Kepe, and J. R. Barrio. 2006. Seeing is believing: Neuroimaging adds to our understanding of cerebral pathology. *Current Opinion in Psychiatry* 29(6)564-569.

Small, G. W., P. Siddarth, V. Kepe, L. M. Ercoli, A. C. Burggren, S. Y. Bookheimer, K. J. Miller, J. Kim, H. Lavretsky, S. C. Huang, and J. R. Barrio. 2012. Prediction of cognitive decline by positron emission tomography of brain amyloid and tau. *Archives of Neurology* 69(2):215-222.

Small, G. W., V. Kepe, P. Siddarth, L. M. Ercoli, D. A. Merrill, N. Donoghue, S. Y. Bookheimer, J. Martinez, B. Omalu, J. Bailes, and J. R. Barrio. 2013. PET scanning of brain tau in retired National Football League players: Preliminary findings. *American Journal of Geriatric Psychiatry* 21(2):138-144.

Smodlaka, V. N. 1984. Medical aspects of heading the ball in soccer. *Physician and Sportsmedicine* 12(2):127-131.

Sortland, O., and A. T. Tysvaer. 1989. Brain damage in former association football players: An evaluation by cerebral computed tomography. *Neuroradiology* 31(1):44-48.

Stephens, R., A. Rutherford, D. Potter, and G. Fernie. 2010. Neuropsychological consequence of soccer play in adolescent U.K. school team soccer players. *Journal of Neuropsychiatry and Clinical Neurosciences* 22(3):295-303.

Stern, R. A., D. O. Riley, D. H. Daneshvar, C. J. Nowinski, R. C. Cantu, and A. C. McKee. 2011. Long-term consequences of repetitive brain trauma: Chronic traumatic encephalopathy. *Physical Medicine and Rehabilitation* 3(10 Suppl 2):S460-S467.

Strain, J., N. Didehbani, C. M. Cullum, S. Mansinghani, H. Conover, M. A. Kraut, J. Hart, and K. B. Womack. 2013. Depressive symptoms and white matter dysfunction in retired NFL players with concussion history. *Neurology* 81(1):25-32.

Straume-Naesheim, T. M., T. Andersen, J. Dvořák, and R. Bahr. 2005. Effects of heading exposure and previous concussions on neuropsychological performance among Norwegian elite footballers. *British Journal of Sports Medicine* 39(Suppl 1):i70-i77.

Sutton, R. L., D. A. Hovda, P. D. Adelson, E. C. Benzel, and D. P. Becker. 1994. Metabolic changes following cortical contusion: Relationships to edema and morphological changes. *Acta Neruchirugica Supplement (Wien)* 60:446-448.

Talvage, T. M., E. Nauman, E. L. Breedlove, U. Yoruk, A. E. Dye, K. Morigaki, H. Feuer, and L. J. Leverenz. 2010. Functionally-detected cognitive impairment in high school football players without clinically-diagnosed concussion. *Journal of Neurotrauma* [epub ahead of print].

Tavazzi, B., R. Vagnozzi, S. Signoretti, A. M. Amorini, M. Cimatti, R. Delfini, V. DiPietro, A. Finocchiaro, and G. Lazzarino. 2007. Temporal window of metabolic brain vulnerability to concussions: Oxidative and nitrosative stresses—Part II. *Neurosurgery* 61(2):390-395.

Teasdale, G. M., G. D. Murray, and J. A. Nicoll. 2005. The association between APOE epsilon4, age and outcome after head injury: A prospective cohort study. *Brain* 128(Pt 11):2556-2561.

Terrell, T. R., R. M. Bostick, R. Abramson, D. Xie, W. Barfield, R. Cantu, M. Stanek, and T. Ewing. 2008. APOE, APOE promoter, and tau genotypes and risk for concussion in college athletes. *Clinical Journal of Sport Medicine* 18(1):10-17.

Thomas, S., M. L. Prins, M. Samii, and D. A. Hovda. 2000. Cerebral metabolic response to traumatic brain injury sustained early in development: A 2-deoxy-D-glucose autoradiographic study. *Journal of Neurotrauma* 17(8):649-665.

Tokuda, T., S. Ikeda, N. Yanagisawa, Y. Ihara, and G. G. Glenner. 1991. Re-examination of ex-boxers' brains using immunohistochemistry with antibodies to amyloid β-protein and tau protein. *Acta Neuropathologica* 82(4):280-285.

Tran, H. T., F. M. LaFerla, D. M. Holtzman, and D. L. Brody. 2011. Controlled cortical impact traumatic brain injury in 3xTg-AD mice causes acute intra-axonal amyloid-β accumulation and independently accelerates the development of tau abnormalities. *Journal of Neuroscience* 31(26):9513-9525.

Tsaudousides, T., J. B. Cantor, and W. A.Gordon. 2011. Suicidal ideation following TBI: Prevalence rates and correlates in adults living in the community. *Journal of Head Trauma Rehabilitation* 26(4):265-275.

Tysvaer, A. T., and E. A. Lochen. 1991. Soccer injuries to the brain. A neuropsychologic study of former soccer players. *American Journal of Sports Medicine* 19(1):56-60.

Uryu, K., H. Laurer, T. McIntosh, D. Pratico, D. Martinez, S. Leight, V. M. Lee, and J. Q. Trojanowski. 2002. Repetitive mild brain trauma accelerates Aβ deposition, lipid peroxidation, and cognitive impairment in a transgenic mouse model of Alzheimer amyloidosis. *Journal of Neuroscience* 22(2):446-454.

Vagnozzi, R., S. Signoretti, B. Tavazzi, M. Cimatti, A. M. Amorini, S. Donzelli, R. Delfini, and G. Lazzarino. 2005. Hypothesis of the postconcussive vulnerable brain: Experimental evidence of its metabolic occurrence. *Neurosurgery* 57(1):164-171.

Vagnozzi, R., B. Tavazzi, S. Signoretti, A. M. Amorini, A. Belli, M. Cimatti, R. Delfini, V. DiPietro, A. Finocchiaro, and G. Lazzarino. 2007. Temporal window of metabolic brain vulnerability to concussions: Mitochondrial-related impairment—Part I. *Neurosurgery* 61(2):379-388.

Vagnozzi, R., S. Signoretti, B. Tavazzi, A. Lucovici, S. Marziali, G. Tarascio, A. M. Amorini, V. DiPietro, R. Delfini, and G. Lazzorino. 2008. Temporal window of metabolic brain vulnerability to concussion: A pilot 1H-magnetic resonance spectropic study in concussed athletes—Part III. *Neurosurgery* 62(6):1286-1295.

Wiese-Bjornstal, D. M., A. M. Smith, S. M. Shaffer, and M. A. Morrey. 1998. An integrated model of response to sport injury: Psychological and sociological dynamics. *Journal of Applied Sport Psychology* 10(1):46-69.

Wilberger, J. E., and J. C. Maroon. 1989. Head injuries in athletes. *Clinics in Sports Medicine* 8(1):1-9.

Wong, M. M., K. J. Brower, and R. A. Zucker. 2011. Sleep problems, suicidal ideation, and self-harm behaviors in adolescents. *Journal of Psychiatric Research* 54(4):505-511.

Yoshino, A., D. A. Hovda, T. Kawamata, and D. P. Becker. 1991. Dynamic changes in local cerebral glucose utilization following cerebral concussion in rats: Evidence of a hyper- and subsequent hypometabolic state. *Brain Research* 561(1):106-119.

Yoshino, A., D. A. Hovda, Y. Katayama, T. Kawamata, and D. P. Becker. 1992. Hippocampal CA3 lesion prevents postconcussive metabolic dysfunction in CA1.*Journal of Cerebral Blood Flow and Metabolism* 12(6):996-1006.

Yoshiyama, Y., K. Uryu, M. Higuchi, L. Longhi, R. Hoover, S. Fujimoto, T. McIntosh, V. M. Lee, and J. Q. Trojanowski. 2005. Enhanced neurofibrillary tangle formation, cerebral atrophy, and cognitive deficits induced by repetitive mild brain injury in a transgenic tauopathy mouse model. *Journal of Neurotrauma* 22(10):1134-1141.

Young, K., P. White, and W. McTeer. 1994. Body talk: Male athletes reflect on sport, injury, and pain. *Sociology of Sport Journal* 11(2):175-194.

Zhang, L., L. D. Ravdin, N. Relkin, R. D. Zimmerman, B. Jordan, W. E. Lathan, and A. M. Ulug. 2003. Increased diffusion in the brain of professional boxers: A preclinical sign of traumatic brain injury. *American Journal of Neuroradiology* 24(1):52-57.

Zhang, L., L. A. Heier, R. D. Zimmerman, B. Jordan, and A. M. Ulug. 2006. Diffusion anisotropy changes in the brains of professional boxers. *American Journal of Neuroradiology* 27(9):2000-2004.

6

Protection and Prevention Strategies

This chapter addresses the portion of the committee's statement of task concerning the effectiveness of protection devices and equipment and sports regulations for the prevention of concussions. The chapter begins with an overview of research on the effectiveness of protective equipment for the prevention and mitigation of sports-related concussions in youth. The committee's information gathering for this section included the commissioning of a paper that reviews the published literature on the ability of helmets to reduce the risk of sports-related concussions in youth (Duma et al., 2013). The chapter then discusses the roles of sports rules, concussion education initiatives, and state concussion legislation in concussion awareness and prevention. The chapter concludes with the committee's findings for this portion of its charge.

There is debate around the words "prevention" and "reduction" relative to concussions in youth sports (Duma et al., 2013). All activity involves some risk of injury. Although it may be impossible to prevent all sports-related concussions in youth, measures can be taken to reduce the risk of these injuries. Similarly, in modern medicine, although preventive measures such as screening examinations and prophylactic use of medications will not avert all disease in all individuals, such measures can decrease the risk for disease.

PROTECTIVE EQUIPMENT

Helmets and Other Headgear

Helmets are designed to mitigate the likelihood of head injuries from an impact to the head by dissipating and distributing the energy of impact and protecting the head from penetration. Early helmets were designed to prevent such injuries as skull fractures as well as moderate to severe brain injuries such as focal contusions and hemorrhages. The typical helmet has a comfort liner, an impact energy attenuating liner, a restraint system, and a shell. Some helmets, such as those used in motor sport, bicycling, and alpine skiing, are designed to attenuate a single impact. Once one of these single-impact helmets has sustained an impact, it must be replaced. Other helmets, such as those used in ice hockey, football, and lacrosse, are designed to withstand multiple impacts over a season of games and practices (Hoshizake and Brien, 2004). Part of the difference between single-impact helmets and multiple-impact helmets lies in the materials used. For example, multiple-impact helmets, such as those for hockey and football, use materials that do not permanently deform but rather compress and return to their original dimensions. Inner shells can be made of vinyl nitrile or expanded polypropylene, and outer shells use lightweight plastics and composites for durability and protection. Single-impact helmets contain materials that are frangible and deform or fracture permanently upon impact as part of their energy management strategy.

Helmet design involves a series of trade-offs between optimal safety and parameters such as the thickness and other characteristics of the attenuation material, the size and mass of the helmet, comfort, and acceptability. A primary goal of the attenuation layer is to decrease the peak deceleration and to increase the time duration over which the deceleration occurs; this can be achieved by a thicker or more compliant layer of material which improves the energy management by reducing the peak linear deceleration upon impact. However, better energy management via an increased thickness results in a large helmet that may be unacceptable from a style, agility, or visibility standpoint. A helmet with increased mass would have reduced linear head acceleration for a given force; however, it may actually increase the rotational acceleration generated from an impact because there would be an increased radius over which the forces are acting.

Review of the Biomechanics of Concussion

In order to determine if helmet design can indeed be protective against concussion, one must first understand what mechanical events lead to concussions and then determine whether the helmet can mitigate those mechanical forces. The key biomechanical principles that define the mechanics of concussion were discussed in detail in Chapter 2 and are only briefly reviewed here. Local brain tissue deformation (i.e., strain) has been shown to cause brain injury as defined by loss of consciousness, white matter injury, hemorrhage, cell death, or some combination of these (Cater et al., 2006; Elkin and Morrison, 2007; LaPlaca et al., 2005; Margulies and Coats,

2013; Monson et al., 2003; Raghupathi and Margulies, 2002; Raghupathi et al., 2004). If the magnitude or rate of tissue strain is high, local tissue damage occurs. The threshold for the amount of strain required to cause a concussion is unknown, as is whether that threshold varies by age, direction, or individual biological and physiological characteristics. Researchers have developed computational models designed to calculate the distortion of brain tissue that results from global head kinematics such as the acceleration or velocity associated with head impacts in sports (e.g., Kleiven, 2007; Post et al., 2011, 2012; Takhounts et al., 2003), but the thresholds used in these studies are not directly applicable to youth concussions as they are often extrapolated from adult human or animal data. Furthermore, the computational models required to make this translation are hampered by a lack of the pediatric-specific brain and skull data needed to ensure that the model adequately mimics a real child.

There are several key mechanical factors that influence brain strain that need to be considered when examining the potential concussion-reducing effect of helmets. These include (1) head-impact versus non-head-impact scenarios, (2) rotational versus linear acceleration, and (3) centroidal versus non-centroidal impacts. Because a concussion is a diffuse injury rather than a focal one, the primary difference between an impact directly to the head and an impact to the body that accelerates or decelerates the head is the overall magnitude of the acceleration. Impacts directly to the head raise the risk of focal injuries such as skull fractures and brain contusions, but they have also been shown to result in head accelerations of greater magnitude (Kimpara and Iwamoto, 2012). Work by Ommaya and colleagues in the 1960s and 1970s demonstrated that loading via direct head impact resulted in unconsciousness at lower input severities (Ommaya and Gennarelli, 1974; Ommaya et al., 1971), and studies of diffuse axonal injury, a severe form of diffuse brain injury, have reported that an impact is likely necessary to decelerate the head quickly enough to cause such injury (Yoganandan et al., 2009). Impacts to the body, which occur frequently in such contact sports as football and ice hockey, can induce a whiplash-like movement of the head which may be able to generate high enough accelerations to cause injury without subsequent head impact, but the impact velocity to the body must be high. A more common concussion-causing scenario occurs when an impact to the body (i.e., person to person) causes the head to hit some other surface (i.e., boards in hockey or the playing surface in football).

An impact to the head can result in both linear and rotational accelerations. These two types of acceleration can at times be very strongly correlated (Newman et al., 1999; Pellman et al., 2003; Viano et al., 2012b), but this is often not the case.

The centricity of the impact—that is, whether the impact is directed through the center of mass of the head (centroid) or not—is critical to understanding the role of rotational versus linear acceleration in concussion mechanics. Post and colleagues (2011, 2012) conducted an experimental and computational study of centroidal and non-centroidal impacts to a helmeted head. In those impacts directed through the center of mass of the head (centroidal impacts), linear acceleration had a strong correlation with rotational acceleration. For non-centroidal impacts (those not directed through the center of mass) the relationship between linear and rotational acceleration was weak. Furthermore, in those non-centroidal impacts rotational acceleration correlated strongly with brain tissue injury metrics such as strain (correlation=0.638) and stress (correlation=0.677), while linear acceleration did not (correlation=–0.238). These findings were replicated in a study of impacts on equestrian helmets (Forero Rueda et al., 2011) and in simulations of National Football League (NFL) concussion cases (Kleiven, 2007). Walsh and colleagues (2011) also reported that linear and rotational acceleration were only moderately correlated especially in noncentroidal impacts.

Chapter 2 highlighted several animal studies that examined the independent role of linear and rotational acceleration in producing concussions. This research suggested that those scenarios in which the head was allowed to rotate resulted in a greater likelihood of concussion and that a pure linear motion of the head was unlikely to produce such injuries (Hardy et al., 2001; King et al., 2003; Ommaya and Gennarelli, 1974; Ommaya et al., 1971).

These laboratory animal studies with controlled loading conditions examined the influence of linear or rotational accelerations on brain injury risk independently. In sports, however, the vast majority of impacts to the head result in a combination of both linear and rotational motions; it is unlikely to have either purely linear or purely rotational acceleration. Recent head impact data collected in athletes on the playing field using helmet-based sensors, such as the Head Impact Telemetry (HIT) system (see Beckwith et al., 2012; Rowson et al., 2009), initially focused on the role of linear acceleration in concussion risk. From these studies it has been proposed that reducing linear acceleration would lead to reductions in concussion risk (Funk et al., 2012; Rowson and Duma, 2011). However, such conclusions are influenced by important design limitations in how these systems collect and process data. For example, the HIT system does not directly measure rotational acceleration or velocity but rather estimates it from linear acceleration using geometrical assumptions. As a result, the rotational kinematic measures provided by the HIT system have less accuracy than its linear measures do (Allison et al., 2013; Jadischke et al., 2013). In the case of head motions that may have both rotational and linear components, researchers would ideally use independent measures of linear and rotational acceleration (e.g., Camarillo et al., 2013) in order to evaluate which of these types of movements are associated with greater concussion risk.

When interpreting data on the safety benefits of helmets or other protective devices, it is important to realize that a particular reduction in either linear or rotational acceleration does not necessarily correspond to a similar reduction in concussion risk. Injury risk curves describe the probability of injury given a specific mechanical input—that is, the risk of concussion given a particular rotational acceleration. This relationship is not linear but rather sigmoid (s-shaped), often in the form of a Weibull distribution or some other cumulative distribution function (see Figure 6-1). As a result, a 25 percent reduction in acceleration, for example, could actually correspond to a very small decrease in the probability of injury if the values of acceleration lie in the early lower left region of the curve. On the other hand, if the 25 percent acceleration reduction is along the steep portion of

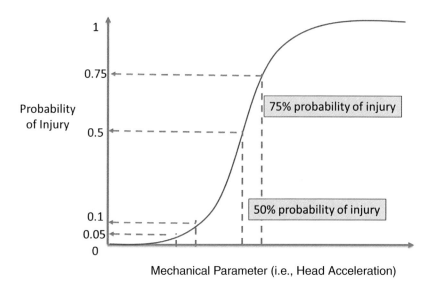

Mechanical Parameter (i.e., Head Acceleration)

FIGURE 6-1 Injury risk curve relating a mechanical parameter such as head acceleration to the probability of injury. Note that a given reduction in the mechanical parameter does not correspond to an equivalent reduction in injury risk due to the sigmoidal shape of the curve. If the reduction in the mechanical parameter is on the left side of the curve, the corresponding reduction in injury risk is rather small (10 percent to 5 percent in the example above). In contrast, if the reduction in the mechanical parameter is in the steep portion of the curve, the actual injury risk reduction could be rather large (75 percent to 50 percent in the example above).

the risk curve, the corresponding reduction in concussion risk may actually be much greater than 25 percent.

Other research attempted to quantify the relationship between head kinematics and concussion risk using injury risk curves. The initial attempts proposed quantitative relationships between concussion risk and linear acceleration; for example, Pellman and colleagues (2003) used reconstructions of impacts in the NFL, and Rowson and Duma (2011) used collegiate data collected with the HIT system. These efforts focused on linear kinematic measures and thus did not include an evaluation of the influence of rotational kinematics on injury risk. Other researchers have developed injury risk curves that incorporate rotational acceleration or velocity; however, these studies are limited by small sample sizes, particularly of the uninjured (Zhang et al., 2004), include estimates of rotational kinematics that have substantial measurement error and incorporate a generic approximation of concussion underreporting (Rowson et al., 2012). More recently, Rowson and Duma (2013) developed a promising concussion risk curve that includes a combination of linear and rotational acceleration; however, this study non-randomly reclassified players who reported no injury to the injured group thus biasing the relationship between acceleration and injury outcome in a way that makes interpretation difficult. None of the risk curves in the literature comprehensively account for parameters such as impact direction, previous concussion history, or other biological or physiological parameters, all of which likely influence the quantitative relationship. Most importantly, all of the existing risk curves are based on data from collegiate or professional football and cannot be directly applied to children and adolescents.

Evidence That Helmets Have the Potential to Mitigate Concussion Risk

Biomechanical evidence Based on the preceding discussion of the mechanics of concussion, devices that reduce both linear acceleration and rotational acceleration or velocity of the head have the potential to reduce the risk of concussion (Benson et al., 2009, 2013). Reductions in linear acceleration with particular helmet designs may help mitigate skull fractures and other focal brain injuries and likely contribute to some reduction in concussion risk. However, due to the decoupling of linear and rotational acceleration under certain impact conditions as described above, reductions of linear acceleration alone do not necessarily translate into a reduced concussion risk in most impact conditions.

There is some evidence, however, that helmets can indeed reduce rotational acceleration. By comparing the impacts of a bare anthropomorphic test device (ATD) head to one fitted with a football helmet, it has been shown that helmets reduce rotational acceleration by approximately 30 percent (Viano and Halstead, 2012). In a follow-up study, Viano described generic changes in football helmet design that led to decreases in rotational acceleration, suggesting that there are aspects of helmet design that can be modified to reduce the angular motion of the head (Viano et al., 2012b). Post and colleagues (2011) studied different hockey helmet designs through physical testing and a computational model. The helmets demonstrated variability in rotational acceleration which corresponded to variations in brain injury metrics such as maximum principal strain and Von Mises stress.[1] Some helmet designs that passed all relevant standards currently based on linear acceleration produced relatively high brain injury metrics (strain) as a result of the angular motion (Post et al., 2011). A similar effect has been observed in speed skating and bicycle helmets (Karton et al., 2012). Rousseau and colleagues (2009) evaluated two different liner materials (vinyl nitrile and expanded polypropylene foam) in hockey helmets and found that while the resulting linear accelerations of the head were similar for the two materials, they differed in the rotational accelerations produced.

In an effort to reduce rotational energy in helmet impacts, several companies have developed a novel helmet design in which a lubricated flexible membrane is placed either on the outside of the helmet or on the inside between the head and the padding. The fundamental idea underlying this new helmet design is the addition of a low-friction layer between the head and the padding that will reduce the rotational acceleration transmitted to the head. Its benefits vary by impact direction. This design concept has been applied, for example, under the MIPS (Multi-directional Impact Protection System) name for equestrian, alpine skiing, snowboarding, and cycling helmets[2] and under the Suspend-Tech name by Bauer for hockey helmets. Recently, Hansen and colleagues described the development of such a system in bicycle helmets that was shown to reduce rotational acceleration in oblique impacts by 34 percent (Hansen et al., 2013). While this design approach is promising and suggests that the characteristics of a helmet can be manipulated to reduce rotational acceleration, until an appropriate injury threshold for concussion can be developed that is age- and direction-specific, it will not be clear what levels of rotational acceleration are acceptable and therefore it will remain impossible to quantify the influence of these design changes on actual concussion risk.

In addition to helmets, several other protective devices have emerged that claim to reduce concussion risk. Soccer head gear is a primary example.

---

[1]Maximum principal strain refers to the maximum value of elongation or stretch along one of the principal axes of strain. Von Mises stress refers to an equivalent stress (force/area) and is used to determine if the stress state would result in failure of the material. These two metrics are used separately or together in brain injury mechanics to assess whether a brain will sustain injury under a certain set of loading conditions.

[2]See http://mipshelmet.com/find-a-helmet (accessed October 7, 2013).

Understanding the role that soccer headgear plays in impacts to the head involves understanding the nature of differences between impacts with hard surfaces, such as other players, goal posts, or the ground, and impacts with the compliant surface of the ball (Niedfeldt, 2011; Spiotta et al., 2012). In an impact between the more compliant ball and a noncompliant head, the ball will deform and absorb the energy of the impact, thus reducing the peak acceleration and increasing the duration of the impact. Headgear has the potential to change the duration of the impact and lower the peak linear acceleration during heading only if it is at least as compliant as the ball and it does not compress fully. Once it compresses fully, it loses its ability to attenuate or reduce the energy transferred to the head. Current headgear compresses fully and rather easily upon impact.

The efficacy of soccer headgear in reducing head acceleration has been tested in the laboratory. Withnall and colleagues (2005) conducted volunteer testing of heading and observed that, because of the amount of ball deformation that occurs during the impact, the linear acceleration of the head did not vary with the use of head gear. When these researchers mimicked head-to-head contact using two ATD headforms, because the head form is not deformable the headgear provided an overall 33 percent reduction in both linear acceleration and a metric that included both linear and rotational acceleration. Their findings likely apply to impacts with other solid objects as well, such as an opponent's elbow, the ground, or the goal post. The findings were confirmed by Naunheim and colleagues (2003), who observed no effect of headgear on impacts from heading but noted attenuation of the impact via the headgear in higher-speed impacts with a noncompliant surface.

Epidemiologic evidence Epidemiological evidence that helmets mitigate concussion primarily comes from the bicycle helmet literature. In a review of five case-control studies from the literature, Thompson and colleagues (2000) concluded that bicycle helmets reduce the risk of head injury (defined as any injury to the brain or skull) by 69 percent, the risk of brain injury by 69 percent, and the risk of more serious brain injury (a score of 3 or more as measured by the Abbreviated Injury Scale score, or AIS) (see AAAM, 1998) by 74 percent as compared with control groups consisting of individuals who visited emergency departments after bicycle accidents in which they were not wearing helmets. Furthermore, when they used a control population of all cyclists who crashed, they documented even stronger benefits (85 percent reduction of head injury, 88 percent reduction in brain injury). Although these studies do not specifically separate out concussion injuries, approximately 70 percent of the brain injury subgroup in the study sustained injuries of an AIS 2 level, most of which were likely concussions. The studies they reviewed did not focus exclusively on children, but about two-thirds of the population studied were children and adolescents. One of the studies (Thompson et al., 1996) found no effect of age on the effectiveness of the helmet in preventing head injury but suggested that there was a trend that the helmet's effectiveness in preventing brain injury decreased with increasing age.

In the sports environment, by contrast, the epidemiological evidence of helmet effectiveness in preventing concussions is not as strong. Collins and colleagues (2006) demonstrated that newer football helmet technology in high school athletes resulted in a 31 percent decrease in the relative risk of concussion compared to older helmet designs, suggesting that some aspects of helmet design can help mitigate concussion. However, the absolute decrease in risk in this study was only 2 percent (7.6 percent versus 5.3 percent), suggesting that these findings were not very robust. In equestrian sports, the use of protective riding helmets has been associated with a fivefold reduction in head injury (Havlik, 2010), and similar benefits have been documented in some studies of skiing and snowboarding helmets (Hagel et al., 2005; Mueller et al., 2008; Sulheim et al., 2006); however, these studies have not specifically looked at concussions.

The most substantial line of research has been in the evaluation of protective headgear in the sport of rugby, where results have been conflicting. In an early study of 16 "under 15" rugby teams, McIntosh and McCrory (2001) found no difference in concussion rates with headgear usage; however, this study suffered from selection bias because the use of headgear was not randomized (McIntosh and McCrory, 2001). Players could chose to wear or not wear headgear, and it is possible that players' perceived risks influenced their decision. A later study involving male rugby players of ages 12 to 19 corrected this flaw by randomizing participants to standard headgear, modified headgear (made from a thicker and denser foam than standard headgear), or no headgear. There was a nonsignificant trend toward wearers of the modified headgear, who have a lower likelihood of missing a game due to concussion, than toward wearers of the standard headgear; however, the subjects in this study showed poor compliance with the headgear use, and there was limited control for such confounding variables as player position and previous concussion history (McIntosh et al., 2009; Navarro, 2011). Kemp and colleagues (2008) prospectively enrolled a cohort of adult rugby players and documented a 57 percent reduction in concussion risk with the use of headgear. Those researchers used a symptom-based definition of concussion which was broader than the definition used by McIntosh and colleagues (2009). In prospective studies, Hollis and colleagues (2009) found that male nonprofessional rugby players (n=3,207) who self-reported that they always wear headgear during games were less likely to sustain a mild traumatic brain injury (mTBI) over one playing season (incidence rate ratio = 0.57; 95% confidence interval [CI],

0.40-0.82). Conversely, in a cohort study of both adult and adolescent male and female rugby players (n=304), Marshall and colleagues (2005) found that rugby headgear had no protective effect on concussions.

In soccer the only formal epidemiological evaluation of headgear in the literature was conducted by Delaney and colleagues (2008), who reported that among Canadian male and female soccer players ages 12 to 17 (n=278) those who did not use headgear were 2.6 times more likely to sustain a concussion than those who did. However, there are important methodological limitations to this study that bias its conclusions. The most important of these is the fact that the use of protective headgear was not randomized so that the headgear may have been used by those who felt they were at risk due to their style of play or occurrence of previous concussions. Furthermore, the outcomes were all obtained via self-report using unvalidated tools (Delaney et al., 2008; Navarro, 2011).

In sum, epidemiological evidence that helmets and other protective devices actually reduce the risk of concussions is lacking. Carefully controlled epidemiological studies are needed to further evaluate these devices' potential for protection.

Helmet Standards

Organizations such as the National Operating Committee on Standards for Athletic Equipment (NOCSAE) and ASTM International (formerly the American Society for Testing and Materials) have developed helmet standards that specify test protocols and quantitative impact criteria such as the Head Injury Criterion or the Severity Index (see Gadd, 1966; Versace, 1971). These standards are performance standards and do not specify materials or design. They are often sport-specific, and some have different tolerance thresholds for youth helmets than for adult helmets. Such standards were developed initially to prevent skull fracture, and at their core they remain true to that mission today. Many of the standards include a drop test of the helmet with a humanoid headform at specified impact locations and velocities and require that the headform experience linear acceleration below a prescribed threshold known to cause fracture. None of these standards incorporate a measure of rotational acceleration, nor do they include a test protocol that would probe the ability of the helmet to mitigate rotational forces that, as described above, have been shown to cause concussion.

There is considerable controversy among experts on the relevance of these test standards for concussion prevention. There are advocates of this testing methodology who claim that reductions in linear acceleration lead to reductions in angular acceleration and therefore holding helmets to a linear acceleration–based standard decreases the risk of concussions (Rowson and

Duma, 2011). There are others who point out that, as highlighted above, linear and rotational acceleration are not always correlated—particularly in the oblique and non-centroidal impacts that occur often on the playing field—and that any helmet standard or rating system that relies solely on reducing linear acceleration will be limited (Forero Rueda et al., 2011; Halldin et al., 2001; McIntosh et al., 2011).

In addition to testing standards for helmets, helmet rating systems have also begun to emerge. One is the STAR rating system, developed by engineers at Virginia Tech. It is a quantitative metric for rating football helmets that combines concussion injury risk and a theoretical distribution of head impact exposure by impact direction and severity with a helmet's linear acceleration response from NOCSAE-like drop tests at various impact locations and drop heights (Rowson and Duma, 2011).

The STAR system is theoretically grounded and represents an intriguing approach to how the injury mitigation properties of a helmet could be assessed. However, the rating system contains several assumptions that limit its generalizability. These include (1) estimates of an average number of head impacts per player per season and a distribution of impact direction based on collegiate data; (2) use of a NOCSAE-like drop test which limits the injury risk curve to linear acceleration alone; (3) a concussion risk curve that does not incorporate injury sensitivity to impact direction which has been shown to be an important parameter in head injury thresholds (Gennarelli et al., 1987; Hodgson et al., 1983; Kleiven, 2003; Margulies et al., 1990); and (4) the use of concussion incidence rates derived from college data to weight the injury and non-injury data including a factor of 50 percent applied universally to the data to account for underreporting.

Because the assumptions outlined above are based on collegiate data, the STAR rating system as currently defined cannot be directly utilized to rate helmets for pre-college-age youth. In order to extend the rating systems like the STAR system to younger populations, the following pediatric-specific data would need to be collected: (1) the number of head impacts and the distribution of impact location per season, (2) the distribution of impact severity by impact location, and (3) an injury risk curve for concussion. These data should be acquired using measurement systems that reliably assess impact direction and impact severity and include both linear and rotational motions. It is important that the rating system incorporate the measurement error of these systems perhaps as a confidence range for injury risk. For example, the measurement error associated with the HIT system, which has been used to generate the data for the current STAR system and is being used to collect pediatric-specific data, has recently been reported to be higher than previously published (Allison et al., 2013; Jadischke et al., 2013). Furthermore, it is likely that several of these data sets will need to be created across the pediatric age range—a rating system for high school helmets is likely not the same as one for youth football helmets. It would also be important that a rating system consider how to incorporate such parameters as helmet fit, helmet condition, and individual variations in style of play or concussion risk and history that are likely to also influence the probability of injury.

In sum, helmet rating systems have the potential to provide useful information to guide consumer decision making. The STAR system is based upon sound principles but is limited by the data available to develop concussion risk curves and thresholds. Through collection of data that could replace some of the assumptions outlined above, its value for widespread application would be increased.

Advances in helmet test standards that incorporate new methods and new injury criteria that evaluate protection in both linear and rotational loading modes are needed before real progress can be made on this issue. NOCSAE, to offer one example, has research under way to develop such test protocols, but the limiting factor may be having sufficiently robust, age-dependent concussion tolerance criteria with which to interpret the results of such tests.

Mouthguards

A mouthguard is a protective device for the mouth that fits over the teeth and gums in order to prevent or reduce the severity of dental and maxillofacial injuries. Research indicates that properly fitted mouthguards reduce the incidence of dental and maxillofacial injuries in sports (Barbic et al., 2005; Daneshvar et al., 2011; Knapik et al., 2007; Labella et al., 2002; Marshall et al., 2005; McNutt et al., 1989; Viano et al., 2012a). One meta-analysis of studies comparing mouthguard users and nonusers showed that the overall risk of orofacial injury is 1.6 to 1.9 times greater when a mouthguard is not worn than when a mouthguard is worn (Knapik et al., 2007). Mouthguards are mandated in several youth contact sports. Both the National Collegiate Athletic Association (NCAA) and the National Federation of State High School Associations (NFHS) require the use of mouthguards in football, ice hockey, field hockey, and lacrosse (Knapik et al., 2007; NFHS, 2011). Some states have passed legislation requiring the use of mouthguards by youth in certain sports. The American Dental Association, although it has no formal authority over youth sports, recommends that individuals who participate in contact sports as well as those who participate in several non-contact sports such as gymnastics, skiing, and track and field, wear a properly fitted mouthguard during practice and competition to prevent dental injuries (ADA, 2004).

There are three broad categories of mouthguards: stock, boil-and-bite, and custom-fitted. Stock mouthguards come ready to wear. Boil-and-bite mouthguards are made of a thermoplastic material that is softened in boiling water and then formed to fit over the teeth as it cools. Both stock and boil-and-bite mouthguards are relatively inexpensive and may be purchased at sporting goods outlets. Custom-fitted mouthguards are made by a dental professional. They are more expensive, but these mouthguards offer the best fit because they are made using a mold of the athlete's mouth. The majority of all mouthguards worn by nonprofessional athletes are of the boil-and-bite type (Barbic et al., 2005; Wisniewski et al., 2004). Some research indicates that custom-fitted mouthguards are better for preventing dental and maxillofacial injuries than are other types of mouthguards (Bemelmanns and Pfeiffer, 2001; Finch et al., 2005; Hoffman et al., 1999).

It has been speculated that mouthguards may reduce the risk of concussions caused by impact to the jaw by positioning the jaw to absorb some of the forces that would otherwise be transferred through the base of the skull to the brain (Knapik et al., 2007; Takeda et al., 2005). One biomechanical study found that when hits to the mandibular undersurface of a mechanical skull were applied, the presence of a mouthguard significantly ($p < .01$) decreased surface distortions related to deformation or fractures to the mandibular bone (by 54.7 percent) and significantly decreased linear acceleration of the head (by 18.5 percent) compared to when a mouthguard was not in place. Nonetheless, the authors of this study acknowledged that further well-designed research is needed on the relationship between mouthguards and concussion risk. Another group of researchers, who worked with a cadaver model, found that having a mouthguard in place reduced by 50 percent the amplitude of bone deformation and intracranial pressure that followed a hit to the chin (Hickey et al., 1967). As noted by McCrory (2001), however, this research does not translate well to live humans because of differences in the compliance of cadaveric and live human tissue, among other reasons.

Several epidemiologic studies have assessed the differences in concussion incidence between users and nonusers of mouthguards as well as between users of custom-made and non-custom-made mouthguards. On the whole, the available research suggests no significant difference in the risk of concussion for athletes who wear mouthguards and those who do not (Benson et al., 2009; Labella et al., 2002). One of the larger, more well-designed studies followed 50 men's NCAA Division I basketball teams over one season and found no significant differences between mouthguard users and nonusers in rates of concussions (0.35 versus 0.55) (Labella et al., 2002). Furthermore, there is no evidence that custom-made mouthguards offer any more protection against concussion than other types of mouthguards. One large prospective study collected data for 87 NCAA Division I-A football teams over a 15-week period. Over the course of all the games and practices, 369 physician-verified concussions were reported.

No statistical difference was observed in either concussion incidence or concussion severity between players who wore custom-made mouthguards and those who wore non-custom-made mouthguards (Wisniewski et al., 2004). Another small longitudinal study evaluated concussion incidence among 28 high school football players before and after implementation of a customized mandibular orthotic. The mean self-reported incidence of concussion/mTBI for the two seasons prior to the use of the orthotic was 2.1 ± 1.4 events per player, which amounted to 59 concussions/mTBIs. Following the implementation of the orthotic, three concussions/mTBIs were reported over three seasons; the number of concussive events per player fell to 0.11 ± 0.31 with an odds ratio (OR) of 38.33 (95% CI, 8.2-178.6) (Singh et al., 2009). This finding was significant but limited by the small sample size and the fact that 23 of the 28 players had a previous history of concussion, suggesting the possibility of self-selection bias. Player compliance with the orthotics was not reported (Navarro, 2011; Singh et al., 2009).

The WIPSS Brain-Pad mouthguard is a two-layered boil-and-bite mouthguard that fits over the upper and lower teeth. It is designed to minimize acceleration forces more than other mouthguards by maintaining a space at the temporomandibular joint (Barbic et al., 2005). At one time the packaging for a version of this mouthguard developed for youth stated that it could reduce the risk of concussions from lower jaw impacts (U.S. Senate Committee on Commerce, Science, and Transportation, 2011). A multicenter, cluster-randomized trial involving 614 male football players and male and female rugby players at universities in Ontario, Canada, found no significant difference in the number of concussions observed between athletes who wore the WIPPS Brain-Pad mouthguard and athletes in the control group who continued to use their mouthguard of choice. There were 22 and 21 concussions in the intervention and in the control group, respectively (Barbic et al., 2005).

Mihalik and colleagues (2007) investigated possible differences in neurocognitive and symptomatic impairments in youth athletes who were concussed while wearing a mouthguard versus those who were concussed while not wearing a mouthguard. Baseline neurocognitive testing was performed before the start of the season using Immediate Post-Concussion Assessment and Cognitive Testing (ImPACT) (see Chapter 3 for a discussion of ImPACT). Among the 152 male and 28 female athletes who sustained a concussion, no significant differences with respect to mouthguard use were observed in neurocognitive deficits for verbal memory, visual memory, visual motor speed, reaction time, or symptom status upon follow-up assessment with ImPACT. Athletes had significantly lower neurocognitive test scores and higher symptom scores following a concussion regardless of mouthguard use (Mihalik et al., 2007).

In summary, over the past decade, although manufacturers have made claims regarding the protective features of mouthguards to reduce or eliminate concussions, the vast majority of studies have consistently failed to link the use of mouthguards to lowered concussion risk (Barbic et al., 2005; Benson et al., 2009; Knapik et al., 2007; Labella et al., 2002; Mihalik et al., 2007; Navarro, 2011; Viano et al., 2012a; Wisniewski et al., 2004).

Ice Hockey Face Shields, Visors, and Cages

A face shield in ice hockey is a protective device made of impact-resistant plastic that is attached to a player's helmet in order to lessen the risk of injury to the face. Full-face shields cover the entire face, and half-face shields (or visors) cover the upper half of the face. Cages, an alternative to the full face shield, cover the entire face and are usually made of metal. NFHS rules mandate full facial protection for high school ice hockey players, and USA Hockey requires facial protection in all age classifications below adult (NFHS, 2013; USA Hockey, 2013). NCAA rules require college-level ice hockey players to wear full facial protection that has met standards set by the Hockey Equipment Certification Council (NCAA, 2012).

Facial protection has been shown to reduce the incidence of ocular, facial, and dental injuries in ice hockey (Asplund et al., 2009; Hendrickson et al., 2008; LaPrade et al., 1995; Stuart et al., 2002). It has been hypothesized that facial protection may also reduce the incidence and severity of head injury in ice hockey by decreasing head acceleration after an impact (Lemair and Pearsall, 2007). One biomechanical study using a surrogate headform showed substantially reduced peak linear acceleration during blunt impacts when facial protection, in combination with a helmet, was in place, with cages showing lower peak acceleration than with visors (Lemair and Pearsall, 2007). However, there is no evidence from epidemiologic research that facial protection reduces concussions in ice hockey. An analysis of injury data from the National Hockey League (NHL) (n=787), which does not require players to wear facial protection, found that athletes wearing visors were no less likely to experience concussions than were those not wearing any facial protection (Stevens et al., 2006).[3] In addition, studies of college and amateur ice hockey players show no significant difference in the occurrence of concussion between ice hockey players who wear half-face protection versus those who wear full-face protection (Apslund et al., 2009; Benson et al., 1999, 2002; Stuart et al., 2002). One study of university ice hockey players who were followed over one season showed that, although there was no significant difference in the overall risk of sustaining a con-

---

[3]Beginning in the 2013-2014 season, the NHL began to grandfather in the mandatory use of visors for new players. Facial protection continues to be optional for athletes who are not new to the league (NHL, 2013).

cussion for players wearing visors (n=323) compared with those wearing full-face protection (n=319), athletes sustaining concussions while wearing visors missed significantly more practices and games per concussion than those sustaining concussions while wearing full-face protection (4.07 sessions; 95% CI, 3.48 to 4.74 versus 1.71 sessions; 95% CI, 1.32 to 2.18) (Benson et al., 2002).

Marketing of Protective Equipment

There are concerns that the makers of sports protective equipment have taken advantage of growing concussion awareness by making unsubstantiated claims that certain products can reduce concussion risk. For example, as discussed at a 2011 hearing on concussions and the marketing of sports equipment before the U.S. Senate Committee on Commerce, Science, and Transportation, packaging and online advertising for particular devices (e.g., mouthguards and soccer headbands) designed specifically for youth athletes have included language that may be construed to mean that the product reduces concussion risk or else they have made explicit claims of reduced concussion risk with use of the product (U.S. Senate Committee on Commerce, Science, and Transportation, 2011). In order to avoid a false sense of security, it is important that athletes, parents, and coaches be aware of—and that marketers of sports equipment accurately convey—the limitations of protective equipment as it relates to concussions. Until a universally accepted injury risk curve for concussions is established, as well as associated variants with age and perhaps direction, claims of reduced concussion risk with protective devices will not be based on fundamentally sound science.

Risk Compensation

One unintended consequence of wearing helmets and other protective devices is that the athlete may be emboldened by the increased protection to take additional risks, thus mitigating any benefits of the protective device. This phenomenon, termed "risk compensation," has been studied extensively in the safety literature; for an excellent review of the topic, the reader is directed to Hedlund (2000), who summarizes the theory and research in this field. The theory of risk compensation is based on the idea that every individual has an acceptable level of risk. If a protective device lowers that risk, the individual's actions will change (i.e., become more risky) in such a way as to re-equilibrate the risk to the maximum acceptable level. Hedlund suggests that there are four factors that influence risk compensation: visibility ("Do I know there has been a safety change?"); effect ("How does the safety change affect me?"); motivation ("What influences my safety behavior?"); and control ("How much control do I have of my behavior?"). Two examples of risk compensation in Hedlund's review are drivers with antilock brakes driving faster and braking harder than those without antilock brakes and loggers working more quickly and more carelessly once protective equipment was required (Hedlund, 2000). It certainly appears that the four factors described above come into play in the area of sports and protective equipment: The use of protective equipment has high visibility; it may appear to adversely affect a person's ability to play at a high level; a person may not be motivated to wear such devices if the person does not perceive a risk; and an individual may sometimes have no control over the use of the protective equipment (i.e., it is required). Hagel and Meeuwisse (2004) summarized the issues of risk compensation in sports and provided several examples: the increase in tackling drill fatalities in football in the 1950s and 1960s after the introduction of mandatory hard shell helmets, an increase in injury rates associated with the introduction of soft core baseballs, and increased helmet usage in fatally injured skiers versus the uninjured skiing population.

There has been limited exploration of the role that risk compensation may play in concussions. Tierney and colleagues (2008) studied both men and women soccer players in a controlled soccer heading scenario both with and without headgear and observed that women attacked the balls more forcefully while wearing headgear. This could be attributed to risk compensation or simply to the perception by the women players that they needed to strike the ball harder to reach the target. In a survey of attitudes and beliefs around protective equipment, two-thirds of adolescent rugby players reported increased confidence and an ability to play harder when wearing headgear (Finch et al., 2001). In a convenience sample of recreational ice hockey players using facial protection (n=152), 69 percent reported that they felt they could play more aggressively with the protection (Woods et al., 2007).

Risk compensation studies are difficult to conduct and analyze because the effects are typically evaluated over a population rather than via individual differences in behavior before and after institution of a safety change. As a result, they must control for other behavioral variations of the populations studied. Still, future work in protective devices in sport must evaluate these potential unintended consequences as policy and equipment changes intended to reduce risk are considered.

Playing Surfaces

Playgrounds are a major source of injury for children. From 2001 through 2008 there were an estimated 1,786,608 emergency department (ED)–treated injuries associated with playground equipment, of which

30,578 (2 percent) were concussions. (The actual number of playground-related injuries, including concussions, is likely much higher, given that many such injuries are not treated in an ED.) The greatest share of playground injuries of all types (44 percent) involved falls from, into, or onto equipment, followed by injuries involving equipment breakage, tip over, or poor design or assembly (23 percent) (CPSC, 2009). To reduce the likelihood of head injuries on playgrounds, it is important to consider the impact-attenuating properties of the surfacing under and around the playground equipment (CPSC, 2010). The Consumer Product Safety Commission (CPSC) and ASTM International have developed guidelines for playground surfacing. The most recent CPSC handbook for public playgrounds states that playground equipment should not be placed over asphalt, concrete, dirt, grass, or carpet not tested to ASTM F1292. ASTM standard F1292 provides a "critical height" rating for playground surfaces that approximates the fall height below which a life-threatening head injury would not be expected to occur. The rating assigned to a given surface should be greater than or equal to the fall height of the highest piece of equipment on the playground. Preferred surfacing includes unitary surfaces (rubber tiles, mats) tested to ASTM F1292; loose fill materials (pea gravel, sand, wood mulch not treated with chemical preservative, and wood chips) maintained at a minimum depth of 9 inches; or shredded or rubber mulch maintained at a minimum depth of 6 inches (CPSC, 2010).[4] Recent nationwide data on the safety conditions of playgrounds are not available. A 2004 survey of 3,000 school, childcare, and park playgrounds in the United States resulted in overall grade of B– for fall surfacing and, within this category, a grade of F for appropriate depth of loose fill materials (National Program for Playground Safety, 2004). There currently are no national safety standards for outdoor play equipment. A few states mandate compliance with the CPSC guidelines.

One organized sport for which the impact-attenuating properties of the playing surface are particularly important is cheerleading. Concussions and other closed-head injuries account for 4 to 6 percent of all cheerleading injuries (Labella and Mjaanes, 2012). Although concussion rates in cheerleading (0.06 per 1,000 exposures) are low compared with other sports, from 1998 to 2008 concussion rates in cheerleading increased by 26 percent each year, which was a greater rate of increase than for any other sport played by female youth at the high school and college levels. This increase is thought to have been due to the increasing difficulty of stunts (Labella and Mjaanes,

---

[4]The recommendations for protective surfacing do not apply to equipment that requires a child to be standing or sitting at ground level, such as sandboxes, playhouses, activity walls at ground level, and any other equipment that children use when their feet remain in contact with the ground surface (CPSC, 2010).

2012; Shields and Smith, 2009a). Falls and stunts that involve interaction with the surface (e.g., tumbling) account for a sizable share of all injuries in cheerleading (Marar et al., 2012; Schulz et al., 2004; Shields and Smith, 2009a). The potential for concussions and other injuries can be minimized by increasing the shock-absorbing capacity of the surface on which cheerleaders practice and perform (Shields and Smith, 2009b).

Daneshvar and colleagues (2011) noted that the momentum transfer and impact associated with collisions increases as the speed of athletes increases. Because the surface on which an athlete plays affects his or her speed, it may also influence the incidence of concussions. Synthetic surfaces are generally harder and result in faster speeds than on natural ones. Artificial turfs (e.g., AstroTurf), which do not require sunlight and regular maintenance, were introduced in the 1960s following the construction of indoor football stadiums. These turfs were made of a hard plastic material and are believed to have led to an increase in injuries, particularly musculoskeletal injuries, among football players. Beginning in 2000 synthetic turfs designed to mimic the properties of natural grass while reducing friction and impact forces were developed and deployed (Williams, 2007). A few epidemiologic studies have evaluated whether athletes sustain more injuries when playing on the newer artificial turfs than when playing on natural grass. Findings have varied across studies and injury type (Dragoo et al., 2012; Fuller et al., 2007; Guskiewicz et al., 2000; Meyers, 2010; Meyers and Barnhill, 2004). An analysis of NCAA Injury Surveillance System data for soccer showed that the three most common injuries on artificial turf for men (ankle lateral ligament complex tear, hamstring tear, concussion) and for women (ankle lateral ligament complex tear, concussion, and anterior cruciate ligament tear) were the same as the most common injuries on grass, but the incidence of head and neck injuries, including concussions, was significantly ($p < .01$) higher on artificial turf than on grass for men (4.31/1,000 player hours [95% CI, 3.03-6.13] on artificial turf versus 2.37/1,000 player hours [95% CI, 1.86-3.02] on natural grass) (Fuller et al., 2007). Meanwhile, a study of college football players showed no significant variation in the incidence of head trauma by field type (Meyers, 2010), and another study found that football players experienced more concussions on natural grass than on artificial turf (Meyers and Barnhill, 2004). In summary, the evidence is inconclusive as to whether concussion risks are higher on synthetic than on natural turf.

SPORTS RULES

The rules of play are the foundation of safe conduct in sports because they set expectations for behavior and define infractions. As noted in the 2013 American Medical Society for Sports Medicine position statement on concussion in sports, promoting fair play encourages respect for opponents and emphasizes safety precautions for athletes (Harmon et al., 2013). Enforcement of the rules by coaches and officials and adherence to rules by players may help to reduce the incidence and severity of sports-related concussions in youth (Cusimano et al., 2013; Harmon et al., 2013; Lincoln et al., 2013; Roberts et al., 1996; Yard et al., 2008). In a 2008 study of athletes in 100 U.S. high schools, 25 percent of the concussions reported were related to illegal play activity as determined by a referee or disciplinary committee (Collins et al., 2008). In contact and collision sports in particular, a shift toward a greater emphasis on player safety will require education and a change in expectations on the part of coaches, officials, and athletes as well as of parents and fans (Harmon et al., 2013).

Some research has been conducted on the relationship between the rules for specific sports and concussion risk. Body checking in ice hockey is a tactic in which a defensive player uses his or her body to legally separate a puck carrier from the puck. Body checks must be done with the trunk of the body (hips and shoulders) and must be above the opponent's knees and below the neck. Although legal body checking is a necessary skill at more advanced levels of play, safety can be jeopardized when players do not have the skills to check in the correct way (USA Hockey, 2009). Body checking is a leading cause of injury in general and of concussion in particular in youth ice hockey (Cusimano et al., 2011; Emery and Meeuwisse, 2006; Emery et al., 2010a; MacPherson et al., 2006; McIntosh and McCrory, 2005). Research from Canada that studied youth ages 10 to 15 in ice hockey leagues in which body checking was permitted and those where it was not found that body checking was associated with an increased risk of concussions (Emery et al., 2010b; MacPherson et al., 2006). In a study comparing rates of concussion in male ice hockey players before and after a Hockey Canada rule change that lowered the legal age of body checking from 11 to 9, the odds of an ED visit due to a body checking–related concussion increased significantly for "Atom" division players (i.e., those 10 and 11 years old). There were four reported concussions prior to rule change and 22 after the rule change (OR 10.08, 95% CI, 2.35-43.29) (Cusimano et al., 2011). These findings support policies that prohibit body checking for younger ice hockey players as a means of reducing the risk of concussions and other injuries. Recognizing that the youngest ice hockey players may not be prepared for body checking in competitive play, USA Hockey delayed the legal age for body checking from 12 to 14 starting with the 2011-2012 season. In older youth for whom body checking is permitted, USA Hockey requires officials to penalize players who engage in illegal body checking, such as checking another player from behind or for the purpose of intimidation (USA Hockey, 2011, 2013).

Using accelerometers to monitor linear and rotational head acceleration, Guskiewicz and colleagues examined the biomechanics of legal and illegal plays in youth ice hockey players. Illegal collisions—those involving elbowing, intentional head contact, or high sticking to the head—made up 17 percent of all body collisions. Illegal collisions resulted in slightly higher linear and rotational acceleration (23 g; 1530 rad/s^2) than did legal collisions (21 g; 1417 rad/s^2). The researchers concluded that athletes and coaches should better conform to game rules and that officials should be more stringent in enforcing and assessing more severe penalties to players who purposefully foul an opponent (Guskiewicz, 2013; Mihalik et al., 2010). It is important to note, however, that these differences are relatively small and their effect on concussion risk is not clear.

Low rates of adherence to fair play policy have been linked to a greater risk of injury in youth soccer (Koutures and Gregory, 2010). Unintentional collisions such as the head-to-head and head-to-elbow contacts that are associated with more aggressive play are frequent mechanisms for concussion in this sport (Boden et al., 1998; Kolodziej et al., 2011).

The responsibilities of officials who preside over sporting events include enforcing game rules, assessing penalties, detecting infractions and signaling other participants and officials when infractions occur, and starting and stopping play when necessary (BLS, 2012). Aside from other players, officials often have the closest view of play and any injuries that occur. Officials therefore have a role to play in both the prevention of sports-related concussions and the identification of players who may have been concussed. At a committee workshop, Jeff Triplette of the National Association of Sports Officials reported that many officials of youth sports have not been educated on the signs and symptoms of concussions, and he noted further that many of them are former athletes from a time when the prevalent mindset was to play through injuries. He also described the sorts of incidents that can lead to a concussion and discussed how enforcement of rules can protect athletes. Triplette noted that greater awareness and reporting of possible concussions in youth sports could be facilitated by

- a requirement that officials and coaches receive concussion training before they can supervise athletic activities;
- education of first responders (i.e., medical personnel) to engage officials in the assessment of injured players;
- the use of video documentation to assess whether officials are enforcing safety rules; and
- the discipline of officials who fail to enforce rules that affect player safety (Triplette, 2013).

In response to concerns about the long-term consequences of repetitive head impacts, several organizations have called for a "hit count" in youth sports—in other words, a limit on the amount of head contacts a particular player experiences over a given amount of time. This concept, most publicly advanced by the Sports Legacy Institute,[5] is similar to the pitch counts that are used in youth baseball to reduce injury to the shoulder and elbow of pitchers. Reflecting concern about the hit count, the NFL and collegiate athletic organizations such as the Ivy League and PAC-12 conference have limited the number of full-contact practices in an effort to reduce the number of head impacts (Council of Ivy League Presidents, 2011, 2012). Similar actions were taken in 2012 by Pop Warner Football, the largest youth football program in the United States. At the high school level there has been no national limit on contact, but some states have taken action. Most notably, Texas passed limits on contact in football practice during the 2013 season (House Bill 887).

Support for such limits is not universal. Some believe that the technology to quantify the number and magnitude of head impacts is not adequately developed and that the science behind setting a specific threshold is not well defined (see discussions earlier in this chapter and in Chapter 2). Furthermore, there is some concern that delaying or reducing contact in practice puts athletes at risk down the road because they have not adequately learned appropriate contact skills at an early age when the ability to acquire skills is at its greatest (Guskiewicz, 2013). These researchers advocate for proper coaching techniques that emphasize fundamentals and the development and enforcement of sport-specific rules to prevent unsafe behavior and to reduce but not eliminate contact.

While the concept of limiting the number of head impacts is fundamentally sound, there is no evidence available at this time to provide a scientific basis for implementing a specific limit on the number of impacts or the magnitude of impacts per week or per season.

CONCUSSION EDUCATION

Knowledge of concussion signs and symptoms has been found to be deficient in some surveys of youth athletes (Bloodgood et al., 2013; Kaut et al., 2003; Kroshus et al., 2013). Studies of the effectiveness of educational interventions, including workshops and lectures, videos, and other programs, show with some consistency that education can improve concussion knowledge in youth (Bagley et al., 2012; Bramley et al., 2012; Cook et al., 2003; Cusimano et al., 2014; Echlin et al., 2010; Miyashita et al., 2013). In one of the larger studies, students ages 9 to 18 (n=599)— who participated in an education workshop lasting 40 to 60 minutes and featuring interactive demonstrations, discussion, and case studies of athletes—displayed significant improvement in concussion knowledge; specifically, the pre- and post-intervention mean scores on a quiz assessing the recognition of signs and symptoms and appropriate responses after a concussion were 43 and 65 percent, respectively. Furthermore, the proportion of students who passed the quiz (i.e., who answered half of the quiz questions correctly) increased from 34 percent to 80 percent (Bagley et al., 2012). Miyashita and colleagues (2013) found that concussion knowledge scores among 70 male and female college soccer and basketball players improved significantly after the athletes participated in an educational lecture describing concussion basics and a question and answer session. A randomized study involving 67 junior ice hockey players ages 16 to 21 showed that participants who viewed a concussion DVD or interactive computer module had greater increases in concussion knowledge than did controls based on the results of pre- and post-intervention knowledge tests (Echlin et al., 2010). Another randomized study of 267 minor league ice hockey players found that players who viewed an ice hockey safety video on concussion had significant increases in concussion knowledge immediately following the video. However, a reassessment 2 months later revealed that in athletes who had viewed the video concussion knowledge had decreased, suggesting that the effect of the intervention was temporary (Cusimano et al., 2014).

Knowledge, although essential to behavior change, does not necessarily translate into changes in behavior. Various factors—including social, attitudinal, and emotional forces—influence whether and how individuals respond to information. Yet little research has evaluated the effect of concussion education on behavior change in youth. One study found a significant reduction in body checking–related penalties (which in other studies have been linked to concussion risk) as well as improvements in concussion knowledge in 75 youth ice hockey players ages 11 to 12 who viewed a video on the mechanisms, consequences, and prevention of brain and spinal cord injury versus a group of controls (Cook et al., 2003). Another study found no effect of an ice hockey safety video on behavior change among minor league ice hockey players (Cusimano et al., 2014). Although not focused specifically on concussions, an evaluation of the "Bike Smart" program—an eHealth software program using video, animations, and still images to teach bicycle safety behaviors to children—found that elementary-school-age children who participated in the program had significant gains in their recognition of safety rules, helmet placement, and hazard discrimination as compared with children who watched a video about childhood safety. One particularly important result was that children viewing the Bike Smart program more often donned a bike helmet correctly (McLaughlin and

Glang, 2010).[6] In a prospective study of 146 NCAA Division 1 ice hockey players from six universities who had received NCAA compliant concussion education, Kroshus and colleagues observed only a small decrease in athletes' reported intention to continue to play while experiencing concussion symptoms. Because the NCAA mandate states only that institutions provide concussion education, the content and form of delivery (e.g., handout, email, lecture, video) of the education varied across schools. Change in intention to continue to play with a concussion was significantly higher among athletes who reported receiving a lecture (p=0.021) and significantly lower among those who reported receiving concussion information via email (Kroshus et al., 2013).

As discussed earlier in the report, the current culture of sports may discourage athletes from reporting their concussion symptoms and removing themselves from play (Kroshus et al., 2013; Torres et al., 2013). A recent study of high school athletes' (n=167, age=15.7±1.4) intentions to report sports-related concussions showed that intention to report was associated with perceptions about concussion reporting, perception of important social referents' beliefs about concussion reporting, and perceived control over concussion reporting. Although reporting intention may not always be an indicator of what an individual's actual concussion reporting behaviors will be, these findings suggest that future concussion education initiatives should focus on improving attitudes and beliefs about concussions among athletes, coaches, and parents (Register-Mihalik et al., 2013b). Greater athlete knowledge about concussions and more favorable attitude toward reporting possible concussion also was associated with increased reporting prevalence of concussion and "bell-ringer" events in these youth (Register-Mihalik et al., 2013a).

A recent online survey of youth athletes (n=252) showed that younger youth (ages 10 to 13) were significantly more likely to view concussions as a "critical issue" than were older youth (ages 16 to 18 years) (Bloodgood et al., 2013), perhaps indicating that existing concussion educational efforts are reaching younger youth more effectively than older youth.

Especially in youth sports, coaches often preside over athletic events without medical personnel present. It is therefore important that youth coaches have a basic knowledge of concussions. A small number of studies have evaluated the effectiveness of concussion education interventions

---

[6]Bicycle crashes are a leading cause of sports- and recreation-related mTBI in youth. Centers for Disease Control and Prevention data from emergency department visits (nonfatal sports- and recreation-related TBI) show that bicycle crashes are the most common cause of concussion among boys 5 to 9 years old and the second most common cause of concussion among boys 10 to 14 and 15 to 19. Bicycle crashes are also the second most common cause of concussion among girls 5 to 9 and the most common cause of concussion among girls 10 to 14 (Gilchrist et al., 2011).

for coaches. The Athletic Concussion Training using Interactive Video Education (ACTive) program was developed to train community coaches of youth ages 10 to 18 about youth sports concussions. Designed using the Health Belief Model (Becker, 1974; Rosenstock et al., 1988) as its conceptual framework, the program offers an interactive video consisting of three modules that cover the prevention, recognition, and management of youth sports concussions using simple graphics and video segments. In one study, 75 coaches (52 males and 23 females) completed the program over the Internet. Post-intervention analysis showed significant overall gains in concussion knowledge compared to baseline among coaches who received the intervention versus coaches in the control group who were sent a link to materials prepared by the Centers for Disease Control and Prevention (CDC) on bicycle and pedestrian safety. The greatest gains were obtained in knowledge about concussion symptoms, followed by general concussion knowledge, knowledge of misperceptions about concussion, perceived self-confidence about taking appropriate action based on scenarios presented, and intention to take action based on the scenarios (Glang et al., 2010). A cross-sectional investigation showed that prior coaching education was predictive of the ability of youth sport coaches (n=157) to recognize concussion signs and symptoms (Valovich-McLeod et al., 2007). In a study involving 20,000 coaches and 4,000 referees of community rugby in New Zealand, Gianotti and colleagues found that a concussion management education program consisting of a film and slide show provided "minimum best practice" for the management of suspected concussions (Gianotti and Hume, 2007). The committee did not identify any studies of the effect of concussion education on changes in coaching behavior, such as the removal of athletes who may have sustained a concussion from play.

Over the past several years, the CDC has developed concussion education materials for a variety of stakeholders. In collaboration with 26 health, sports, and national organizations, the CDC created the "Heads Up: Concussion in Youth Sports" initiative in 2007. The initiative is centered on a toolkit designed to provide coaches, school administrators, athletes, and parents with practical and easy-to-read information on concussions from a reliable source. The toolkit includes fact sheets tailored for coaches, parents, and athletes; a clipboard; a magnet; and a quiz to test concussion knowledge. An online concussion training module for coaches is also available via the campaign's website[7] (CDC, 2009, 2012a).

Despite relatively low response rates, survey assessments of the Heads Up campaign concerning changes in knowledge and attitudes about concussions among youth coaches indicated that after reviewing the Heads Up

---

[7]The toolkit materials are available in English and Spanish and may be downloaded from http://www.cdc.gov/concussion/HeadsUp/youth.html (accessed January 15, 2014).

materials the coaches viewed concussions more seriously and were better able to identify athletes who may have had a concussion. Many of the coaches surveyed said that they had learned something new about concussions from the materials and that they would continue to use the materials (Covassin et al., 2012; Sarmiento et al., 2010; Sawyer et al., 2010).

"Heads Up: Brain Injury in Your Practice" is a CDC initiative that provides materials on mTBI and concussion for physicians, including a booklet with information on concussion diagnosis and management, a patient assessment tool, a care plan, concussion prevention fact sheets, a palm card for on-field management, and a CD-ROM with downloadable kit materials and other resources (CDC, 2011).[8] An analysis of the effect of the toolkit on concussion knowledge in a random sample of physicians showed no difference in general concussion knowledge between an intervention group who received the materials (183 physicians) and a control group that did not (231 physicians). However, physicians who received the toolkit were significantly less likely to recommend next-day return to play (OR .31, 95% CI, .12-.76) (Chrisman et al., 2011), suggesting that continuing medical education on concussion may improve the management of patients with concussions.

As discussed earlier in the report, youth often experience deficits in concentration and in short-term and working memory after a concussion. These deficits can interfere with school performance and may require school personnel to make academic accommodations. For example, a student who has difficulty concentrating after a concussion may need to be given more time to take tests or to complete assignments. Thus, school personnel need to receive education on the effects that a concussion may have on a student and on his or her school performance, the role of schools in concussion management, and the potential long-term consequences of returning to activity too soon (Sady et al., 2011). The CDC developed a toolkit, the "Heads Up to Schools: Know Your Concussion ABCs," to aid in the dissemination of concussion information to school personnel who are not directly involved in athletics, such as principals, school counselors, teachers, and school nurses. The toolkit highlights concussion signs, effects, and what schools should watch for when a student returns to school after a concussion. The materials provide a starting point for concussion education for school personnel (CDC, 2012b; Sady et al., 2011). Thus far, there does not appear to have been a peer-reviewed evaluation of the effect of the Heads Up to Schools program on concussion knowledge or on concussion management by schools.

The literature on concussion education in medical schools is sparse. In a Canadian survey of medical schools, only 4 of the 14 schools that responded to the survey (out of a total of 17 medical schools) indicated that

---

[8]Materials are available for download at http://www.cdc.gov/concussion/headsup/physicians_tool_kit.html (accessed January 15, 2014).

concussion education is included in the curriculum for medical students (Burke et al., 2012). In a study in the United States, practicing pediatric primary care and emergency medicine physicians cited inadequate training on how to provide concussion education as an important barrier to educating families about concussion (Zonfrillo et al., 2012). Furthermore, these doctors demonstrated by their actions that they did not completely understand the cognitive limitations that follow a concussion. While they gave general return-to-activity instructions to more than half of their concussion patients (52 percent of first visits and 53 percent of follow-up visits), they provided instructions about returning to school to far fewer (28 percent first visits, 43 percent on follow-up) (Arbogast et al., 2013). Increasing concussion awareness in the medical community may be accomplished by targeting the medical school and residency curriculums as well as through continuing education through the various academies for board-certified physicians.

Content analyses of social media sites such as Facebook and Twitter show that people use these sites not only to share and discuss news stories about concussions but also to share personal experiences and to seek and offer advice. These content analysis studies highlight the capacity of social media to serve as a broadcast medium for sports concussion information and education (Ahmed et al., 2010; Sullivan et al., 2012).

STATE CONCUSSION LEGISLATION

Washington State House Bill 1824, also known as the Zackery Lystedt law, was signed into law in May 2009 and is widely recognized as the first statewide advocacy effort focused on concussion prevention to formally result in the passage of legislation. As discussed in Chapter 1, most states have since followed suit, which has resulted in a proliferation of laws addressing concussions in youth sports across the United States. In fact, since 2009 all 50 states and the District of Columbia have had bills introduced before their legislatures with language addressing youth concussions. Consideration of these bills has resulted in either codified statute or statewide administrative regulation in 49 states and the District of Columbia. The one exception is Mississippi; concussion legislation was last introduced in the Mississippi legislature in January 2013, but it did not pass through committee (USA Football, 2013).[9] Although state concussion laws do not focus on the primary prevention of concussion, they do aim to increase awareness about concussion signs, symptoms, and outcomes and to reduce the risk and consequences of multiple concussions (e.g., second impact syndrome) and potentially to promote quicker recovery (Harvey, 2013).

---

[9] See http://legiscan.com/gaits/search?state=MS&keyword=concussion (accessed January 15, 2014).

Requirements of State Concussion Laws[10]

A committee review of state concussion laws, including review of the text from the laws as well as previously published analyses of these laws, shows that most states require (1) education or training of athletes, coaches, and parents about the nature and risk of concussions in sports, with parents signing a form acknowledging receipt of the information; (2) removal from play of any youth athlete suspected of having sustained a concussion; and (3) clearance for return to play by a licensed health care professional. However, state laws vary somewhat along several important dimensions that may influence the effect that they actually have on concussion prevention, diagnosis, and recovery, such as the extent of education and training required, the expertise of the health care providers who are permitted to clear athletes for return to play, and the entities that are covered by the law.

In most states, coaches are required to receive education on concussion recognition, sequelae, treatment, and return-to-play criteria. However, the extent of education that is required varies widely across states. Laws in some states require that coaches complete formal concussion training at specific time intervals, while laws in other states require that coaches be provided with concussion information materials. For example, as a condition of the issuance and renewal of a coaching permit, Connecticut's law (Senate Bill 456) mandates that coaches of intramural and interscholastic athletics complete an initial training course on concussions and head injuries prior to coaching and every 5 years thereafter and that coaches review relevant information on concussions and head injuries each year that the course is not required. In contrast, legislation in Illinois (House Bill 200) states that educational materials describing the nature and risk of concussions and head injuries should be made available to school districts in order to educate coaches as well as parents and student athletes.

States also vary on their education and release requirements for parents and youth athletes. Although laws in the majority of states require that parents be provided with concussion education materials, several states do not require parents to read and sign an information sheet describing the nature and risks of concussion as a prerequisite to their children's participation in sports. Many states' laws do not require youth athletes themselves to read and sign a concussion information sheet (Tomei et al., 2012). CDC's Heads Up initiative materials are explicitly mentioned in some state's laws as the guideline for creating educational materials for parents and athletes.

Some states' laws identify a specific entity, such as a state agency, to implement training and education provisions, while others are less specific.

---

[10]For detailed information on each state's concussion legislation, please see NCSL, 2013, and Sun, 2013.

State and local boards of education are the governing bodies most commonly cited as responsible for implementation of concussion laws across the country. Interscholastic athletic associations, independently or in collaboration with a board of education, are the organizations next most likely to be identified in legislation as having an implementation role, especially in the education and training of coaches and adult volunteers. Health departments are generally given supportive responsibility, although in Massachusetts, Missouri, New York, and Pennsylvania, the legislative language gives health departments primary responsibility for the development of concussion training. The only example of an academic entity that has been given the lead responsibility for the development of concussion safety training programs is the Sport-Related Traumatic Brain Injury Research Center at the University of North Carolina at Chapel Hill, which leads a coalition that is developing such programs for the state of North Carolina.

Current guidelines for the management of sports-related concussions suggest that athletes who may have sustained a concussion be removed from practice or play (see Giza et al., 2013; Harmon et al., 2013; McCrory et al., 2013). Similarly, laws in the majority of states require that a youth athlete be removed from play when a concussion is suspected. In a handful of states, the laws are more specific, stating that athletes should be removed from play when signs, symptoms, or behaviors consistent with concussion are observed (Tomei et al., 2012). North Carolina's law (House Bill 792), for example, states that "if a student participating in an interscholastic athletic activity exhibits signs or symptoms consistent with concussion," he or she should be removed from the activity at that time. Some states' laws name coaches, officials, or athletic trainers as the parties responsible for removal of an athlete from play, while most say nothing about who has this authority. Texas law specifies that parents and guardians are among the individuals who may call for the removal of a youth athlete from play (House Bill 2038). The removal-from-play requirements of concussion laws highlight the importance of education on signs, symptoms, behaviors, and other indicators (e.g., a hard impact to the head or body) of concussion for coaches, athletes, parents, and others who participate in or attend youth sporting events.

Another way in which states vary considerably is the types of health care providers who can provide clearance for return to play. Laws in several states specify that a licensed health care provider trained in concussion diagnosis and management may provide clearance for athletes to return to play. Other states allow any licensed health care provider to make such decisions, and still others say nothing about who is allowed to evaluate concussions. In states that are more specific about the types of health care providers who may make return-to-play decisions, all allow physicians to evaluate concussions, and many allow physician assistants and nurse practitioners to do so. Some states allow athletic trainers, psychologists with training in neuropsychology, or physical therapists to provide clearance for return to play. Figure 6-2 shows the types of providers who were permitted to clear youth athletes for return to play according to a review of state laws as of December 2012 (Tomei et al., 2012). As these laws are continually being updated, there may have been some shift in states' provisions regarding the types of providers who may make return-to-play decisions since the review was published.

Although a provider would need experience managing concussions in order to provide clearance for return to play, there is no consensus regarding why a particular health professional should perform this function or whether one type of professional should be preferred over another (Harvey, 2013). A qualitative assessment of concussion laws in Washington state and Massachusetts (discussed in the following section) noted that parents and athletes in rural and low-income communities face greater barriers than do those in other communities to accessing experts in concussion assessment and management services who can provide medical clearance (CDC, 2013). This finding suggests that there is a need for broader concussion education so that more providers can deliver these services and

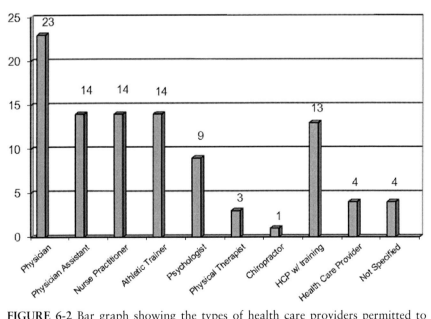

FIGURE 6-2 Bar graph showing the types of health care providers permitted to make return-to-play decisions, according to state laws as of December 2012.
NOTE: HCP = health care provider.
SOURCE: Adapted from Tomei et al., 2012.

also a need for the creation of mechanisms that local providers can use to remotely coordinate with providers with concussion expertise.

States also differ somewhat in the entities that are covered by concussion laws. In the District of Columbia, the law applies to all public, charter, parochial, and private schools, as well as athletic programs sponsored by the Department of Parks and Recreation and nonprofit and for-profit organizations (Athletic Concussions Protection Act of 2011). However, state concussion laws often cover only school athletic teams and include no specific requirements or guidelines for recreational leagues (CDC, 2013). College athletes are not affected by state concussion legislation, which leaves organizations such as the NCAA to implement concussion management policies at this level.

As discussed in Chapter 3, baseline neurocognitive testing may be a useful tool in the evaluation of concussion. Currently, a small number of states (e.g., Pennsylvania and Rhode Island) recommend baseline testing. Other states, such as Massachusetts, have recently introduced legislation to mandate baseline neurocognitive testing for youth athletes.

Implementation and Efficacy of State Concussion Laws

Of the 47 fully enacted and adopted state laws, 39 of them (83 percent) were passed between 2011 and 2013 and are in the early stages of implementation; many of them have already been or are in the process of being amended and revised. No comprehensive evaluation of the implementation and efficacy of these laws or their specific provisions has yet been published. While undertaking such an analysis will be necessary, it will be challenging in the absence of pre-legislation baseline data, especially for those provisions directed at assessing public awareness and professional education.

Investigators at the University of Washington administered a survey to youth soccer parents, coaches, and adult volunteers 1 year after the passage of the Lystedt Law (House Bill 1824) to assess knowledge about concussion and the return-to-play guidelines contained in the legislation (Shenouda et al., 2012). The law specifically requires that athletes, coaches, and parents be educated about concussions and annually sign an information sheet before the start of practice or competition. In Washington State, local boards of education in collaboration with the interscholastic activities association are responsible for developing the educational materials and for the administration of the signed information forms. The law also explicitly states that all youth athletes suspected of sustaining a concussion must be immediately removed from play and receive written medical clearance from a licensed health care provider before returning to play. The survey by Shenouda and colleagues was electronically distributed over 2 consecutive months at the beginning of the 2010 soccer season to a convenience sample of adults receiving the electronic newsletter of the Washington Youth Soccer association. Of the 391 survey respondents, 63 percent were parents, 20 percent were coaches, and 17 percent were non-coach volunteers. Almost all respondents (>90 percent) had good general knowledge about concussions (e.g., knew that a concussion is a type of traumatic brain injury, that concussions may occur without loss of consciousness, and that identifying and treating a first concussion may prevent further injury). Ninety percent appropriately said that they would elect to delay return to play in the face of a neurologic symptoms scenario. Eighty-five percent were aware that the Lystedt Law requires that a youth athlete be evaluated by a trained professional before he or she can return to play. However, only 73 percent were aware that the return-to-play provisions of the law require written clearance from a licensed health care provider, and 80 percent were unaware that the health care provider could be a volunteer (Shenouda et al., 2012).

Oklahoma's concussion law (Senate Bill 1700), which was passed in May 2010, requires school districts to work with the Oklahoma Secondary School Activities Association (OSSAA) to develop concussion guidelines and educational materials for coaches, youth athletes, and parents. To reinforce the law, OSSAA worked with the Oklahoma State Department of Health Injury Prevention Service to disseminate CDC Heads Up campaign materials to YMCAs and schools. Thirty-four YMCAs, 958 schools, and 205 martial arts schools received the information. An evaluation of this effort showed that of 163 schools that received the materials and responded to a survey, all reported that they were aware of the law, and 79 percent reported that their schools had strengthened their return-to-play policies in response to the law. All but one school responded that its coaches had been notified about the law and return-to-play guidelines (Langthorn and Wendling, 2012).

An online survey of high school varsity football coaches in Connecticut evaluated the effectiveness of mandatory concussion education for coaches required under the state's concussion law. The survey included three knowledge questions that were part of the coaching education. Seventy-six of 143 coaches responded to the survey, and most (>70 percent) responded correctly to concussion knowledge questions relating to concussion risk factors and signs and symptoms, and most (>85 percent) also responded correctly to questions about when to remove an athlete from play. Sixty-six percent of the coaches responded that the mandatory concussion education required in the law was "definitely" or "probably" useful, but only half responded that they felt the mandatory concussion education increased their knowledge of concussions. Although the survey had no information about what concussion knowledge these coaches possessed prior to receiving the mandatory coaching education, the authors noted that after the coaches had received the education, the accuracy of their responses to some questions was lower than in a previous survey of high school football coaches in New England (Guilmette et al., 2007). The low overall response rate (53 percent) for this study was a major limitation, as coaches who responded may have viewed the concussion education more positively or gained more from the education (Trojian and Hoey, 2012).

Because state concussion laws do not always provide guidance on how they should be carried out, implementers are sometimes required to make decisions after the law has passed that can influence the success of the implementation (CDC, 2013). CDC's National Center for Injury Prevention and Control conducted a case study evaluation of the implementation of legislation in Washington state and Massachusetts, two of the first states to adopt concussion legislation. Using information from interviews with stakeholders at the state level (health departments and statewide Inter-scholastic Athletic Associations) and at the school level (athletic directors and coaches), the evaluation assessed implementation efforts and related challenges and successes in order to inform implementation in other states (CDC, 2013). The evaluation identified the following factors as important for successful implementation of state concussion laws:

- the involvement of a wide range of stakeholders in the imple-mentation planning process in order to identify various barriers and facilitators to implementation and to improve outreach and education;
- the development of a comprehensive and specific implementation plan early on to support the consistent and complete implementa-tion of the law by the various stakeholders;
- the consideration of a broad approach to injury prevention, such as combining the return-to-play protocols for concussion with those for other sports-related injuries;
- communication with and provision of resources to recreational leagues to whom the state law does not apply by, for example, providing public access to resources developed for entities that are covered under the law;
- continuing education for individuals involved in the diagnosis and management of sports-related concussions to ensure that they stay up to date on the latest science; and
- consideration of the importance of educating teachers about con-cussions and "return to academics" in order to increase their un-derstanding of the symptoms and management of concussions.

The case study also highlighted the importance of planning ahead to as-sess the effects of a law. In addition to determining what types of evaluation should be conducted (e.g., evaluations of the implementation or the impact of the law), it is important to take into account staff time and capacity to conduct the evaluations and also to consider potential sources of additional funding for the evaluations. The data elements needed to respond to the questions of interest also should be considered. Data may be available through existing administrative databases or collected via instruments developed specifically for the evaluation (CDC, 2013).

Although no definitive conclusions can be drawn from the experiences of these states, with similar legislation being broadly implemented across the country there is ample opportunity for impact analysis and evaluation. Ultimately, as educators, advocates, providers, parents, and researchers all learn from one another about what works best in terms of legislation, a set of model provisions may be identified that can then be applied with uniformity, minimizing state-to-state variability and objectively informing policy makers as they move forward in dealing with youth concussions.

It is important to note that state concussion legislation is only one of several policy layers that shape concussion education and management. Sports clubs, school districts, and even individual schools may have their own policies. Health care provider protocols and standing orders also may influence how concussions are managed. Exactly how these various levels of policy will interact remains a question.

FINDINGS

The committee offers the following findings concerning protection and prevention strategies aimed at youth concussions:

- There is little evidence that current helmet designs reduce the risk of sports-related concussions in young athletes. However, there is evidence that helmets reduce the risk of other injuries, such as skull fractures, and thus the use of properly fitted helmets should be promoted.
- There is currently no evidence that mouthguards or facial protection, such as face masks worn in ice hockey, reduce concussion risk. These devices are known to reduce the risk of other sports-related injuries—such as those to the eyes, face, mouth, and teeth—and their use is important for this reason.
- The marketing of some protective devices designed for youth athletes, such as mouthguards and soccer head gear, has included statements that these devices reduce concussion risk without sufficient scientific foundation to support such claims.
- Reductions in a specific biomechanical parameter, such as head acceleration, by a particular protective device do not correspond to

an equivalent reduction in concussion risk because of the nonlinear relationship between the mechanical input and injury risk.

- Current testing standards and rating systems for protective devices do not incorporate measures of rotational head acceleration or velocity and therefore do not comprehensively evaluate a particular device's ability to mitigate concussion risk.
- While the concept of limiting the number of head impacts is fundamentally sound, implementing a specific threshold for the number of impacts or for the magnitude of impacts per week or per season is without scientific basis based on the evidence available at this time.
- While additional research across a variety of sports is needed, some studies involving youth ice hockey and soccer players have shown that the enforcement of rules and fair play policies contributes to reductions in the incidence of sports-related injuries, including concussions.
- Research indicates that concussion education programs are effective in improving concussion knowledge, although there is a lack of research concerning the effect of these interventions on behavior. Preliminary evidence suggests a need for additional research to evaluate the effectiveness of educational programs that emphasize improving attitudes and beliefs about concussions among athletes, coaches, and parents in order to improve concussion reporting among youth athletes.
- Most state concussion laws include requirements for concussion education, criteria for removal from play, and standards for health care providers who make return-to-play decisions. There is variation across states in the specific educational requirements for coaches, student athletes, and parents; the qualifications of providers who are permitted to make return-to-play decisions; and the populations to which the legislation applies. Given that most states are in the early stages of implementing these laws, there is so far very little evidence of their efficacy.

REFERENCES

AAAM (Association for the Advancement of Automotive Medicine). 1998. The Abbreviated Injury Scale, 1998 revision (AIS-98) Des Plaines, Illinois.

ADA (American Dental Association). 2004. The importance of using mouthguards: Tips for keeping your smile safe. *Journal of the American Dental Association* 135(7):1061.

Ahmed, O. H., S. J. Sullivan, A. G. Schneiders, and P. McCrory. 2010. iSupport: Do social networking sites have a role to play in concussion awareness? *Disability and Rehabilitation* 32(22):1877-1883.

Allison, M. A., Y. S. Kang, M. R. Maltese, J. H. Bolte, and K. B. Arbogast. 2013. Validation of a helmet-based system to measure head impact biomechanics in ice hockey. *Medicine and Science in Sports and Exercise* 46(1):115-123.

Arbogast, K. B., A. D. McGinley, C. L. Master, M. F. Grady, R. L. Robinson, and M. R. Zonfrillo. 2013. Cognitive rest and school-based recommendations following pediatric concussion: The need for primary care support tools. *Clinical Pediatrics* 52(5):397-402.

Asplund, C., S. Bettcher, and J. Borcher. 2009. Facial protection and head injuries in ice hockey: A systematic review. *British Journal of Sports Medicine* 43(13):993-999.

Bagley, A. F., D. H. Daneshvar, B. D. Shanker, D. Zurakowski, C. A. d'Hemecourt, C. J. Nowinski, R. C. Cantu, and K. Goulet. 2012. Effectiveness of the SLICE Program for youth concussion education. *Clinical Journal of Sport Medicine* 22(5):385-389.

Barbic, D., J. Pater, and R. J. Brison. 2005. Comparison of mouth guard designs and concussion prevention in contact sports. *Clinical Journal of Sport Medicine* 15(5):294-298.

Becker, M. H. 1974. The Health Belief Model and personal health behavior. *Health Education Monographs* 2:324-473.

Beckwith, J. G., R. M. Greenwald, and J. J. Chu. 2012. Measuring head kinematics in football: Correlation between the head impact telemetry system and Hybrid III headform. *Annals of Biomedical Engineering* 40(1):237-248.

Bemelmanns, P., and P. Pfeiffer. 2001. Shock absorption capabilities of mouthguards in different types and thicknesses. *International Journal of Sports Medicine* 22(2):149-153.

Benson, B. W., N. G. H. Mohtadi, M. S. Rose, and W. H. Meeuwisse. 1999. Head and neck injuries among ice hockey players wearing full face shields vs. half face shields. *JAMA* 292(24):2328-2332.

Benson, B. W., M. S. Rose, and W. H. Meeuwisse. 2002. The impact of face shield use on concussions in ice hockey: A multivariate analysis. *British Journal of Sports Medicine* 36(1):27-32.

Benson, B. W., G. M. Hamilton, W. H. Meeuwisse, P. McCrory, and J. Dvořák. 2009. Is protective equipment useful in preventing concussion? A systematic review of the literature. *British Journal of Sports Medicine* 43(Suppl 1):i56-i57.

Benson, B. W., A. S McIntosh, D. Maddocks, S. A. Herring, M. Raftery, and J. Dvořák. 2013. What are the most effective risk-reduction strategies in sport concussion? *British Journal of Sports Medicine* 47(5):321-326.

Bloodgood, B., D. Inokuchi, W. Shawver, K. Olson, R. Hoffman, E. Cohen, K. Sarmiento, and K. Muthuswamy. 2013. Exploration of awareness, knowledge, and perceptions of traumatic brain injury among American youth athletes and their parents. *Journal of Adolescent Health* 53(1):34–39.

BLS (Bureau of Labor Statistics). 2012. What umpires, referees, and other sports officials do. http://www.bls.gov/ooh/entertainment-and-sports/umpires-referees-and-other-sports-officials.htm#tab-2 (accessed August 5, 2013).

Boden, B. P., D. T. Kirkendall, and W. E. Garrett. 1998. Concussion incidence in elite college soccer players. *American Journal of Sports Medicine* 26(2):238-241.

Bramley, H., K. Patrick, E. Lehman, and M. Silvis. 2012. High school soccer players with concussion education are more likely to notify their coach of a suspected concussion. *Clinical Pediatrics (Phila)* 51(4):332-336.

Burke, M. J., J. Chundamala, and C. H. Tator. 2012. Deficiencies in concussion education for Canadian medical students. *Canadian Journal of Neurological Sciences* 39(6):763-766.

Camarillo, D. B., P. B. Shull, J. Mattson, R. Shultz, and D. Garza. An instrumented mouthguard for measuring linear and angular head impact kinematics in American football. *Annals of Biomedical Engineering* 41(9):1939-1949.

Cater, H. L., L. E. Sundstrom, and B. Morrison. 2006. Temporal development of hippocampal cell death is dependent on tissue strain but not strain rate. *Journal of Biomechanics* 39(15):2810-2818.

CDC (Centers for Disease Control and Prevention). 2009. *Heads Up: Concussion in Youth Sports. Activity Report, 2007–2008.* Atlanta, GA: U.S. Department of Health and Human Services, Centers for Disease Control and Prevention. http://www.cdc.gov/concussion/pdf/Heads_Up_Activity_Report_Final-a.pdf (accessed August 5, 2013).

CDC. 2011. Heads Up: Brain injury in your practice. http://www.cdc.gov/concussion/headsup/physicians_tool_kit.html (accessed August 5, 2013).

CDC. 2012a. Heads Up: Concussion in youth sports. http://www.cdc.gov/concussion/HeadsUp/youth.html (accessed August 5, 2013).

CDC. 2012b. Heads Up to schools: Know your concussion ABCs. http://www.cdc.gov/concussion/headsup/schools.html#3 (accessed August 5, 2013).

CDC. 2013. Implementing return to play: Learning from the experiences of early implementers. http://www.cdc.gov/concussion/policies/rtp_implementation.html (accessed August 5, 2013).

Chrisman, S. P., M. A. Schiff, and F. P. Rivara. 2011. Physician concussion knowledge and the effect of mailing the CDC's "Heads Up" toolkit. *Clinical Pediatrics (Phila)* 50(11):1031-1039.

Collins, C. L., S. K. Fields, and R. D. Comstock. 2008. When the rules of the game are broken: What proportion of high school sports-related injuries are related to illegal activity? *Injury Prevention* 14(1)34-38.

Collins, M., M. R. Lovell, G. L. Iverson, T. Ide, and J. Maroon. 2006. Examining concussion rates and return to play in high school football players wearing newer helmet technology: A three-year prospective cohort study. *Neurosurgery* 58(3):275-286.

Cook, D. J., M. D. Cusimano, C. H. Tator, and M. L. Chipman. 2003. Evaluation of the ThinkFirst Canada, Smart Hockey, brain and spinal injury prevention video. *Injury Prevention* 9(4):361-366.

Council of Ivy League Presidents. 2011. Ivy League presidents approve concussion-curbing measures for football. http://www.ivyleaguesports.com/sports/fball/2011-12/releases/Ivy_League_Presidents_Approve_Concussion-Curbing_Measures_for_Football (accessed August 5, 2013).

Council of Ivy League Presidents. 2012. Ivy League presidents approve concussion recommendations for lacrosse and soccer. http://www.ivyleaguesports.com/information/gen-releases/2012-13/releases/Ivy_League_Presidents_Approve_Concussion_Recommendations_for_Lacrosse_and_Soccer (accessed August 5, 2013).

Covassin, T., R. J. Elbin, and K. Sarmiento. 2012. Educating coaches about concussion in sports: Evaluation of the CDC's "Heads Up: Concussion in Youth Sports" initiative. *Journal of School Health* 82(5):233-238.

CPSC (Consumer Product Safety Commission). 2009. Injuries and investigated deaths associated with playground equipment, 2001–2008. http://www.cpsc.gov//PageFiles/108596/playground.pdf (accessed August 5, 2013).

CPSC. 2010. *Public Playground Safety Handbook.* Bethesda, MD: U.S. Consumer Product Safety Commission. http://www.cpsc.gov//PageFiles/122149/325.pdf (accessed August 5, 2013).

Cusimano, M. D., N. A. Taback, S. R. McFaull, R. Hodgins, T. M. Bekele, and N. Elfeki. 2011. Effect of bodychecking on rate of injuries among minor hockey players. *Open Medicine* 5(1):E57-E64.

Cusimano, M. D., S. Nastis, and L. Zuccaro. 2013. Effectiveness of interventions to reduce aggression and injuries among ice hockey players: A systematic review. *Canadian Medical Association Journal* 185(1):E57-E69.

Cusimano, M. D., M. Chipman, P. Donnelly, and M. G. Hutchison. 2014. Effectiveness of an educational video on concussion knowledge in minor league hockey players: A cluster randomized controlled trial. *British Journal of Sports Medicine* 48(2):141-146.

Daneshvar, D. H., C. M. Baugh, C. J. Nowinski, A. C. McKee, R. A. Stern, and R. C. Cantu. 2011. Helmets and mouth guards: The role of personal equipment in preventing sport-related concussions. *Clinics in Sports Medicine* 30(1):145-163.

Delaney, J. S., A. Al-Kashmiri, R. Drummond, and J. A. Correa. 2008. The effect of protective headgear on head injuries and concussions in adolescent football (soccer) players. *British Journal of Sports Medicine* 42(2):110-115.

Dragoo, J. L., H. J. Braun, J. L. Durham, M. R. Chen, and A. H. Harris. 2012. Incidence and risk factors for injuries to the anterior cruciate ligament in National Collegiate Athletic Association football: Data from the 2004–2005 through 2008–2009 National Collegiate Athletic Association Injury Surveillance System. *American Journal of Sports Medicine* 40(5):990-995.

Duma, S. M., S. Rowson, B. Cobb, A. MacAllister, T. Young, and R. Daniel. 2013. Effectiveness of Helmets in the Reduction of Sports-Related Concussions in Youth. Commissioned Paper. Committee on Sports-Related Concussions in Youth.

Echlin, P. S., A. M. Johnson, S. Riverin, C. H. Tator, R. C. Cantu, M. D. Cusimano, J. E. Taunton, R. E. G. Upshur, C. R. Hall, L. A. Forwell, and E. N. Skopelja. 2010. A prospective study of concussion education in 2 junior ice hockey teams: Implications for sports concussion education. *Neurosurgery Focus* 29(5):E6.

Elkin, B. S., and B. Morrison. 2007. Region-specific tolerance criteria for the living brain. *Stapp Car Crash Journal* 51:127-138.

Emery, C. A., and W. J. Meeuwisse. 2006. Injury rates, risk factors, and mechanisms of injury in minor hockey. *American Journal of Sports Medicine* 34(12):1960-1969.

Emery, C. A., B. Hagel, M. Cecloe, and C. McKay. 2010a. Risk factors for injury and severe injury in youth ice hockey: A systematic review of the literature. *Injury Prevention* 16(2):113-118.

Emery, C. A., J. Kang, I. Shrier, C. Goulet, B. E. Hagel, B. W. Benson, A. Nettel-Aguirre, J. R. McAllister, G.M. Hamilton, and W. H. Meeuwisse. 2010b. Risk of injury associated with body checking among youth ice hockey players. *JAMA* 303(22):2265-2272.

Finch, C. F., A. S. McIntosh, and P. McCrory. 2001. What do under 15 year old schoolboy rugby union players think about protective headgear? *British Journal of Sports Medicine* 35(2):89-94.

Finch, C., R. Braham, A. McIntosh, P. McCrory, and R. Wolfe. 2005. Should football players wear custom fitted mouthguards? Results from a group randomized controlled trial. *Injury Prevention* 11(4):242-246.

Forero Rueda, M. A., L. Cui, and M. D. Gilchrist. 2011. Finite element modeling of equestrian helmet impacts exposes the need to address rotational kinematics in future helmet designs. *Computer Methods in Biomechanics and Biomedical Engineering* 14(12):1021-1031.

Fuller, C. W., R. W. Dick, J. Corlette, and R. Schmalz. 2007. Comparison of the incidence, nature and cause of injuries sustained on grass and new generation artificial turf by male and female football players. Part 1: Match injuries. *British Journal of Sports Medicine* 41(Suppl I):i20-i26.

Funk, J. R., S. Rowson, R. W. Daniel, and S. M. Duma. 2012. Validation of concussion risk curves for collegiate football players derived from HITS data. *Annals of Biomedical Engineering* 40(1):79-89.

Gadd, C. W. 1966. Use of a weighted-impulse criterion for estimating injury hazard. In *Proceedings of the 10th Stapp Car Crash Conference*. New York: Society of Automotive Engineers. Pp. 164-174.

Gennarelli, T., L. Thibault, G. Tomei, R. Wiser, D. Graham, and J. Adams. 1987. Directional dependence of axonal brain injury due to centroidal and non-centroidal acceleration. In *Proceedings of the 31st Stapp Car Crash Conference*. New York: Society of Automotive Engineers.

Gianotti, S., and P. A. Hume. 2007. Concussion sideline management intervention for rugby union leads to reduced concussion claims. *NeuroRehabilitation* 22(3):181-189.

Gilchrist, J., K. E. Thomas, L. Xu, L. C. McGuire, and V. Coronado. 2011. Nonfatal traumatic brain injuries related to sports and recreation activities among persons ≤19 years—United States, 2001–2009. *Morbidity and Mortality Weekly Report* 60(39):1337-1342.

Giza, C. C., J. S. Kutcher, S. Ashwal, J. Barth, T. S. D. Getchius, G. A. Gioia, G. S. Gronseth, K. Guskiewicz, S. Mandel, G. Manley, D. B. McKeag, D. J. Thurman, and R. Zafonte. 2013. Summary of evidence-based guideline update: Evaluation and management of concussion in sports. *Neurology* 80(24):2250-2257.

Glang, A., M. C. Koester, S. Beaver, J. Clay, and K. McLaughlin. 2010. Online training in sports concussion for youth sports coaches. *International Journal of Sports Science and Coaching* 5(1):1-12.

Guilmette, T. J., L. A. Malia, and M. D. McQuiggan. 2007. Concussion understanding and management among New England high school football coaches. *Brain Injury* 21(10): 1039-1047.

Guskiewicz, K. 2013. The Role of Sports Rules and Training in the Prevention of Sports-Related Concussions in Youth. Presentation before the committee, Washington, DC, February 25.

Guskiewicz, K. M., N. L. Weaver, D. A. Padua, and W. E. Garrett. 2000. Epidemiology of concussion in collegiate and high school football players. *American Journal of Sports Medicine* 28(5):643-650.

Hagel, B., and W. Meeuwisse. 2004. Risk compensation: A "side effect" of sport injury prevention? *Clinical Journal of Sport Medicine* 14(4):193-196.

Hagel, B. E., I. B. Pless, C. Goulet, R.W. Platt, and Y. Robitaille. 2005. Effectiveness of helmets in skiers and snowboarders: Case-control and case crossover study. *British Medical Journal* 330(7486):281-283.

Halldin, P., A. Gilchrist, and N. J. Mills. 2001. A new oblique impact test for motorcycle helmets. *International Journal of Crashworthiness* 6(1):53-64.

Hansen, K., N. Dau, F. Feist, C. Deck, R. Willinger, S. M. Madey, and M. Bottlang. 2013. Angular Impact Mitigation system for bicycle helmets to reduce head acceleration and risk of traumatic brain injury. *Accident Analysis and Prevention* 59:109-117.

Hardy, W. N., C. D. Foster, M. J. Mason, K. H. Yang, A. I. King, and S. Tashman. 2001. Investigation of head injury mechanisms using neutral density technology and high-speed biplanar x-ray. *Stapp Car Crash Journal* 45:337-368.

Harmon, K. G., J. A. Drezner, M. Gammons, K. M. Guskiewicz, M. Halstead, S. A. Herring, J. S. Kutcher, A. Pana, M. Patukian, and W. O. Roberts. 2013. American Medical Society for Sports Medicine position statement: Concussion in sport. *British Journal of Sports Medicine* 47(1):15-26.

Harvey, H. H. 2013. Reducing traumatic brain injuries in youth sports: Youth sports traumatic injury state laws, January 2009-December 2012. *American Journal of Public Health* 103(7):1249-1254.

Havlik, H. S. 2010. Equestrian sport-related injuries: A review of current literature. *Current Sports Medicine Reports* 9(5):299-302.

Hedlund, J. 2000. Risky business: Safety regulations, risk compensation, and individual behavior. *Injury Prevention* 6(2):82-90.

Hendrickson, C. D., K. Hill, and J. E. Carpenter. 2008. Injuries to the head and face in women's collegiate field hockey. *Clinical Journal of Sport Medicine* 18(5):399-402.

Hickey, J., A. Morris, L. Carlson, and T. E. Seward. 1967. The relation of mouth protectors to cranial pressure and deformation. *Journal of the American Dental Association* 74(4):735-740.

Hodgson, V., L. Thomas, and T. Khali. 1983. The role of impact location in reversible cerebral concussion. In *Proceedings of the 27th Stapp Car Crash Conference*. New York: Society of Automotive Engineers.

Hoffman, J., G. Alfter, and N. K. Rudolph. 1999. Experimental comparative study of various mouthguards. *Endodontics and Dental Traumatology* 15(4):157-163.

Hollis, S. J., M. R. Stevenson, A. S. McIntosh, E. A. Shores, M. W. Collins, and C. B. Taylor. 2009. Incidence, risk, and protective factors of mild traumatic brain injury in a cohort of Australian nonprofessional male rugby players. *American Journal of Sports Medicine* 37(12):2328-2333.

Hoshizake, T. B., and S. E. Brien. 2004. The science and design of head protection in sport. *Neurosurgery* 55(4):956-967.

Jadischke R., D. C. Viano, N. Dau, A. I. King, and J. McCarthy. 2013. On the accuracy of the Head Impact Telemetry (HIT) System used in football helmets. *Journal of Biomechanics* 46(13):2310-2315.

Karton, C., P. Rousseau, M. Vassilyadi, and T. B. Hoshizake. 2012. The evaluation of speed skating helmet performance through peak linear acceleration and rotational acceleration. *British Journal of Sport Medicine*. January 11 [Epub ahead of print.]

Kaut, K. P., R. DePompei, J. Kerr, and J. Congeni. 2003. Reports of head injury and symptom knowledge among college athletes: Implications for assessment and educational intervention. *Clinical Journal of Sports Medicine* 13(4):213-221.

Kemp, S. P. T., Z. Hudson, J. H. M. Brooks, and C. W. Fuller. 2008. The epidemiology of head injuries in English professional rugby union. *Clinical Journal of Sport Medicine* 18(3):227-234.

Kimpara, H., and M. Iwamoto. 2012. Mild traumatic brain injury predictors based on angular accelerations during impacts. *Annals of Biomechanical Engineering* 40(1):114-126.

King, A. I., K. H. Yang, L. Zhang, W. Hardy, and D. C. Viano. 2003. Is head injury caused by linear or angular acceleration? IRCOBI Conference–Lisbon (Portugal). http://snell-helmets.org/docs/articles/hic/King_IRCOBI_2003.pdf (accessed August 5, 2013).

Kleiven, S. 2003. Influence of impact direction on the human head in prediction of subdural hematoma. *Journal of Neurotrauma* 20(4):365-379.

Kleiven, S. 2007. Predictors of traumatic brain injuries evaluated through accident reconstructions. *Stapp Car Crash Journal* 51:81-114.

Knapik, J. J., S. W. Marshall, R. B. Lee, S. S. Drakjy, S. B. Jones, T. A. Mitchener, G. G. dela Cruz, and B. H. Jones. 2007. Mouthguards in sport activities. History, physical properties and injury prevention effectiveness. *Sports Medicine* 37(2)117-144.

Kolodziej, M. A., S. Koblitz, C. Nimsky, and D. Hellwig. 2011. Mechanisms and consequences of head injures in soccer: A study of 451 patients. *Neurosurgery Focus* 31(5):E1.

Koutures, C. G., and A. J. M. Gregory. 2010. Injuries in youth soccer. *Pediatrics* 125(2):410-414.

Kroshus, E., D. Daneshvar, C. M. Baugh, C. J. Nowinski, and R. C. Cantu. 2013. NCAA concussion education in ice hockey: An ineffective mandate. *British Journal of Sports Medicine* 48(2):135-140.

Labella, C. R., and Mjaanes, J. 2012. Cheerleading injuries: Epidemiology and recommendations for prevention. *Pediatrics* 130(5):966-971.

Labella, C. R., B. W. Smith, and A. Sigurdsson. 2002. Effects of mouthguards on dental injuries and concussions in college basketball. *Medicine and Science in Sports and Exercise* 34(1):41-44.

Langthorn, L., and T. Wendling. 2012. Young athletes protected by concussion law. *Journal of Safety Research* 43(4):311-312.

LaPlaca, M. C., D. Kacy Cullen, J. J. McLoughlin, and R. S. Cargill. 2005. High rate shear strain of three-dimensional neural cell cultures: A new in vitro traumatic brain injury model. *Journal of Biomechanics* 38(5):1093-1105.

LaPrade, R. F., Q. M. Burnett, R. Zarzour, and R. Moss. 1995. The effect of the mandatory use of face masks on facial lacerations and head and neck injuries in ice hockey. A prospective study. *American Journal of Sports Medicine* 23(6):773-775.

Lemair, M., and D. J. Pearsall. 2007. Evaluation of impact attenuation of facial protectors in ice hockey helmets. *Sports Engineering* 10(2):65-74.

Lincoln, A. E., S. V. Caswell, J. L. Almquist, R. E. Dunn, and R. Y. Hinton. 2013. Video incident analysis of concussions in boys' high school lacrosse. *American Journal of Sports Medicine* 41(4):756-761.

MacPherson, A., L. Rothman, and A. Howard. 2006. Body-checking rules and childhood injuries in ice hockey. *Pediatrics* 117(2):e143-e147.

Marar, M., N. M. McIlvain, S. K. Fields, and R. D. Comstock. 2012. Epidemiology of concussions among United States high school athletes in 20 sports. *American Journal of Sports Medicine* 40(4):747-755.

Margulies, S., and B Coats. 2013. Experimental injury biomechanics of the pediatric head and brain. In *Pediatric Injury Biomechanics*, edited by J. R. Crandall, B. S. Myers, D. F. Meaney, and S. Zellers Schmidtke. New York: Springer. Pp. 157-189.

Margulies, S. S., L. E. Thibault, and T. A. Gennarelli. 1990. Physical model simulations of brain injury in the primate. *Journal of Biomechanics* 23(8):823-836.

Marshall, S. W., D. P. Loomis, A. E. Waller, D. J. Chalmers, Y. N. Bird, K. L. Quarrie, and M. Feehan. 2005. Evaluation of protective equipment for prevention of injuries in rugby union. *International Journal of Epidemiology* 34(1):113-118.

McCrory, P. 2001. Do mouthguards prevent concussion? *British Journal of Sports Medicine* 35(2):81-82.

McCrory, P., W. H. Meeuwisse, M. Aubry, B. Cantu, J. Dvořák, R. J. Echemendia, L. Engebretsen, K. Johnston, J. S. Kutcher, M. Raftery, A. Sills, B.W. Benson, G. A. Davis, R. G. Ellenbogen, K. Guskiewicz, S. A. Herring, G. L. Iverson, B. D. Jordan, J. Kissick, M. McCrea, A. S. McIntosh, D. Maddocks, M. Makdissi, L. Purcell, M. Putukian, K. Schneider, C. H. Tator, and M. Turner. 2013. Consensus statement on concussion in sport: The 4th International Conference on Concussion in Sport held in Zurich, November 2012. *British Journal of Sports Medicine* 47(5):250-258.

McIntosh, A. S., and P. McCrory. 2001. Effectiveness of headgear in a pilot study of under 15 rugby union football. *British Journal of Sports Medicine* 35(3):167-169.

McIntosh, A. S., and P. McCrory. 2005. Preventing head and neck injury. *British Journal of Sports Medicine* 39(6):314-318.

McIntosh, A. S., P. McCrory, C. F. Finch, J. P. Best, D. J. Chalmers, and R. Wolfe. 2009. Does padded headgear prevent head injury in rugby union football? *Medicine and Science in Sports and Exercise* 41(2):306-313.

McIntosh, A. S., T. E. Andersen, R. Bahr, R. Greenwald, S. Kleiven, M. Turner, M. Varese, and P. McCrory. 2011. Sports helmets now and in the future. *British Journal of Sports Medicine* 45(16):1258-1265.

McLaughlin, K. A., and A. Glang. 2010. The effectiveness of a bicycle safety program for improving safety-related knowledge and behavior in young elementary students. *Journal of Pediatric Psychology* 35(4):343-353.

McNutt, T., S. W. Shannon, J. T. Wright, and R. A. Feinstein. 1989. Oral trauma in adolescent athletes: A study of mouth protectors. *Pediatric Dentistry* 11(3):209-213.

Meyers, M. C. 2010. Incidence, mechanisms, and severity of game-related college football injuries on FieldTurf versus natural grass: A 3-year prospective study. *American Journal of Sports Medicine* 38(4):687-697.

Meyers, M. C., and B. S. Barnhill. 2004. Incidence, causes, and severity of high school football injuries on FieldTurf versus natural grass: A 5-year prospective study. *American Journal of Sports Medicine* 32(7):1626-1638.

Mihalik, J. P., M. A. McCaffrey, E. M. Rivera, J. E. Pardini, K. M. Guskiewicz, M. W. Collins, and M. R. Lovell. 2007. Effectiveness of mouthguards in reducing neurocognitive deficits following sports-related cerebral concussion. *Dental Traumatology* 23(1):14-20.

Mihalik, J. P., R. M. Greenwald, J. T. Blackburn, R. C. Cantu, S. W. Marshall, and K. M. Guskiewicz. 2010. Effect of infraction type on head impact severity in youth ice hockey. *Medicine and Science in Sports and Exercise* 42(8):1431-1438.

Miyashita, T. L., W. M. Timpson, M. A. Frye, and G. W. Gloeckner. 2013. The impact of an educational intervention on college athletes' knowledge of concussions. *Clinical Journal of Sport Medicine* 23(5):349-353.

Monson, K. L., W. Goldsmith, N. M. Barbaro, and G. T. Manley. 2003. Axial mechanical properties of fresh human cerebral blood vessels. *Journal of Biomechanical Engineering* 225(2):288-294.

Mueller, B. A., P. Cummings, F. P. Rivara, M. A. Brooks, and R. D. Terasaki. 2008. Injuries of the head, face, and neck in relation to ski helmet use. *Epidemiology* 19(2):270-276.

National Program for Playground Safety. 2004. State report cards. http://playgroundsafety.org/research/state-report-cards (accessed April 1, 2013).

Naunheim, R. S., A. Ryden, J. Standeven, G. Genin, L. Lewis, P. Thompson, and P. Bayly. 2003. Does soccer headgear attenuate the impact when heading a soccer ball? *Academy of Emergency Medicine* 10(1):85-90.

Navarro, R. R. 2011. Protective equipment and the prevention of concussion: What is the evidence? *Current Sports Medicine Reports* 10(1):27-31.

NCAA (National Collegiate Athletic Association). 2012. NCAA 2012-13 and 2013-14 Rules and Interpretations. http://www.ncaapublications.com/productdownloads/IH14.pdf (accessed October 9, 2013).

NCSL (National Conference of State Legislatures). 2013. Traumatic brain injury legislation. http://www.ncsl.org/issues-research/health/traumatic-brain-injury-legislation.aspx (accessed March 28, 2013).

Newman, J. A., M. C. Beusenberg, E. Fournier, N. Shewchenko, C. Withnall, A. I. King, K. Yang, L. Zhang, J. McElhaney, L. Thibault, and G. McGinnes. 1999. A new biomechanical assessment of mild traumatic brain injury: Part 1: Methodology. In *International Research Council on Biomechanics of Injury*. Pp. 17-36.

NFHS (National Federation of State High School Associations). 2011. Position statement and recommendations for mouthguard use in sports. http://www.nfhs.org/search.aspx?searchtext=mouthguard (accessed August 5, 2013).

NFHS. 2013. NFHS rules changes affecting risk, 1982–2013. www.nfhs.org/WorkArea/DownloadAsset.aspx?id=5760 (accessed September 6, 2013).

NHL (National Hockey League). 2013. NHL, NHLPA agree on mandatory visors. http://www.nhl.com/ice/news.htm?id=672983#&navid=nhl-search (accessed September 16, 2013).

Niedfeldt, M. W. 2011. Head injuries, heading, and the use of headgear in soccer. *Current Sports Medicine Reports* 10(6):324-329.

Ommaya, A. K., and T. A. Gennarelli. 1974. Cerebral concussion and traumatic unconsciousness. Correlation of experimental and clinical observations of blunt head injuries. *Brain* 97(4):633-654.

Ommaya, A. K., R. L. Grubb, and R. A. Naumann. 1971. Coup and contre-coup injury: Observations on the mechanics of visible brain injuries in the rhesus monkey. *Journal of Neurosurgery* 35(5):503-516.

Pellman, E. J., D. C. Viano, A. M. Tucker, I. R. Casson, and J. F. Waeckerle. 2003. Concussion in professional football: Reconstruction of game impacts and injuries. *Neurosurgery* 53(4):799-812.

Post, A., A. Oeur, B. Hoshisake, and M. D. Gilchrist. 2011. Examination of the relationship between peak linear and angular accelerations to brain deformation metrics in hockey helmet impacts. *Computer Methods in Biomechanics and Biomedical Engineering* 16(5):511-519.

Post, A., A. Oeur, B. Hoshisake, and M. D. Gilchrist. 2012. The influence of centric and non-centric impacts to American football helmets on the correlation between commonly used metrics in brain injury research. IRCOBI Conference Proceedings. http://ircobi.org/downloads/irc12/pdf_files/52.pdf (accessed August 5, 2013).

Raghupathi, R., and S. S. Margulies. 2002. Traumatic axonal injury after closed head injury in the neonatal pig. *Journal of Neurotrauma* 19(7):843-853.

Raghupathi, R., M. F. Mehr, M. A. Helfaer, and S. S. Margulies. 2004. Traumatic axonal injury is exacerbated following repetitive closed head injury in the neonatal pig. *Journal of Neurotrauma* 21(3):307-316.

Register-Mihalik, J. K., K. M. Guskiewicz, T. C. McLeod, L. A. Linnan, F. O. Mueller, and S. W. Marshall. 2013a. Knowledge, attitude, and concussion-reporting behaviors among high school athletes: A preliminary study. *Journal of Athletic Training* 48(5):645-653.

Register-Mihalik, J. K., L. A. Linnan, S. W. Marshall, T. C. McLeod, F. O. Meuller, and K. M. Guskiewicz. 2013b. Using theory to understand high school aged athletes' intentions to report sport-related concussion: Implications for concussion education initiatives. *Brain Injury* 27(7-8):878-886.

Roberts, W. O., J. D. Brust, B. Leonard, and B. J. Hebert. 1996. Fair-play rules and injury reduction in ice hockey. *Archives of Pediatric and Adolescent Medicine* 150(2):140-145.

Rosenstock, I. M., V. J. Strecher, and M. H. Becker. 1988. Social Learning Theory and the Health Belief Model. *Health Education Quarterly* 15(2):175-183.

Rousseau, P., A. Post, and T. B. Hoshizaki. 2009. The effects of impact management materials in ice hockey helmets on head injury criteria. *Journal of Sports Engineering and Technology* 223(4):159-165.

Rowson, S., and S. Duma. 2011. Development of the STAR evaluation system for football helmets: Integrating player head impact exposure and risk of concussion. *Annals of Biomedical Engineering* 39(8):2130-2140.

Rowson, S., and S. Duma. 2013. Brain injury prediction: Assessing the combined probability of concussion using linear and rotational head acceleration. *Annals of Biomechanical Engineering* 41(5):873-882.

Rowson, S., G. Brolinson, M. Goforth, D. Dietter, and S. Duma. 2009. Linear and angular head acceleration measurements in collegiate football. *Journal of Biomechanical Engineering* 131(6):061016 doi:10.1115/1.3130454.

Rowson, S., S. M. Duma, J. G. Beckwith, J. J. Chu, R. M. Greenwald, J. J. Crisco, P. G. Brolinson, A. C. Duhaime, T. W. McAllister, and A. C. Maerlender. 2012. Rotational head kinematics in football impacts: An injury risk function for concussion. *Annals of Biomedical Engineering* 40(1):1-13.

Sady, M. D., C. G. Vaughan, and G. A. Gioia. 2011. School and the concussed youth: Recommendations for concussion education and management. *Physical Medicine and Rehabilitation Clinics of North America* 22(4):701-719.

Sarmiento, K., J. Mitchko, C. Klein, and S. Wong. 2010. Evaluation of the Centers for Disease Control and Prevention's concussion initiative for high school coaches: "Heads Up: Concussion in High School Sports." *Journal of School Health* 80(3):112-118.

Sawyer, R. J., M. Hamdallah, D. White, M. Pruzan, J. Mitchko, and M. Huitric. 2010. High school coaches' assessments, intentions to sue, and use of a concussion prevention toolkit: Centers for Disease Control and Prevention's Heads Up: Concussion in high school sports. *Health Promotion Practice* 11(1):34-43.

Schulz, M. R., S. W. Marshall, J. Yang, F. O. Mueller, N. L. Weaver, and J. M. Bowling. 2004. A prospective cohort study of injury incidence and risk factors in North Carolina high school competitive cheerleaders. *American Journal of Sports Medicine* 32(2):396-405.

Shenouda, C., P. Hendrickson, K. Davenport, J. Barber, and K. R. Bell. 2012. The effects of concussion legislation one year later—What have we learned: A descriptive pilot survey of youth soccer player associates. *Physical Medicine and Rehabilitation* 4(6):427-435.

Shields, B. J., and G. A. Smith. 2009a. Cheerleading-related injuries in the United States: A prospective surveillance study. *Journal of Athletic Training* 44(6):567-577.

Shields, B. J., and G. A. Smith. 2009b. The potential for brain injury on selected surfaces used by cheerleaders. *Journal of Athletic Training* 46(6):595-602.

Singh, G. D., G. J. Maher, and R. R. Padilla. 2009. Customized mandibular orthotics in the prevention of concussion/mild traumatic brain injury in football players: A preliminary study. *Dental Traumatology* 25(5):515-521.

Spiotta, A. M., A. J. Bartsch, and E. C. Benzel. 2012. Heading in soccer: Dangerous play? *Neurosurgery* 70(1):1-11.

Stevens, S. T., M. Lassonde, L. deBeaumont, and J. P. Keenan. 2006. The effect of visors on head and facial injury in National Hockey League players. *Journal of Science and Medicine in Sport* 9(3):238-242.

Stuart, M. J., A. M. Smith, S. A. Malo–Ortiguera, T. L. Fischer, and D.R. Larson. 2002. A comparison of facial protection and the incidence of head, neck, and facial injuries in Junior A hockey players. A function of individual playing time. *American Journal of Sports Medicine* 30(1):39-44.

Sulheim, S., I. Holme, A. Ekeland, and R. Bahr. 2006. Helmet use and risk of head injuries in alpine skiers and snowboarders. *JAMA* 295(8):919-924.

Sullivan, S. J., A. G. Schneiders, C. Cheang, E. Kitto, H. Lee, J. Redhead, S. Ward, O. H. Ahmed, and P. R. McCrory. 2012.What's happening? A content analysis of concussion-related traffic on Twitter. *British Journal of Sports Medicine* 46(4):258-263.

Sun, J. F. 2013. See where your state stands on concussion law. http://usafootball.com/news/featured-articles/see-where-your-state-stands-concussion-law (accessed July 17, 2013).

Takeda, T., K. Ishigami, S. Hoshina, T. Ogawa, J. Handa, K. Nakajima, A. Shimada, T. Nakajima, and C. W. Regner. 2005. Can mouthguards prevent mandibular bone fractures and concussions? A laboratory study with an artificial skull model. *Dental Traumatology* 21(3):134-140.

Takhounts, E. G., R. H. Eppinger, J. Q. Campbell, R. E. Tannous, E. D. Power, and L. S. Shook. 2003. On the development of the SIMon Finite Element Head Model. *Stapp Car Crash Journal* 47:107-133.

Thompson, D. C., F. P. Rivara, and R. S. Thompson. 1996. Effectiveness of bicycle safety helmets in preventing head injuries: A case-control study. *JAMA* 276(24):1968-1973.

Thompson, D. C., F. Rivara, and R. Thompson. 2000. Helmets for preventing head and facial injuries in bicyclists. *Cochrane Database of Systematic Reviews* 2:CD001855.

Tierney, R. T., M. Higgins, S. V. Caswell, J. Brady, K. McHardy, J. B. Driban, and K. Darvish. 2008. Sex differences in head acceleration during heading while wearing soccer headgear. *Journal of Athletic Training* 43(6):578-584.

Tomei, K. L., C. Doe, C. J. Prestigiacomo, and C. D. Gandhi. 2012. Comparative analysis of state-level concussion legislation and review of current practices in concussion. *Neurosurgery Focus* 33(6):E11.

Torres, D. M., K. M. Galetta, H. W. Phillips, et al. 2013. Sports-related concussion: Anonymous survey of a collegiate cohort. *Neurology Clinical Practice* 3(4):279-287.

Triplette, J. 2013. Perspectives of Families, Coaches, and Officials. Presentation at the IOM Committee on Sports-Related Concussions in Youth Workshop, February 25. Washington, DC.

Trojian, T. H., and P. R. Hoey. 2012. Connecticut high school football coaches and concussion law CT PA 10–62. *Connecticut Medicine* 76(8):495-498.

U.S. Senate Committee on Commerce, Science, and Transportation. 2011. Concussions and the marketing of sports equipment. http://www.gpo.gov/fdsys/pkg/CHRG-112shrg73514/pdf/CHRG-112shrg73514.pdf (accessed September 6, 2013).

USA Football. 2013. See where your state stands on concussion law. http://usafootball.com/news/featured-articles/see-where-your-state-stands-concussion-law (accessed August 7, 2013).

USA Hockey. 2009. Checking the right way for youth hockey. http://www.usahockey.com/uploadedFiles/USAHockey/Menu_Coaches/Menu_Coaching_Materials/Menu_Checking_materials/Checking%20Manual_FINAL.pdf (accessed August 5, 2013).

USA Hockey. 2011. *2011–2013 Official Rules of Ice Hockey.* http://www.usahockey.com/uploadedFiles/USAHockey/Menu_Officials/Menu_RulesEquipment/2011%20-%2013%20Rulebook.pdf (accessed August 5, 2013).

USA Hockey. 2013. *2013–2017 Official Rules of Ice Hockey.* http://wwa.usahockey.com/uploadedFiles/USAHockey/Menu_Officials/Menu_RulesEquipment/2013-17%20USAH%20Rulebook.pdf (accessed September 6, 2013).

Valovich-McLeod, T., C. Schwartz, R.C. Bay, and R. Curtis. 2007. Sport-related concussion misunderstandings among youth coaches. *Clinical Journal of Sport Medicine* 17(2):140-142.

Versace, J. 1971. A review of the severity index. In *Proceedings of the 15th Stapp Car Crash Conference.* New York: Society of Automotive Engineers. Pp. 771-796.

Viano, D. C., and D. Halstead. 2012. Change in size and impact performance of football helmets from the 1970s to 2010. *Annals of Biomechanical Engineering* 40(1):175-184.

Viano, D. C., C. Withnall, and M. Wonnacott. 2012a. Effect of mouthguards on head responses and mandible forces in football helmet impacts. *Annals of Biomedical Engineering* 40(1):47-69.

Viano, D. C., C. Withnall, and D. Halstead. 2012b. Impact performance of modern football helmets. *Annals of Biomedical Engineering* 40(1):160-174.

Walsh, E. S., P. Rousseau, and T. B. Hoshizaki. 2011. The influence of impact location and angle on the dynamic response of the Hybrid III headform. *Sports Engineering* 13(3):135-143.

Williams, J. H. 2007. How safe are the new artificial turf fields? http://filebox.vt.edu/users/jhwms/SOS/Turf%20Field%20Research.pdf (accessed August 5, 2013).

Wisniewski, J. F., K. Guskiewicz, M. Trope, and A. Sigurdsson. 2004. Incidence of cerebral concussions associated with type of mouthguard used in college football. *Dental Traumatology* 20(3):143-149.

Withnall, C., N. Shewchenko, M. Wonnacott, and J. Dvořák. 2005. Effectiveness of headgear in football. *British Journal of Sports Medicine* 39(Suppl 1):40-48.

Woods, S. E., E. Zabat, M. Daggy, J. Diehl, A. Engel, and R. Okragly. 2007. Face protection in recreational hockey players. *Family Medicine* 39(7):473-476.

Yard, E. E., M. J. Schroeder, S. K. Fields, C. L. Collins, and R. D. Comstock. 2008. The epidemiology of United States high school soccer injuries, 2005–2007. *Sports Medicine* 36(10):1930-1937.

Yoganandan, N., T. A. Gennarelli, J. Zhang, F. A. Pintar, E. Takhounts, and S. A. Ridella. 2009. Association of contact loading in diffuse axonal injuries from motor vehicle crashes. *Journal of Trauma* 66(2):309-315.

Zhang, L., K. H. Yang, and A. I. King. 2004. A proposed injury threshold for mild traumatic brain injury. *Journal of Biomechanical Engineering* 126(2):226-236.

Zonfrillo, M. R., C. L. Master, M. F. Grady, F. K. Winston, J. M. Callahan, and K. B. Arbogast. 2012. Pediatric providers' self-reported knowledge, practices, and attitudes about concussion. *Pediatrics* 130(6):1120-1125.

7

Conclusions and Recommendations

SURVEILLANCE

• There is currently insufficient data to accurately estimate the incidence of sports-related concussions in youth and in subpopulations of youth. Existing surveillance systems, including the National Collegiate Athletic Association Injury Surveillance System and the High School RIO™ surveillance system, provide data for collegiate and high school–level athletes in select sports. There are very limited data on the incidence of sports-related concussions among pre-high-school-age youth and among those playing in youth clubs and recreational sports. There is also inadequate collection of data on potential concussion risk factors and modifiers. Understanding of the epidemiology of sports-related concussions is further hindered by variations in terminology and the data elements employed in relevant research. Federal interagency initiatives to identify common data elements for traumatic brain injury research, including research on concussions, and to develop the Federal Interagency Traumatic Brain Injury Research (FITBIR) informatics system may help to advance such research through the use of common definitions and standards. Incomplete data limits understanding of not only the incidence of sports-related concussions in youth overall and in specific sports but also of where there might be disparities and a need for targeted interventions. More complete epidemiological data would better enable researchers to assess the effectiveness of legislation and other interventions in reducing the incidence of sports-related concussions in youth.

Recommendation 1. The Centers for Disease Control and Prevention, taking account of existing surveillance systems and relevant federal data collection efforts, should establish and oversee a national surveillance system to accurately determine the incidence of sports-related concussions, including those in youth ages 5 to 21. The surveillance data collected should include, but not be limited to, demographic information (e.g., age, sex, race and ethnicity), preexisting conditions (e.g., attention deficit hyperactivity disorder, learning disabilities), concussion history (number and dates of prior concussions), the use of protective equipment and impact monitoring devices, and the qualifications of personnel making the concussion diagnosis. Data on the cause, nature, and extent of the concussive injury also should be collected, including

- Sport or activity
- Level of competition (e.g., recreational or competitive level)
- Event type (e.g., practice or competition)
- Impact location (e.g., head or body) and nature (e.g., contact with playing surface, another player, equipment)
- Signs and symptoms consistent with a concussion

EVIDENCE-BASED GUIDELINES FOR CONCUSSION DIAGNOSIS AND MANAGEMENT

- Research involving animals and individuals with more severe head injuries has provided a limited understanding of neurophysiological changes that take place following a concussion and of potential biomarkers of concussion. As the diagnosis of concussion is currently based primarily on symptoms, there is a major need for objective diagnostic markers of concussion as well as for objective markers of recovery. Neuropsychological tests used alone will not be appropriate for the identification of concussions or for diagnosis until better studies are conducted that can provide more accurate and valid information about the relation of test scores to cognitive impairment after a concussion.
- Existing guidelines for the treatment and management of concussions and their short- and long-term sequelae in youth are based primarily on clinical experience rather than on scientific evidence. Additional prospective studies that include children and adolescents are needed in order to be able to define typical and atypical recovery from sports-related concussion. Randomized controlled trials or

other appropriately designed studies on the management of concussion and on post-concussion syndrome in youth are needed in order to develop empirically based clinical guidelines, including studies to determine the efficacy of physical and cognitive rest following concussion, the optimal period of rest, and the best protocol for returning individuals to full physical activity as well as to inform the development of evidence-based protocols and appropriate accommodations for students returning to school. Prospective studies to delineate individual differences in concussion symptomatology and course as well as the predictors of recovery and persistence in children and adolescents with sports-related concussions are also needed in order to identify individuals who are likely to have persistent symptoms and therefore to be in need of intervention.

Recommendation 2. The National Institutes of Health and the Department of Defense should support research to (1) establish objective, sensitive, and specific metrics and markers of concussion diagnosis, prognosis, and recovery in youth and (2) inform the creation of age-specific, evidence-based guidelines for the management of short- and long-term sequelae of concussion in youth.

SHORT- AND LONG-TERM CONSEQUENCES OF CONCUSSIONS AND REPETITIVE HEAD IMPACTS

- Epidemiological studies of the neurocognitive effects of repetitive head impacts (i.e., head impacts that do not result in symptoms of concussion) and multiple concussions in high school and collegiate athletes have had mixed results, and many are limited by small sample sizes and methodological weaknesses. There are limited data from imaging research indicating that repetitive head impacts result in changes to the integrity of brain white matter. Research involving retired professional football players provides preliminary evidence of a positive association between the number of concussions an athlete has sustained and the risk of depression; however, data on the relationship between the number of concussions and the risk of suicide are not available. Whether repetitive head impacts and multiple concussions sustained in youth increases the risk for long-term neurodegenerative diseases, such as chronic traumatic encephalopathy (CTE) and Alzheimer's disease, remains unclear. Additional research is needed to determine whether CTE represents a distinct disease entity or is part of a spectrum of disease manifestations that share a common finding of tau pathology, as well as to identify biomarkers for the in vivo diagnosis of CTE and the early detection of neurodegeneration in athletes that may be related to repetitive head impacts and multiple concussions.

Recommendation 3. The National Institutes of Health and the Department of Defense should conduct controlled, longitudinal, large-scale studies to assess the short- and long-term cognitive, emotional, behavioral, neurobiological, and neuropathological consequences of concussions and repetitive head impacts over the life span. Assessments should also include an examination of the effects of concussions and repetitive head impacts on quality of life and activities of daily living. It is critical that such studies identify predictors and modifiers of outcomes, including the influence of socioeconomic status, race and ethnicity, sex, and comorbidities. To aid this research, the National Institutes of Health should maintain a national brain tissue and biological sample repository to collect, archive, and distribute material for research on concussions.

AGE-APPROPRIATE RULES AND PLAYING STANDARDS

- Rules are the foundation for safe play in sports and have the potential to discourage player behaviors that may increase the risk of injury and to advance a culture in which youth athletes are not pressured to play through their injuries or return to activity before they have fully recovered. There is some evidence from studies of youth ice hockey and soccer that the modification and enforcement of rules to promote player safety and fair play policies contribute to a reduction in practices that contribute to sports-related injuries, including concussions. Although this evidence is promising, more rigorous research is needed to measure the effectiveness of rules, regulations, and playing standards across a variety of sports and among youth athletes at different ages for fostering changes in norms and beliefs (e.g., among athletes, coaches, officials, and parents) and reducing the occurrence of concussions and other injuries. Such research also is needed to inform the development of effective standards for return to physical and cognitive (e.g., school, work) activity.

Recommendation 4. The National Collegiate Athletic Association, in conjunction with the National Federation of State High School Associations, national governing bodies for youth sports, and youth sport organizations, should undertake a rigorous scientific evaluation of the effectiveness of age-appropriate techniques, rules, and playing and practice standards in reducing sports-related concussions and sequelae.

The Department of Defense should conduct equivalent research for sports and physical training, including combatives, at military service academies and for military personnel.

BIOMECHANICS, PROTECTIVE EQUIPMENT, AND SAFETY STANDARDS

- Available studies of head injury biomechanics are based on models that have limited applicability to concussions in youth or to concussions that occur in sports environments. Thus there is currently inadequate data to determine the thresholds associated with sports-related concussive injuries in youth. In addition, it is unclear if or when the threshold of injury for a second concussion might be lower than for an initial injury. Research is needed to identify biomechanical thresholds and risk curves specifically for sports-related concussions in youth to better inform the development of protective equipment, head-impact-monitoring devices, athletic training programs, and sports rules in an effort to reduce sports-related concussions in youth. Given the potential physiological differences in concussion risk between males and females and youth of different ages, this research should explicitly take into account both age and sex.

Recommendation 5. The National Institutes of Health and the Department of Defense should fund research on age- and sex-related biomechanical determinants of injury risk for concussion in youth, including how injury thresholds are modified by the number of and time interval between head impacts and concussions. These data are critical for informing the development of rules of play, effective protective equipment and equipment safety standards, impact-monitoring systems, and athletic and military training programs.

CULTURE CHANGE

- Acknowledgment of the seriousness of sports-related concussions has initiated a culture change, as evidenced by campaigns to educate athletes, coaches, physicians, and parents of young athletes about concussion recognition and management; by rule changes designed to reduce the risk of head injury; and by the enactment of legislation designed to protect young athletes suspected of having a concussion. Despite such efforts, there are indications that the culture shift is not complete. Athletes profess that the game and the team are more important than their individual health and that they may play through a concussion to avoid letting down their teammates, coaches, schools, and parents. Given the serious nature of concussions and the potential for additional injury during recovery, it is important to foster a culture of acceptance that encourages the reporting of concussive injury and compliance with appropriate concussion management plans, including restrictions aimed at preventing athletes from returning to play before being fully recovered.

Recommendation 6. The National Collegiate Athletic Association and the National Federation of State High School Associations, in conjunction with the Centers for Disease Control and Prevention, the Health Resources and Services Administration, the National Athletic Trainers' Association, and the Department of Education, should develop, implement, and evaluate the effectiveness of large-scale efforts to increase knowledge about concussions and change the culture (social norms, attitudes, and behaviors) surrounding concussions among elementary school through college-age youth and their parents, coaches, sports officials, educators, athletic trainers, and health care professionals. These efforts should take into account demographic variations (e.g., socioeconomic status, race and ethnicity, and age) across population groups. The Department of Defense should conduct equivalent research for military personnel and their families.

PARTNERSHIPS

- Efforts to increase concussion knowledge and to change behavior among young athletes might include the development by the Department of Education, the Centers for Disease Control and Prevention, the National Athletic Trainers Association, or other organizations of evidence-based curricula with which to educate elementary, middle, and high school students about concussions, including sports-related concussions. It will be important to evaluate the effectiveness of concussion education programs on students' knowledge of concussions and on their attitudes toward and compliance with guidelines for removal from play and return to physical and cognitive activity following concussion. Parallel efforts perhaps involving the National Collegiate Athletic Association (NCAA), the National Federation of State High School Associations, national governing bodies for youth sports, and youth sports organizations might be undertaken for collegiate athletes, coaches, and officials.

- There is a need for school administrators, teachers, guidance counselors, and school nurses or student health services to receive evidence-based education about the potential effects of concussions on cognitive function and behavior and for them to provide appropriate academic and emotional support for students recovering from concussion. The NCAA and the Department of Education could fund research to develop evidence-based curricula and procedures to assist local school districts and other institutions in implementing such education efforts.
- It is important for health care professional credentialing bodies to incorporate evidence-based standards for concussion diagnosis and management into the core curricula for students in medicine, nursing, and other health professions and to provide continuing medical education on concussion diagnosis and management to practicing professionals.

Appendix A

Public Workshop Agendas

Workshop on Sports-Related Concussions in Youth (Workshop 1)

Hosted by the IOM-NRC Committee on
Sports-Related Concussions in Youth

February 25, 2013

Room 120
National Academy of Sciences
2101 Constitution Ave., NW
Washington, DC

AGENDA

9:00 a.m.   **Welcome and Introductory Remarks**
             Robert Graham, M.D., George Washington University
             (Committee Chair)

9:10 a.m.   **The Roles of Pediatric Neurologists and Family and
             Rehabilitation Medicine Physicians in the Diagnosis and
             Management of Sports-Related Concussions in Youth**

             Paul Graham Fisher, M.D., M.H.S., Chief, Division of
             Child Neurology, Department of Neurology, Stanford
             University (10 min)

             Yvette Rooks, M.D., Executive Vice Chair and Residency
             Director, Department of Family and Community
             Medicine, University of Maryland (10 min)

Stanley Herring, M.D., Clinical Professor, Departments of Rehabilitation Medicine, Orthopedics and Sports Medicine, and Neurological Surgery, University of Washington (10 min)

DISCUSSION

10:00 a.m.   **Perspectives on Management of Students' Return to School**

Gerard Gioia, Ph.D., Chief, Division of Pediatric Neuropsychology; Director, Safe Concussion Outcome, Recovery and Education (SCORE) Program, Children's National Medical Center (10 min)

Brenda Eagan Brown, M.S.Ed., CBIS, Coordinator, Child & Adolescent Brain Injury School Re-entry Program, Brain Injury Association of Pennsylvania (10 min)

Lisa Boarman, M.S., Coordinator, School Counseling and Related Services, Howard County Public Schools, Maryland (10 min)

DISCUSSION

10:50 a.m.   **Break**

11:05 a.m.   **Sports- and Physical Training–Related Concussion in Military Personnel and Their Dependents**

Tim Kelly, M.A., ATC, Head Athletic Trainer, U.S. Military Academy (10 min)

Capt. Jack Tsao, M.D., D.Phil., Director, Traumatic Brain Injury Programs, U.S. Navy Bureau of Medicine and Surgery (10 min)

Maj. Sarah Goldman, Ph.D., OTR/L, CHT, Traumatic Brain Injury Program Manager, Rehabilitation and Reintegration Division, Army Office of the Surgeon General (10 min)

DISCUSSION

12:00 p.m.   Lunch

1:00 p.m.   Safety Standards for Protective Equipment Used in Youth Sports

              Michael Oliver, Executive Director, National Operating Committee on Standards for Athletic Equipment (10 min)

              Alan Ashare, M.D., President, Hockey Equipment Certification Council (10 min)

              DISCUSSION

1:30 p.m.   The Effectiveness of Protective Equipment for the Prevention of Sports-Related Concussions in Youth

              Stefan Duma, Ph.D., Professor and Department Head, School of Biomedical Engineering and Sciences, Virginia Tech–Wake Forest University (20 min)

              DISCUSSION

2:00 p.m.   The Role of Sports Rules and Training in the Prevention of Sports-Related Concussions in Youth

              Kevin Guskiewicz, Ph.D., ATC, FACSM, Chair, Department of Exercise and Sport Science; Director, Matthew Gfeller Sport-Related Traumatic Brain Injury Research Center, University of North Carolina at Chapel Hill (20 min)

              DISCUSSION

2:30 p.m.   Break

2:45 p.m.   Perspectives of Families, Coaches, and Officials

              Katherine Price Snedaker, M.S.W., Founder and Editor-in-Chief, SportsCAPP.com (10 min)

Michael Gray, Ed.D., 2nd Vice President, Board of Directors, National/International Alliance for Youth Sports (10 min)

Jeff Triplette, Vice Chair, National Association of Sports Officials (10 min)

DISCUSSION

3:35 p.m.   Public Comment

4:25 p.m.   **Closing Remarks**
             Robert Graham, M.D., George Washington University
             (Committee Chair)

4:30 p.m.   Adjourn

Workshop on Sports-Related Concussions in Youth (Workshop 2)

Hosted by the IOM-NRC Committee on
Sports-Related Concussions in Youth

April 15, 2013

Renaissance Seattle Hotel
Madison Ballroom, Salon B
515 Madison Street
Seattle, Washington

AGENDA

9:00 a.m.   **Welcome and Introductory Remarks**
             Robert Graham, M.D., George Washington University
             (Committee Chair)

9:05 a.m.   **Emerging Science in Concussion Risk, Diagnosis, and
             Management**

Genetic and Neurogenetic Sources of Increased Risk for Concussion and Outcome Variation Post Concussion
Thomas McAllister, M.D., Millennium Professor of Psychiatry and Neurology, Geisel School of Medicine, Dartmouth (10 min)

Concussion Biomarkers
Jeffrey Bazarian, M.D., M.P.H., Associate Professor, Departments of Emergency Medicine, Neurology, Neurosurgery, and Public Health Sciences, University of Rochester (10 min)

Concussion Imaging Technologies
Inga Koerte, M.D., Psychiatry Neuroimaging Laboratory, Harvard Medical School (10 min)

DISCUSSION

9:50 a.m.   **Mental Health Outcomes of Concussion in Children and Adolescents**

Jeffrey Max, M.D., Professor, Department of Psychiatry, University of California, San Diego, and Director, Neuropsychiatric Research, Rady Children's Hospital, San Diego (15 min)

DISCUSSION

10:15 a.m.   **Summary of American Academy of Neurology Sport Concussion Guidelines**

Christopher Giza, M.D., Associate Professor of Pediatric Neurology and Neurosurgery, Brain Injury Research Center, David Geffen School of Medicine, University of California, Los Angeles (15 min)

DISCUSSION

10:40 a.m.   Break

10:50 a.m.   **Perspectives of Youth Sports Organizations**

                    Brian Hainline, M.D., Chief Medical Officer, National
                    College Athletic Association (10 min)

                    Bob Colgate, Assistant Director, National Federation of
                    State High School Associations (10 min)

                    Carrie O'Hara-Gutierrez, Registrar, Inland Empire
                    District, Amateur Athletic Union (10 min)

                    DISCUSSION

11:35 a.m.   **Perspective of the Athlete**

                    Chris Coyne, Yale University student (15 min)

                    DISCUSSION

12:00 p.m.   **Public Comment**

12:15 p.m.   **Adjourn**

Appendix B

Biographical Sketches of Committee Members

Robert Graham, M.D. (*Chair*), is the national program director of Aligning Forces for Quality, the cornerstone of the Robert Wood Johnson Foundation's multiyear, $300 million commitment to improve the quality and equality of health care nationwide. Dr. Graham also holds an appointment as a research professor of Health Policy at George Washington University (GWU) School of Public Health and Health Services. GWU serves as the national program office of the Aligning Forces for Quality program. After receiving his medical degree, Dr. Graham began a distinguished career in health policy administration. He served as administrator of the Health Resources and Services Administration in the U.S. Public Health Service, held senior positions with the Agency for Healthcare Research and Quality and the Health Services and Mental Health Administration, and was chief executive officer of the American Academy of Family Physicians. He is currently chair of the board of the Alliance for Health Reform and a member of the Institute of Medicine (IOM). He is also a faculty member at the University of Cincinnati College of Medicine as an adjunct professor in the Department of Family and Community Medicine. Dr. Graham has served as a member of the IOM Roundtable on Environmental Health Sciences, Research, and Medicine and was on the IOM Membership Committee for Section 8 (Family Medicine, Emergency Medicine, and Physical Medicine and Rehabilitation). Dr. Graham has also chaired the IOM Committee on Lesbian, Gay, Bisexual, and Transgender Health Issues (2010-2011) and the Committee on Contributions for the Behavioral and Social Sciences in Reducing and Preventing Teen Motor Vehicle Crashes (2005-2007). He received his medical degree from the University of Kansas.

Frederick P. Rivara, M.D., M.P.H. (*Vice Chair*), is the Seattle Children's Guild Endowed Chair in Pediatrics and a professor in pediatrics at the University of Washington. He is also adjunct professor of epidemiology, chief of the Division of General Pediatrics, and vice chair of the Department of Pediatrics in the School of Medicine. He is editor-in-chief of *JAMA Pediatrics*. Dr. Rivara's career has been devoted to the study of methods to control injuries. He is founding director of the Harborview Injury Prevention and Research Center in Seattle and served as its director from 1987 until 2000, and he is founding president of the International Society for Child and Adolescent Injury Prevention. He has received numerous honors, including the Charles C. Shepard Science Award from the Centers for Disease Control and Prevention (CDC); the American Public Health Association Injury Control and Emergency Health Services Section Distinguished Career Award; the American Academy of Pediatrics, Section on Injury and Poison Prevention, Physician Achievement Award; and the University of Washington School of Public Health Distinguished Alumni Award. Dr. Rivara's contributions to the field of injury control have spanned 30 years. His interests have included the efficacy and promotion of bicycle helmets, prevention of pedestrian injuries, youth violence, epidemiology of firearm injuries, intimate partner violence, interventions for alcohol abuse in trauma patients, and the effectiveness of trauma systems in the care of pediatric and adult trauma patients. Dr. Rivara was elected a member of the IOM in 2005. He chaired the IOM Committee on Oral Health Access to Services (2010-2011) and was a member of the IOM Committee on Adolescent Health Care Services and Models of Care for Treatment, Prevention, and Healthy Development (2006-2009). He received his medical degree from the University of Pennsylvania School of Medicine and his M.P.H. from the University of Washington.

Kristy B. Arbogast, Ph.D., is the engineering core director for the Center for Injury Research and Prevention at the Children's Hospital of Philadelphia and a research associate professor of pediatrics and member of the Graduate Group of Bioengineering at the University of Pennsylvania. Currently, she is also the site director for the National Science Foundation (NSF)-sponsored Center for Child Injury Prevention Studies at Children's Hospital of Philadelphia. She heads multiple projects on motor vehicle injuries in children as well as diverse topics in pediatric biomechanics. She was a co-investigator on the Partners for Child Passenger Safety project, a 10-year national study on child passenger safety funded by State Farm Insurance, which received the CDC Health Impact Award. Dr. Arbogast's current research efforts include the biomechanics of pediatric injury for the development of new safety designs and biofidelic child anthropomorphic dummies. Both nationally and internationally, she has given many invited lectures on the biomechanics of unintentional injury to children, and has been recognized by the Society of Automotive Engineers and the Automotive Occupants Restraints Council for her work. She received her Ph.D. in bioengineering from the University of Pennsylvania.

David A. Brent, M.D., is academic chief of child and adolescent psychiatry at Western Psychiatric Institute and Clinic and professor of psychiatry, pediatrics, and epidemiology at the University of Pittsburgh School of Medicine, and he holds an endowed chair in suicide studies. His work has focused on the risk factors, genetics, treatment, and prevention of adolescent suicide and depression. His work has helped to clarify the role of firearms, substance abuse, and mood disorders as risk factors for youth suicide; has demonstrated the familial transmission of suicidal behavior; and has helped shape best practice for the management of adolescent suicidal behavior and depression. He cofounded and now directs Services for Teens at Risk (STAR), a Commonwealth of Pennsylvania–funded program for suicide prevention, the education of professionals, and the treatment of at-risk youth and their families. He was elected a member of the IOM in 2005, served on the IOM Committee on the Pathophysiology and Prevention of Adolescent and Adult Suicide (2000-2002), and currently serves on the IOM-National Research Council (NRC) Board on Children, Youth, and Families. He received his medical degree from Thomas Jefferson University Medical College and also holds an M.S. Hyg. from the University of Pittsburgh School of Public Health.

B. J. Casey, Ph.D., is the Sackler Professor of Developmental Psychobiology and director of the Sackler Institute for Developmental Psychobiology at Weill Medical College of Cornell University. She is a pioneer in novel uses of neuroimaging methodologies to examine behavioral and brain development. Her program of research focuses on attention and affect regulation, particularly their development, disruption, and neurobiological basis. She has been examining the normal development of brain circuitry involved in attention and behavioral regulation and how disruptions in these brain systems (prefrontal cortex, basal ganglia and cerebellum) can give rise to a number of developmental disorders. Using a mechanistic approach she has dissociated attentional deficits observed across the disorders of attention deficit hyperactivity disorder, obsessive compulsive disorder, Tourette syndrome, and childhood onset schizophrenia. Furthermore, Dr. Casey and her colleagues have developed marker tasks that appear to tap the integrity of specific parallel basal ganglia thalamocortical circuits implicated across these disorders and to addiction. Most recently Dr. Casey and her colleagues have begun to examine the effects of gene–environment interactions on the development of affect and behavioral regulation and related brain systems. Dr. Casey received her Ph.D. in experimental psychology from the University of South Carolina, Columbia. She served on the IOM Committees on the Science of Adolescent Risk Taking (2008-2011) and on Assessing Juvenile Justice Reform (2010-2013), and is a former member of the IOM-NRC Board on Children, Youth, and Families.

Tracey Covassin, Ph.D., ATC, is an associate professor and certified athletic trainer at Michigan State University (MSU) in the departments of Kinesiology and Intercollegiate Athletics. At MSU, she is also the undergraduate athletic training program director. Her research in sports-related concussion includes sex and age differences in concussion outcomes, neurocognitive impairments, and issues associated with multiple concussions. Dr. Covassin currently directs a multisite high school and college sport-concussion outreach program in the mid-Michigan area. Dr. Covassin has more than 40 professional publications and 70 professional presentations, and has received funding as a principal investigator or co–principal investigator from external sources including the National Operating Committee on Standards for Athletic Equipment, the Department of Defense, and CDC. She received her Ph.D. in kinesiology from Temple University.

Joe Doyle is former regional manager, American Development Model, Rocky Mountains and Pacific Districts, at USA Hockey. In this role he oversaw the provision of age-appropriate curriculum to hockey associations to help coaches more effectively coach hockey players and allow players to excel at hockey. A graduate of the U.S. Air Force Academy (AFA) and inaugural inductee into AFA's Hockey Hall of Fame, Mr. Doyle was an assistant hockey coach and recruiting coordinator for the AFA on three different occasions: 1989-1990, 1994-1998, and 2002-2006.

Eric J. Huang, M.D., Ph.D., is a professor of pathology and neuropathology in the Department of Pathology at the University of California, San Francisco (UCSF). He is also director of the UCSF Pediatric Neuropathology Research Lab and staff pathologist at the San Francisco VA Medical Center. Dr. Huang's research and clinical interests include developmental neurobiology, pediatric neuropathology, and genetic mechanisms and animal models of adult-onset neurodegenerative diseases, including Parkinson's disease, frontotemporal dementia, and amyotrophic lateral sclerosis. He received his medical degree from the National Taiwan University in Taipei and his Ph.D. in molecular biology from Cornell University.

Arthur C. Maerlender, Ph.D., is a neuropsychologist and director of Pediatric Neuropsychological Services at Geisel School of Medicine at Dartmouth and Dartmouth-Hitchcock Medical Center, and is an assistant professor of psychiatry. He is the sports neuropsychologist for Dartmouth Athletics, as well as for youth, high school, college, and professional teams. He serves as the co-leader, Ivy League Concussion Research Collaboration with the Big Ten. He is on the board of governors of the Academy of Brain Injury Specialists for the U.S. Brain Injury Association. He also serves as the chair of the New Hampshire Advisory Council for Sports Concussion and is a board member of the Brain Injury Association of New Hampshire. His research and publications are in the areas of sports-related concussions and brain injury, developmental disorders, and learning disorders. He is a former representative-level rugby player and has coached Division I rugby teams. Dr. Maerlender holds a Ph.D. in counseling psychology from the University of Notre Dame and completed his postdoctoral residency in neuropsychology at Dartmouth Medical School.

Susan S. Margulies, Ph.D., is the George H. Stephenson Professor in the department of bioengineering at the University of Pennsylvania. She is an international leader in biomechanics of traumatic head injury and in ventilator-associated lung injuries. Dr. Margulies has more than 30 years of experience in the area of traumatic brain injury research: integrating mechanical properties, animal models, instrumented dolls, patient data, and computational models to identify injury mechanisms that are unique to children and to develop clinical management and therapeutic strategies. She also has experience measuring assessments of cognition, memory, and behavior in immature large animals models of traumatic brain injury. With funding from the National Institutes of Health (NIH), NSF, CDC, and the Department of Transportation, she has published over 118 peer-reviewed papers. She has served or is on the editorial boards of the *Journal of Physiology*, the *Journal of Biomechanical Engineering*, the *Journal of Biomechanics*, *American Journal of Physiology-Lung Cell and Molecular*, and the *Journal of Neurotrauma*. She has served on grant review panels for NSF, NIH, and CDC, and has chaired the NIH Respiratory Integrative Biology and Translational Research study section. Dr. Margulies is a fellow of the American Society of Mechanical Engineers, Biomedical Engineering Society, and American Institute for Medical and Biological Engineering. Dr. Margulies holds a Ph.D. in bioengineering from the University of Pennsylvania.

Dennis L. Molfese, Ph.D., is Mildred Frances Thompson Professor and Director, Center for Brain, Biology, and Behavior, in the Department of Psychology at the University of Nebraska, Lincoln. Dr. Molfese is an internationally recognized expert on the use of brain recording techniques to study the emerging relationships among brain development, language, and cognitive processes. His broad research interests include work on such projects as developmental changes in brain, language, and cognitive processes across the lifespan; the identification of risk for concussion in high school and college athletes; prediction of recovery from concussion following injury; predicting subsequent cognitive and linguistic skills from infancy; cognitive functions in and interventions for head injured adults; factors underlying lateralization of language and cognitive functions; and phonological and semantic confusions by aphasics. Dr. Molfese served as the chair of a number of national panels in the United States on learning disabilities. He is co-director of 1 of 15 national laboratories that make up the NIH Reading and Learning Disabilities Research Network. He is the recipient of a number of honors for outstanding research contributions from societies such as Sigma Xi and Phi Kappa Phi and received the Kentucky Psychologist of the Year Award. His research has been continuously funded since 1975 through grants from NIH, NSF, the Department of Education, the National Foundation/March of Dimes, the MacArthur Foundation, the Kellogg Foundation, the North Atlantic Treaty Organization, and the National Aeronautics and Space Administration. Dr. Molfese has published some 150 books, journal articles, and book chapters on the relationship between developing brain functions, language, and cognitive processes. Dr. Molfese received his Ph.D. in psychology from Penn State University.

Mayumi L. Prins, Ph.D., is associate professor in residence and director of the education program at the Brain Injury Research Center in the David Geffen School of Medicine, University of California, Los Angeles (UCLA). Her research interests include understanding the changes in brain metabolism that occur after pediatric traumatic brain injury and how alternative fuels can be used as therapeutic options for the young brain after head injury. In addition to this main focus, she is interested in repeat mild head injuries as they apply to both children and young adult athletes. Dr. Prins received a Ph.D. degree in neurobiology from UCLA. She completed a postdoctoral fellowship in the Division of Neurosurgery at UCLA and a fellowship in anatomy and cell biology at the Medical College of Virginia.

Neha P. Raukar, M.D., M.S., FACEP, is an assistant professor of emergency medicine and director of the Division of Sports Medicine at the Brown University Warren Alpert School of Medicine. She has managed concussions in the Brown University athletes since 2009 and serves on the Ivy League Athletic Medical Association. Dr. Raukar founded and serves as the medical director for the Center for Sports Medicine, which oversees the majority of concussions in the state of Rhode Island. An advocate for legislation to protect athletes from returning to play before they are ready, Dr. Raukar testified at the state senate hearings in favor of passing a concussion law. Dr. Raukar specializes in the medical management of athletic and musculoskeletal injuries. As an emergency physician with further training in sports medicine, she is uniquely trained to care for the acutely injured athlete. Her relevant research interests include the effects of concussion on the young driver, acute biomarkers to diagnose concussion, and the identification of imaging markers to predict concussion recovery. Dr. Raukar received her medical degree from Howard University.

Nancy R. Temkin, Ph.D., is a professor in the Department of Biostatistics and the Department of Neurological Surgery and an adjunct professor in the Department of Rehabilitation Medicine at the University of Washington (UW). She is currently the principal investigator for the UW Post Traumatic Stress Disorder/Traumatic Brain Injury Clinical Consortium Study Site for the Department of Defense and is a principal investigator and executive committee member for the Transforming Research and Clinical Knowledge in Traumatic Brain Injury (TRACK-TBI) consortium for the National Institute of Neurological Disorders and Stroke (NINDS). Dr. Temkin has devoted her career as a biostatistician to the study of TBI, its consequences, and potential treatments to ameliorate them. These studies have resulted in extensive experience in study design, data management, clinical trial protocol development and implementation, data quality control, and data analyses. Dr. Temkin is a fellow of the American Statistical Association and recipient of Service Award from the American Epilepsy Society. She has been on several TBI expert working groups, scientific advisory boards, and data and safety monitoring boards for CDC and NINDS. Dr. Temkin served on the IOM Committee on Gulf War and Health: Long-Term Consequences of Traumatic Brain Injury (2007-2008). She received her Ph.D. in statistics from the State University of New York (Buffalo).

Kasisomayajula Viswanath, Ph.D., is an associate professor in the Department of Social and Behavioral Sciences at the Harvard School of Public Health and in the McGraw-Patterson Center for Population Sciences at the Dana-Farber Cancer Institute. His primary research is in documenting the relationship between communication inequalities, poverty and health disparities, and knowledge translation to address health disparities. He has written more than 150 journal articles and book chapters concerning communication inequalities and health disparities, knowledge translation, public health communication campaigns, e-health and digital divide, public health preparedness and the delivery of health communication interventions to underserved populations. He is the co-editor of three books: *Mass Media, Social Control and Social Change* (Iowa State University Press, 1999), *Health Behavior and Health Education: Theory, Research & Practice* (Jossey Bass, 2008), and *The Role of Media in Promoting and Reducing Tobacco Use* (National Cancer Institute, 2008). He was also the editor of the Social and Behavioral Research section of the 12-volume *International Encyclopedia of Communication* (Blackwell Publishing, 2008). In recognition of his academic and professional achievements, Dr. Viswanath received several awards, including Outstanding Health Communication Scholar Award (2010), jointly given out by the International Communication Association and the National Communication Association, and the Mayhew Derryberry Award from the American Public Health Association for his contribution to health education research and theory (2009). He delivered the 23rd Annual Aubrey Fisher Lecture at University of Utah in 2009. He was elected Fellow of the International Communication Association (2011), the Society for Behavioral Medicine (2008), and the Midwest Association for Public Opinion Research (2006). He was also the chair of the Board of Scientific Counselors for the National Center for Health Marketing at CDC, from 2007-2010. He has served as a member of the IOM Committee on Gulf War and Health: Treatment of Chronic Multisymptom Illness (2011-2013). He is a member of the National Vaccine Advisory Committee of the U.S. Department of Health and Human Services. His research is supported by funding from private and public agencies, including NIH and CDC.

Kevin D. Walter, M.D., FAAP, is an associate professor in the Department of Orthopaedic Surgery and the Department of Pediatrics at the Medical College of Wisconsin. Board certified in pediatrics and sports medicine, Dr. Walter is currently the program director of Pediatric and Adolescent Primary Care Sports Medicine at Children's Hospital of Wisconsin and also practices at the Children's Hospital of Wisconsin Clinics-Greenway location. He is a co-founder of The Medical College of Wisconsin Sports Concussion Program. Dr. Walter has published articles and given many national presentations on a variety of sports medicine topics. He was a coauthor on "Sport-Related Concussion in Children and Adolescents" published in *Pediatrics* in 2010. He is a co-editor and author for the book *Pediatric Handbook of Concussion*. Dr. Walter's clinical interests include sports injuries in the young athlete, concussion, back pain in the adolescent athlete, and throwing injuries in the young athlete. He also has a special interest in injury prevention, sport specialization, and the culture of youth sports. He has provided medical coverage for a wide range of events and has been a team physician for several high schools and colleges. Since 2006, Dr. Walter has been a member of the Wisconsin Interscholastic Athletic Association Sports Medicine Advisory Committee where he has helped to create guidelines for the safe participation of Wisconsin's high school athletes. He was appointed to the National Federation of State High School Associations Sports Medicine Advisory Committee in 2008. He is also the vice chair of the Wisconsin Chapter of the American Academy of Pediatrics Council on Sports Medicine and Fitness, and he is a fellow of the American Academy of Pediatrics and an active member of the Council on Sports

Medicine and Fitness. Dr. Walter attended medical school at the University of Illinois at Chicago.

Joseph L. Wright, M.D., M.P.H., is senior vice president for Community Affairs and head of the Child Health Advocacy Institute, a newly established center of excellence at Children's National Medical Center in Washington, DC, the nation's third-oldest children's hospital. In that capacity, Dr. Wright provides strategic leadership for the organization's advocacy mission, public policy positions, and community partnership initiatives. Academically, Dr. Wright is professor and vice chairman in the Department of Pediatrics, as well as professor of emergency medicine and health policy at the GWU Schools of Medicine and Public Health and is among the original cohort of board-certified pediatric emergency physicians in the United States. He provides regional leadership as state medical director for pediatrics within the Maryland Institute for Emergency Medical Services Systems and national leadership as principal investigator of the federally funded Emergency Medical Services (EMS) for Children National Resource Center. Dr. Wright's major scholarly interests include emergency medical services for children, youth violence prevention, and the needs of underserved communities, areas in which he has contributed to more than 70 peer-reviewed articles, reviews, and book chapters in the scientific literature. Dr. Wright has been recognized for his advocacy work throughout his career, including the Shining Star award from the Los Angeles–based Starlight Foundation, the Fellow Achievement Award from the American Academy of Pediatrics (AAP) for exceptional contributions in injury prevention, the Distinguished Service Award from the AAP Section on Emergency Medicine, and induction into Delta Omega, the nation's public health honor society. He served as a member of the IOM Committee on Palliative and End-of-Life Care for Children and Their Families (2001-2003). He is currently a sitting member of the AAP Committee on Pediatric Emergency Medicine. Dr. Wright serves on several national advisory bodies, including as an inaugural appointee to the Department of Transportation's National EMS Advisory Council, the Board of Trustees of the National Children's Museum, the March of Dimes Public Policy Advisory Council, and recently as an Obama administration appointee to the Pediatric Advisory Committee of the Food and Drug Administration. Dr. Wright regularly delivers invited expert testimony before Congress and state and municipal legislative bodies, and has made numerous media appearances and lectures widely to both professional and lay audiences. Dr. Wright earned a B.A. from Wesleyan University in Middletown, Connecticut, his M.D. from Rutgers Biomedical and Health Sciences/New Jersey Medical School, and an M.P.H. in administrative medicine and management from GWU.

Appendix C

Clinical Evaluation Tools

CONCUSSION ASSESSMENT TOOLS

Glasgow Coma Scale

Originally developed by Teasdale and Jennett (1974), the Glasgow Coma Scale (GCS) (see Table C-1) is a scoring scale for eye opening, motor, and verbal responses that can be administered to athletes on the field to objectively measure their level of consciousness. A score is assigned to each response type for a combined total score of 3 to 15 (with 15 being normal). An initial score of less than 5 is associated with an 80 percent chance of a lasting vegetative state or death. An initial score of greater than 11 is associated with a 90 percent chance of complete recovery (Teasdale and Jennett, 1974). Because most concussed individuals score 14 or 15 on the 15-point scale, its primary use in evaluating individuals for sports-related concussions is to rule out more severe brain injury and to help determine which athletes need immediate medical attention (Dziemianowicz et al., 2012).

Standardized Assessment of Concussion

The Standardized Assessment of Concussion (SAC) (see Figure C-1) provides immediate sideline mental status assessment of athletes who may have incurred a concussion (Barr and McCrea, 2001; McCrea et al., 1998, 2000). The test contains questions designed to assess athletes' orientation, immediate memory, concentration, and delayed memory. It also includes an exertion test and brief neurological evaluation. The SAC takes approxi-

TABLE C-1 Glasgow Coma Scale

Response Type	Response	Points
Eye Opening	Spontaneous: Eyes open, not necessarily aware	4
	To speech: Nonspecific response, not necessarily to command	3
	To pain: Pain from sternum/limb/supraorbital pressure	2
	None: Even to supraorbital pressure	1
Motor Response	Obeys commands: Follows simple commands	6
	Localizes pain: Arm attempts to remove supraorbital/chest pressure	5
	Withdrawal: Arm withdraws to pain, shoulder abducts	4
	Flexor response: Withdrawal response or assumption of hemiplegic posture	3
	Extension: Shoulder adducted and shoulder and forearm internally rotated	2
	None: To any pain; limbs remain flaccid	1
Verbal Response	Oriented: Converses and oriented	5
	Confused: Converses but confused, disoriented	4
	Inappropriate: Intelligible, no sustained sentences	3
	Incomprehensible: Moans/groans, no speech	2
	None: No verbalization of any type	1

mately 5 minutes to administer and does not require a neuropsychologist to evaluate test scores. The test is scored out of 30 with a mean score of 26.6 (McCrea et al., 1996).

Studies have found the SAC to have good sensitivity and specificity (McCrea, 2001; McCrea et al., 2003), making it a useful tool for identifying the presence of concussion (Giza et al., 2013). Significant differences in scores have been reported for males and females in healthy young athletes (9 to 14 years of age), suggesting the need for separate norms for males and females in this age group (Valovich McLeod et al., 2006) as well as in high school athletes (Barr, 2003).

Sport Concussion Assessment Tool 3

The Sport Concussion Assessment Tool 3 (SCAT3) is a concussion evaluation tool designed for individuals 13 years and older. Due to its demonstrated utility, the SAC has been incorporated into this tool, which also includes the GCS, modified Maddocks questions (Maddocks et al., 1995), a neck evaluation and balance assessment, and a yes/no symptom checklist as well as information on the mechanism of injury and background information, including learning disabilities, attention deficit hyperactivity disorder,

1) ORIENTATION:		
Month: _____	0	1
Date: _____	0	1
Day of week: _____	0	1
Year: _____	0	1
Time (within 1 hr): _____	0	1
Orientation Total Score _____	/	5

2) IMMEDIATE MEMORY: (all 3 trials are completed regardless of score on trial 1 & 2; total score equals sum across all 3 trials)

List	Trial 1		Trial 2		Trial 3	
Word 1	0	1	0	1	0	1
Word 2	0	1	0	1	0	1
Word 3	0	1	0	1	0	1
Word 4	0	1	0	1	0	1
Word 5	0	1	0	1	0	1
Total						

Immediate Memory Total Score _____ / 15
(Note: Subject is not informed of delayed recall testing of memory)

NEUROLOGIC SCREENING:

Loss of Consciousness: (occurrence, duration)

Retrograde & Posttraumatic Amnesia:
(recollection of events pre- and post-injury)

Strength:

Sensation:

Coordination:

3) CONCENTRATION:

Digits Backward (If correct, go to next string length. If incorrect, read trial 2. Stop after incorrect on both trials.)

4-9-3	6-2-9	_____	0	1
3-8-1-4	3-2-7-9	_____	0	1
6-2-9-7-1	1-5-2-8-6	_____	0	1
7-1-8-4-6-2	5-3-9-1-4-8	_____	0	1

Months in Reverse Order: (entire sequence correct for 1 point)

Dec-Nov-Oct-Sep-Aug-Jul Jun-May-Apr-Mar-Feb-Jan	_____	0	1
Concentration Total Score	_____	/	5

EXERTIONAL MANEUVERS
(when appropriate):

5 jumping jacks	5 push-ups
5 sit-ups	5 knee bends

4) DELAYED RECALL:

Word 1		0	1
Word 2		0	1
Word 3		0	1
Word 4		0	1
Word 5		0	1
Delayed Recall Total Score	_____	/	5

SUMMARY OF TOTAL SCORES:

ORIENTATION	_____	/	5
IMMEDIATE MEMORY	_____	/	15
CONCENTRATION	_____	/	5
DELAYED RECALL	_____	/	5
OVERALL TOTAL SCORE	_____	/	30

FIGURE C-1 Standardized assessment of concussion.
SOURCE: McCrea, 2001, Table 2, p. 2276.

and history of concussion, headaches, migraines, depression, and anxiety (McCrory et al., 2013c). The precursor SCAT2 had been standardized as an easy-to-use tool with adequate psychometric properties for identifying concussions within the first 7 days (Barr and McCrea, 2001). The SCAT3 was developed from the original SCAT to help in making return-to-play decisions (McCrory et al., 2009, 2013b). This concussion evaluation tool can be used on the sideline or in the health care provider's office. The SCAT3 takes approximately 15 to 20 minutes to complete.

Because the SCAT3 was recently published (McCrory et al., 2013a), normative data and concussion cutoff scores are not yet available. However, a recent study to determine baseline values of the SCAT2 in normal male and female high school athletes found a high error rate on the concentration portion of the assessment in non-concussed athletes, suggesting the need for baseline testing in order to understand post-injury results (Jinguji et al., 2012). The study also showed significant sex differences, with females scoring higher on the balance, immediate memory, and concentration components of the assessment.

Findings similar to those of Jinguji and colleagues (2012) were reported in a study of youth ice hockey players who demonstrated an average total score of 86.9 out of 100 points (Blake et al., 2012). In the largest assessment of the SAC/SCAT2, Valovich McLeod and colleagues (2012) assessed 1,134 high school students. Male high school athletes and male and female ninth graders were found to have significantly lower SAC and total SCAT2 scores than did female athletes and upperclassmen, respectively (Valovich McLeod et al., 2012). A self-reported history of previous concussion[1] did not have a significant effect on SAC scores, but it did affect the symptom and total SCAT2 scores. The authors recommended baseline assessments in order to understand post-injury results for individual athletes. Schneider and colleagues (2010) tested more than 4,000 youth hockey players with the original SCAT and reported baseline scores showing absolute differences with age and sex. However, because no parametric statistics were provided, the significance of the observed differences is not known.

The Child SCAT3 is a newly developed concussion evaluation tool designed for children ages 5 to 12 years (McCrory et al., 2013a). It is similar to the SCAT3 except that tests such as the SAC and Maddocks questions are age appropriate for younger children. The Child SCAT3 includes versions of the SAC and Maddocks questions, the GCS, a medical history completed by the parent, child and parent concussion symptom scales, neck evaluation, and balance assessment. As is the case with the SCAT3 for adults, the Child SCAT3 has yet to be validated, so no normative data are available, nor are there concussion cutoff scores.

Military Acute Concussion Evaluation

The military currently employs the Military Acute Concussion Evaluation (MACE) tool for concussion screening and initial evaluation (DVBIC, 2012). The first section of the MACE collects data regarding the nature of the concussive event and the signs and symptoms of concussion. The second "examination" portion of the MACE is a version of the SAC. The MACE was first employed in Iraq for determining concussions in theater (French et al., 2008). Coldren and colleagues (2010) examined concussed and control U.S. Army soldiers who were administered the MACE 12 hours after their injury. The researchers concluded that the MACE lacks the sensitivity and specificity necessary to determine a concussive event 12 hours post injury. However, a recent study by Kennedy and colleagues (2012) indicated that the MACE can be effective in serial concussion evaluation if originally administered within 6 hours of the injury.

---

[1]Information on the time elapsed since the previous concussions was not reported.

King-Devick Test

The King-Devick test is designed to assess saccadic eye movements, measuring the speed of rapid number naming as well as errors made by the athlete, with the goal of detecting impairments of eye movement, attention, and language as well as impairments in other areas that would be indicative of suboptimal brain function (Galetta et al., 2011a). The King-Devick test includes a demonstration and three test cards with rows of single-digit numbers that are read aloud from left to right (see Figure C-2). The participant is asked to read the numbers as quickly as possible without making any errors. The administrator records the total time to complete the three cards and the total number of errors made during the test. The results are compared to a personal baseline. The King-Devick test usually takes approximately 2 minutes to complete (King-Devick, 2013).

Studies of the King-Devick test involve 10 or fewer concussed athletes (Galetta et al., 2011a,b, 2013; King et al., 2012, 2013), which is too small

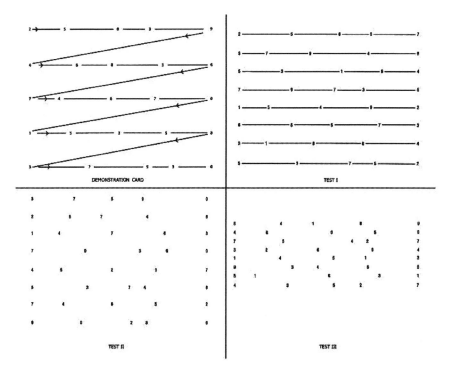

FIGURE C-2 Demonstration and test cards for King-Devick (K-D) test.
SOURCE: King-Devick, 2013.

a sample size to determine the test's effectiveness in evaluating a concussion. Currently, there is not enough evidence to determine whether the test is effective in diagnosing or monitoring a concussion (Giza et al., 2013).

Clinical Reaction Time Test

Eckner and colleagues (2010) have developed a simple tool for measuring clinical reaction time (RT_{clin}). The test involves a systematic approach to dropping a weighted stick that is calibrated to reflect speed of reaction for catching it. The athlete holds his or her hand around, but not touching, a rubber piece at the bottom of the stick, then the test administrator drops the stick, and the athlete catches it on the way down. Several studies document the initial development of this tool and demonstrate its concurrent and predictive validity (Eckner et al., 2010, 2011a,b).

A 2010 pilot study established convergent validity of RT_{clin} with the CogSport simple reaction time measure (Eckner et al., 2010). The Pearson correlation for 68 of the 94 athletes who completed both RT_{clin} and CogSport was .445 (p < .001). The other 26 athletes did not meet the validity criteria on CogSport. For those individuals, the correlations between the two tests were nonsignificant. A 2011 study looked at the test-retest reliability of RT_{clin} at a 1-year interval as well as the same reliability statistic for CogSport reaction time (Eckner et al., 2011a). The researchers used a two-way random effects analysis of variance model for intraclass correlation coefficient analysis for each test. This means that each subject was assessed by each rater, and the raters were *randomly selected*. The RT_{clin} intraclass correlation coefficient was above .60. One might argue that a two-way mixed effects analysis should be used, which would actually increase the coefficient. There was also significant improvement in the absolute reaction times from time one to time two for the RT_{clin} but not for CogSport (here the CogSport analysis only included valid responders).

Eckner and colleagues (2013) have also assessed the diagnostic utility of the RT_{clin}. They compared 28 concussed athletes to 28 controls. Concussed athletes were tested within 48 hours of injury and a control was selected at the same time interval. Post-injury tests were compared to baseline scores and reliable change indices were calculated using the control group means and standard error of difference from the two time-points. Using a 60 percent confidence interval (one-tailed significance), the authors calculated sensitivity at 79 percent and specificity at 61 percent for a score difference of –3. Thirty-three of the 56 athletes obtained this score; of the 33, 22 were concussed and 11 were not, and therefore were misidentified. The sensitivity and specificity were improved somewhat by adjusting the cutoff score to a difference of zero seconds (75 percent sensitivity; 68 percent specificity). This correlated with a 68 percent (one-sided) confidence interval. Of note, more stringent cutoff values lowered sensitivity but increased specificity, meaning that improvements in scores beyond 11 points increased the probability that the athlete did not have a concussion, which can be useful clinical information.

The RT$_{clin}$ is a simple-to-use and low-cost test of reaction time. The initial test of reliability at 1-year intervals is promising, and the diagnostic statistics indicate adequate utility. Further independent validation is needed, and it would be valuable to determine the increase in diagnostic efficiency if the test were combined with other tools because multimodal diagnostic test batteries have been recommended in the literature.

BALANCE TESTS

Balance Error Scoring System

The Balance Error Scoring System (BESS) is a quantifiable version of a modified Romberg test for balance (Guskiewicz, 2001; Riemann et al., 1999). It measures postural stability or balance and consists of six stances, three on a firm surface and the same three stances on an unstable (medium density foam) surface (Guskiewicz, 2001; Riemann et al., 1999). All stances are done with the athlete's eyes closed and with his or her hands on the iliac crests for 20 seconds. The three stances are: feet shoulder width apart, a tandem stance (one foot in front of the other), and a single-leg stance on the person's nondominant leg (Guskiewicz, 2001; Riemann et al., 1999). For every error made—lifting hands off the iliac crests, opening the eyes, stepping, stumbling, or falling, moving the hip into more than a 30 degree of flexion or abduction, lifting the forefoot or heel, or remaining out of the testing position for more than 5 seconds—1 point is assessed. The higher the score, the worse the athlete has performed.

The BESS test has very good test-retest reliability (0.87 to 0.97 intraclass correlations) (Riemann et al., 1999). The test's sensitivity for diagnosis was 0.34 to 0.64, which is considered low to moderate, while specificity is high (0.91) (Giza et al., 2013). Using the BESS test in conjunction with the SAC and a graded symptom checklist increases the sensitivity (Giza et al., 2013). The BESS has only been found to be useful within the first 2 days following injury (Giza et al., 2013; McCrea et al., 2003).

Sensory Organization Test

The Sensory Organization Test (SOT) uses six sensory conditions to objectively identify abnormalities in the patient's use of somatosensory, visual, and vestibular systems to maintain postural control. The test conditions systematically eliminate useful visual and proprioceptive information in order to assess the patient's vestibular balance control and adaptive responses of the central nervous system (NeuroCom, 2013). Broglio and colleagues (2008) examined the sensitivity and specificity of the SOT using the reliable change technique. A baseline and one follow-up assessment were performed on healthy and concussed young adults. Post-injury assessment in the concussed group occurred within 24 hours of diagnosis. An evaluation for change on one or more SOT variables resulted in the highest combined sensitivity (57 percent) and specificity (80 percent) at the 75 percent confidence interval. The low sensitivity of the SOT suggests the need to use additional evaluation tools to improve identification of individuals with concussion.

SYMPTOM SCALES

Acute Concussion Evaluation

The Acute Concussion Evaluation (ACE) tool is a physician/clinician form used to evaluate individuals for a concussion (see Figure C-3; Gioia and Collins, 2006; Gioia et al., 2008a). The form consists of questions about the presence of concussion characteristics (i.e., loss of consciousness, amnesia), 22 concussion symptoms, and risk factors that might predict prolonged recovery (i.e., a history of concussion) (Gioia et al., 2008a). The ACE can be used serially to track symptom recovery over time to help inform clinical management decisions (Gioia et al., 2008a).

Concussion Symptom Inventory

The Concussion Symptom Inventory (CSI) (see Figure C-4) is a derived symptom scale designed specifically for tracking recovery. Randolph and colleagues (2009) analyzed a large set of data from existing scales obtained from three separate case-control studies. Through a series of analyses they eliminated overlapping items that were found to be insensitive to concussion. They collected baseline data from symptom checklists, including a total of 27 symptom variables from a total of 16,350 high school and college athletes. Follow-up data were obtained from 641 athletes who subsequently incurred a concussion. Symptom checklists were administered at baseline (pre-season), immediately post concussion, postgame, and at 1, 3, and 5 days following injury. Effect-size analyses resulted in the retention of only 12 of the 27 variables. Receiver-operating characteristic analyses (non-parametric approach) were used to confirm that the reduction in items did not reduce sensitivity or specificity (area under the curve at day 1 post injury=0.867). Because the inventory has a limited set of symptoms,

---

ACUTE CONCUSSION EVALUATION (ACE)
PHYSICIAN/CLINICIAN OFFICE VERSION
Gerard Gioia, PhD[1] & Micky Collins, PhD[2]
[1]Children's National Medical Center
[2]University of Pittsburgh Medical Center

Patient Name:_____
DOB: _____ Age:_____
Date:_____ ID/MR#_____

A. Injury Characteristics Date/Time of Injury_____Reporter: __Patient __Parent __Spouse __Other_____

1. Injury Description _____

1a. Is there evidence of a forcible blow to the head (direct or indirect)? __Yes __No __Unknown
1b. Is there evidence of intracranial injury or skull fracture? __Yes __No __Unknown
1c. Location of Impact: __Frontal __Lft Temporal __Rt Temporal __Lft Parietal __Rt Parietal __Occipital __Neck __Indirect Force
2. Cause: __MVC __Pedestrian-MVC __Fall __Assault __Sports (specify)_____ Other_____
3. Amnesia Before (Retrograde) Are there any events just BEFORE the injury that you/ person has no memory of (even brief)? __ Yes __No Duration
4. Amnesia After (Anterograde) Are there any events just AFTER the injury that you/ person has no memory of (even brief)? __ Yes __No Duration
5. Loss of Consciousness: Did you/ person lose consciousness? __ Yes __No Duration
6. EARLY SIGNS: __Appears dazed or stunned __Is confused about events __Answers questions slowly __Repeats Questions __Forgetful (recent info)
7. Seizures: Were seizures observed? No__ Yes___ Detail_____

B. Symptom Check List * Since the injury, has the person experienced any of these symptoms any more than usual today or in the past day?
Indicate presence of each symptom (0=No, 1=Yes). *Lovell & Collins, 1998 JHTR*

PHYSICAL (10)			COGNITIVE (4)			SLEEP (4)			
Headache	0	1	Feeling mentally foggy	0	1	Drowsiness	0	1	
Nausea	0	1	Feeling slowed down	0	1	Sleeping less than usual	0	1	N/A
Vomiting	0	1	Difficulty concentrating	0	1	Sleeping more than usual	0	1	N/A
Balance problems	0	1	Difficulty remembering	0	1	Trouble falling asleep	0	1	N/A
Dizziness	0	1	COGNITIVE Total (0-4) ____			SLEEP Total (0-4) ____			
Visual problems	0	1	EMOTIONAL (4)						
Fatigue	0	1	Irritability	0	1	**Exertion:** Do these symptoms worsen with:			
Sensitivity to light	0	1	Sadness	0	1	Physical Activity __Yes __No __N/A			
Sensitivity to noise	0	1	More emotional	0	1	Cognitive Activity __Yes __No __N/A			
Numbness/Tingling	0	1	Nervousness	0	1	**Overall Rating:** How different is the person acting			
PHYSICAL Total (0-10) ____			EMOTIONAL Total (0-4) ____			compared to his/her usual self? (circle)			
(Add Physical, Cognitive, Emotion, Sleep totals) Total Symptom Score (0-22) ____						Normal 0 1 2 3 4 5 6 Very Different			

C. Risk Factors for Protracted Recovery (check all that apply)

Concussion History? Y ___ N___	√	Headache History? Y ___ N___	√	Developmental History	√	Psychiatric History
Previous # 1 2 3 4 5 6+		Prior treatment for headache		Learning disabilities		Anxiety
Longest symptom duration Days__ Weeks__ Months__ Years__		History of migraine headache __ Personal __ Family		Attention-Deficit/ Hyperactivity Disorder		Depression
						Sleep disorder
If multiple concussions, less force caused reinjury? Yes__ No__		_____		Other developmental disorder_____		Other psychiatric disorder _____

List other comorbid medical disorders or medication usage (e.g., hypothyroid, seizures)_____

D. RED FLAGS for acute emergency management: Refer to the emergency department with sudden onset of any of the following:
* Headaches that worsen	* Looks very drowsy/ can't be awakened	* Can't recognize people or places	* Neck pain
* Seizures	* Repeated vomiting	* Increasing confusion or irritability	* Unusual behavioral change
* Focal neurologic signs	* Slurred speech	* Weakness or numbness in arms/legs	* Change in state of consciousness

E. Diagnosis (ICD): __Concussion w/o LOC 850.0 __Concussion w/ LOC 850.1 __Concussion (Unspecified) 850.9 __Other (854) _____
__No diagnosis

F. Follow-Up Action Plan Complete *ACE Care Plan* and provide copy to patient/family.
___ No Follow-Up Needed
___ Physician/Clinician Office Monitoring: Date of next follow-up _____
___ Referral:
  ___ Neuropsychological Testing
  ___ Physician: Neurosurgery____ Neurology____ Sports Medicine____ Physiatrist____ Psychiatrist____ Other_____
  ___ Emergency Department

ACE Completed by:_____   © Copyright G. Gioia & M. Collins, 2006

This form is part of the "Heads Up: Brain Injury in Your Practice" tool kit developed by the Centers for Disease Control and Prevention (CDC).

FIGURE C-3 Page one of the acute concussion evaluation form.
SOURCE: Gioia and Collins, 2006, p. 1.

Concussion Symptom Inventory (CSI) Randolph, Millis, Barr, McCrea, Guskiewicz, & Kelly (2008)					
Player Name:_____ Date of Injury:_____ Date of Exam:_____					
	absent 0	*mild* 1 2	*moderate* 3 4	*severe* 5 6	Score
Headache					
Nausea					
Balance Problems/Dizziness					
Fatigue					
Drowsiness					
Feeling like "in a fog"					
Difficulty concentrating					
Difficulty remembering					
Sensitivity to light					
Sensitivity to noise					
Blurred vision					
Feeling slowed down					
TOTAL:					
Other symptoms evident since injury?:					

FIGURE C-4 Concussion symptom inventory.
SOURCE: Randolph et al., 2009, Appendix, p. 227.

Randolph and colleagues note the need for a complete symptom inventory for other problems associated with concussion.

Graded Symptom Checklist and Graded Symptom Scale

The Graded Symptom Checklist (GSC) (see Figure C-5) and Graded Symptom Scale (GSS) are self-report measures of concussion symptoms derived from the longer Head Injury Scale (Janusz et al., 2012). The symptoms are rated on their severity. The evidence is much stronger to support the use of such self-report symptom measures in youth ages 13 and older. Test-retest reliability has not been reported, but a three factor solution (cognitive, somatic, neurobehavioral) has been reported, although a bet-

Graded Symptom Checklist (GSC)					
Symptom	Time of injury	2-3 Hours postinjury	24 Hours postinjury	48 Hours postinjury	72 Hours postinjury
Blurred vision					
Dizziness					
Drowsiness					
Excess sleep					
Easily distracted					
Fatigue					
Feel "in a fog"					
Feel "slowed down"					
Headache					
Inappropriate emotions					
Irritability					
Loss of consciousness					
Loss of orientation					
Memory problems					
Nausea					
Nervousness					
Personality change					
Poor balance/ coordination					
Poor concentration					
Ringing in ears					
Sadness					
Seeing stars					
Sensitivity to light					
Sensitivity to noise					
Sleep disturbance					
Vacant stare/glassy eyed					
Vomiting					

NOTE: The GSC should be used not only for the initial evaluation but for each subsequent follow-up assessment until all signs and symptoms have cleared at rest and during physical exertion. In lieu of simply checking each symptom present, the [certified athletic trainer] ATC can ask the athlete to grade or score the severity of the symptom on a scale of 0-6, where 0=not present, 1=mild, 3=moderate, and 6=most severe.

FIGURE C-5 Graded symptom checklist.
SOURCE: Guskiewicz et al., 2004, Appendix A, p. 296.

ter solution contained only nine items (Piland et al., 2006). Evidence of convergent validity includes parallel recovery on the GSC and measures of balance and neurocognitive function and correlation with the presence of posttraumatic headaches (McCrea et al., 2003; Register-Mihalik et al., 2007), and discriminant validity between higher and lower impact force (McCaffrey et al., 2007).

Health and Behavior Inventory

The Health and Behavior Inventory (HBI) is a 20-item instrument, with parent and child self-report forms, that has been validated on youth ages 8 to 15 years and their parents (Ayr et al., 2009; Janusz et al., 2012). Test-retest reliability has not been reported. A factor structure was reported (cognitive, somatic, and emotional) that is consistent across parent and child reports and both at baseline and at 3-month follow-up. Parent and child reports are moderately inter-correlated, internal consistency has been reported, and there is evidence of both convergent (correlation with quality of life, family burden, educational and social difficulties) and discriminant (from those with non-head orthopedic injuries, moderate to severe traumatic brain injury) validity. Finally, the measures shows reliable change in 8- to 15-year-olds with mild traumatic brain injury (mTBI) followed over 12 months, and these increases in symptomatology related to orthopedic controls were related to injury characteristics, abnormalities on neuroimaging, the need for educational intervention, and pediatric quality of life (Yeates et al., 2012).

Post-Concussion Symptom Inventory

The Post-Concussion Symptom Inventory (PCSI) has self-report forms for youth ages 5 to 7 years (13 items), 8 to 12 years (25 items), and 13 to 18 years (26 items) as well as reports for parents and teachers (26 items). The forms focus on symptoms in the cognitive, emotional, sleep, and physical domains. Interrater reliability on the child reports was moderate to high (r's ranging from 0.62 to 0.84) (Schneider and Gioia, 2007; Vaughan et al., 2008), as was internal consistency for all three reports (Gioia et al., 2008b; Vaughan et al., 2008). There was moderate agreement among the reporters (r=0.4 to r=0.5) in one of the two studies (see Gioia et al., 2009, Table 2); and evidence of predictive and discriminant validity (Diver et al., 2007; Vaughan et al., 2008). It would appear that the strongest data for adolescents supports the use of the Post-Concussion Symptom Scale (PCSS) (discussed in the following section) and, for children and adolescents, the HBI or the PCSI.

Post-Concussion Symptom Scale

The PCSS is a 21-item self-report measure that records symptom severity using a 7-point Likert scale of severity (see Figure C-6; Lovell and Collins, 1998). The measure has not been studied in youth under the age of 11. In contrast to several of the other measures, evidence of moderate test-retest reliability has been reported (pre- to post-season intraclass correlation was 0.55; test-retest, r=0.65) (Iverson et al., 2003), and the scale is able to detect reliable change (Iverson et al., 2003). Recently, a revised factor structure has been reported in adolescents ranging from ages 13 to 22 years, which showed, post concussion, a four factor solution—cognitive-fatigue-migraine, affective, somatic, and sleep—and higher scores in female than in male participants (Kontos et al., 2012). The PCSS is able to discriminate between concussed and non-concussed athletes (Echemendia et al., 2001; Field et al., 2003; Iverson et al., 2003; Lovell et al., 2006; Schatz et al., 2006); shows greater abnormalities in those with multiple concussions (Collins et al., 1999); and shows convergent validity with measures of neurocognitive performance and regional hyper-activation on functional magnetic resonance imaging during a working memory task (Collins et al., 2003; Pardini et al., 2010). Although a consistent relationship between neuropsychological outcomes and the PCSS has been reported, persistent neurocognitive abnormalities have been reported even in "asymptomatic" athletes who have recovered clinically and on the basis of their scores on the PCSS (Fazio et al., 2007).

Rivermead Post-Concussion Symptoms Questionnaire

The Rivermead Post-Concussion Symptoms Questionnaire (RPCSQ) is a 16-item self-report measure of symptom severity that asks individuals to compare the presence and severity of symptoms they have experienced within the past 24 hours relative to their experience of the same symptoms prior to the injury. One study showed discriminant validity between concussed and non-concussed youth ages 12 and under, but no reliability or factor structure was reported (Gagnon et al., 2005). In adolescents, high internal consistency but low test-retest reliability has been reported (Iverson and Gaetz, 2004) as well as strong discriminant validity between concussed and non-concussed youth (Wilde et al., 2008).

322

Player's Name: _____ Team: _____ Position: _____

SYMPTOM	RATING None Mod. Severe	BASELINE Date:	TESTING 2 Date:	TESTING 3 Date:	TESTING 4 Date:	TESTING 5 Date:
Headache	0 1 2 3 4 5 6					
Nausea	0 1 2 3 4 5 6					
Vomiting	0 1 2 3 4 5 6					
Balance problems	0 1 2 3 4 5 6					
Dizziness	0 1 2 3 4 5 6					
Fatigue	0 1 2 3 4 5 6					
Trouble falling asleep	0 1 2 3 4 5 6					
Sleeping more than usual	0 1 2 3 4 5 6					
Sleeping less than usual	0 1 2 3 4 5 6					
Drowsiness	0 1 2 3 4 5 6					
Sensitivity to light	0 1 2 3 4 5 6					
Sensitivity to noise	0 1 2 3 4 5 6					
Irritability	0 1 2 3 4 5 6					
Sadness	0 1 2 3 4 5 6					
Nervousness	0 1 2 3 4 5 6					
Feeling more emotional	0 1 2 3 4 5 6					
Numbness or tingling	0 1 2 3 4 5 6					
Feeling slowed down	0 1 2 3 4 5 6					
Feeling mentally "foggy"	0 1 2 3 4 5 6					
Difficulty concentrating	0 1 2 3 4 5 6					
Difficulty remembering	0 1 2 3 4 5 6					
TOTAL SCORE						

FIGURE C-6 Post-concussion scale.
NOTE: More recent versions of this instrument include "visual problems" in the list of symptoms rated.
SOURCE: Lovell and Collins, 1998, Figure 1, p. 20.

COMPUTERIZED NEUROCOGNITIVE TESTS

Automated Neuropsychological Assessment Metrics

Automated Neuropsychological Assessment Metrics (ANAM) is a computer-based neuropsychological assessment tool designed to detect the accuracy and efficiency of cognitive processing in a variety of situations (Levinson and Reeves, 1997). ANAM measures attention, concentration, reaction time, memory, processing speed, and decision making (Cernich et al., 2007). Test administration takes approximately 20 minutes.

Recently ANAM has published normative data for sex and age using more than 100,000 military service members 17 to 65 years of age (Vincent et al., 2012). Researchers have also investigated the sensitivity, validity, and reliability of the ANAM test battery. Levinson and Reeves (1997) investigated the sensitivity of ANAM in traumatic brain injury patients who were classified as marginally impaired (n=8), mildly impaired (n=7), or moderately impaired (n=7). The ANAM test battery was administered on two occasions separated by a 2- to 3-month interval in order to examine its ability to classify the patients by comparing accuracy and efficiency scores on the tests to appropriate normative data. At the first administration, the efficiency scores on the ANAM classified 91 percent of the patients into groups accurately; 100 percent classification was obtained in the second administration when the mild and moderately impaired patients were combined as one group. At the second administration, the efficiency scores accurately classified 86.36 percent of the patients. This study revealed the sensitivity of ANAM in distinguishing the severity of traumatic brain injury.

Bleiberg and colleagues (2000) investigated the construct validity of ANAM by examining the relationship between ANAM and a set of traditional clinical neuropsychological tests (Trail Making Test Part B, Consonant Trigrams total score, Paced Auditory Serial Addition test, the Hopkins Verbal Learning test, and the Stroop Color and Word test). The strongest correlation for mathematical processing, Sternberg memory procedure, and spatial processing were found with the Paced Auditory Serial Addition test (0.663, 0.447, and 0.327, respectively). The strongest correlation for matching to sample was found with Trail Making Test Part B (–0.497). This study indicated good construct validity between ANAM and traditional neuropsychological measures.

The ANAM sports medicine battery is a specialized subset designed for serial concussion testing. The ANAM sports medicine battery assesses attention, mental flexibility, cognitive processing efficiency, arousal and fatigue level, learning, and recall and memory (Reeves et al., 2007). Segalowitz and colleagues (2007) examined the test-retest reliability of ANAM sports medicine battery in a group of 29 adolescents. The researchers administered ANAM twice during the same time of day over a 1-week interval. The highest intra-class correlations were reported in matching to sample (0.72), followed by continuous performance test (0.65), mathematical processing (0.61), code substitution (0.58), simple reaction time 2 (0.47), and simple reaction time (0.44). The highest Pearson correlation coefficient was reported in code substitution (0.81), followed by matching to sample (0.72), continuous performance test (0.70), code substitution delayed (0.67), simple reaction time 2 (0.50), and simple reaction time (0.48). The results suggest that there is variability of test-retest reliability for individual subtests of ANAM.

Another study assessed the reliability of ANAM sports medicine battery through test-retest methods using a military sample (Cernich et al., 2007). The average test-retest interval for this study was 166.5 days. Results revealed a wide range of intra-class correlations for each subtest with the highest being in mathematical processing (0.87), followed by matching to sample (0.66), spatial processing (0.60), continuous performance test (0.58), Sternberg memory procedure (0.48), and simple reaction time (0.38). Both of these studies suggest that there are low intraclass correlations values for reaction time subtest scores (Cernich et al., 2007; Segalowitz et al., 2007).

As with all computerized neuropsychological test batteries, it is important to determine whether multiple test sessions result in practice effects. Eonta and colleagues (2011) examined practice effects of ANAM in two groups of military personnel. In the first study, 38 U.S. marines were administered four tests back-to-back on 1 day and on consecutive days. In the second study, 21 New Zealand military personnel were administered the ANAM test battery eight times across 5 days. Individuals demonstrated practice effects on five of six subtests in the two studies.

Bryan and Hernandez (2012) examined military service members who presented with mTBI to a military clinic in Iraq. The findings of the study indicated that on five out of the six ANAM subtests, a larger proportion of mTBI patients than control patients without TBI demonstrated significant declines in speed at 2 days post injury. The one exception was accuracy, which showed no difference between the mTBI and the control groups.

Finally, Coldren and colleagues (2012) examined concussed U.S. Army soldiers at 72 hours and 10 days post injury using the ANAM test battery. Concussed soldiers showed impairment at 72 hours compared to a control group; however, at 10 days the concussed group showed no significant impairments on the ANAM subtests when compared to the control group. Although the researchers concluded that the ANAM lacks utility as a diagnostic or screening tool 10 days following a concussion, they did not report whether the concussed soldiers were also asymptomatic and reporting a normal clinical exam. Thus, more research is warranted to determine whether the ANAM test battery is effective in the long-term assessment of concussed patients.

CogSport/AXON

CogSport is a computerized neuropsychological test battery developed by CogState that measures psychomotor function, speed of processing, visual attention, vigilance, and verbal and visual learning and memory (Falleti et al., 2006). The battery employs a series of eight "card games" to examine cognitive function including simple reaction time, complex reaction time, and one-back and continuous learning. Axon Sports is a recently launched company within CogState that has developed the Computerized Cognitive Assessment Tool (CCAT). Like Cogsport, the CCAT employs a "card game" to evaluate cognitive domains, including processing speed, attention, learning, and working memory. This test specifically examines reaction time and accuracy.

Collie and colleagues (2003) determined the reliability of CogSport by calculating intraclass correlation coefficients on serial data collected in 60 healthy youth volunteers at intervals of 1 hour and 1 week. In the same study, construct validity was determined by calculating intraclass correlation coefficients between CogSport and performance on traditional paper-and-pencil assessment tools (the Digit Symbol Substitution test and the Trail Making Test Part B) in 240 professional athletes competing in the Australian Football League. The results indicated high to very high intraclass correlations in CogSport speed indices at intervals of 1 hour and 1 week (0.69 to 0.90), while CogSport accuracy indices displayed lower and more variable intraclass correlations (0.08 to 0.51). Construct validity between CogSport and the Digit Symbol Substitution test were found to be the highest in decision making ($r=0.86$), followed by working memory speed (0.76), psychomotor speed (0.50), and learning speed (0.42). Smaller and less variable correlation coefficients between CogSport and the Trail Making Test Part B were observed with the highest in psychomotor speed (0.44), decision making (0.34), working memory speed (0.33), and learning speed (0.23).

Broglio and colleagues (2007) examined the test-retest reliability of three computerized neuropsychological testing batteries: Immediate Post-Concussion Assessment and Cognitive Testing (ImPACT), Concussion Resolution Index (CRI), and Concussion Sentinel, which is an earlier version of CogSport. In this study, these computerized neuropsychological test batteries were administered to 73 participants successively (the order of administration was not specified) on three occasions: at baseline, and at 45 days and 50 days after baseline. Based on seven neuropsychological tests, Concussion Sentinel develops five output scores: reaction time, decision making, matching, attention, and working memory. When baseline and day 45 were compared, the highest intraclass correlation was observed for working memory (0.65), followed by reaction time (0.60), decision making (0.56), attention (0.43), and matching (0.23). When days 45 and 50 were compared, the highest correlation was reported for matching (0.66), followed by working memory (0.64), decision making (0.62), reaction time (0.55), and attention (0.39). However, the effect on the participants' performance of successively administering three neuropsychological testing batteries was identified as a possible methodological flaw, potentially contributing to the low intraclass correlation scores.

Makdissi and colleagues (2010) conducted a prospective study that tracked the recovery of 78 concussed male Australian football players using the Axon Sport CCAT and traditional paper-and-pencil tests (the Digit Symbol Substitution Test and the Trail Making Test Part B). Although concussion-associated symptoms lasted an average of 48.6 hours (95 percent CI, 39.5-57.7 hours), and cognitive deficits on the traditional paper-and-pencil test had for the most part resolved at 7 days post injury, 17.9 percent of the athletes still demonstrated significant cognitive decline on the Axon sport CCAT. This study implied that the Axon sport CCAT has greater sensitivity to cognitive impairment following concussion than the Digit Symbol Substitution test and the Trail Making Test Part B. Because Axon Sport is a new computerized neuropsychological test battery, more research is warranted on this test battery to determine whether it is effective in assessing concussion outcomes.

Concussion Resolution Index

The CRI, developed by HeadMinder, Inc., is a Web-based computerized neuropsychological assessment battery composed of six subtests: reaction time, cued reaction time, visual recognition 1 and 2, animal decoding, and symbol scanning (Erlanger et al., 2003). Symbol scanning measures simple and complex reaction time, visual scanning, and psychomotor speed. These six subtests form three CRI indices: Psychomotor, Speed Index, Simple Reaction Time (Erlanger et al., 2003). In addition to cognitive testing, the CRI collects demographic information, medical history, concussion history, and symptom report.

Concurrent validity was established using traditional neuropsychological paper-and-pencil tests. Correlations for CRI Psychomotor Speed Index were 0.66 for the Single Digit Modality Test, 0.60 and 0.57 for the Grooved Pegboard Test dominant and nondominant hand respectively, and 0.58 for the WAIS-III Symbol Search subtest (Erlanger et al., 2001). Correlations for CRI Complex Reaction Time Index were 0.59 and 0.70 for the Grooved Pegboard test for dominant and nondominant hand, respectively (Erlanger et al., 2001). Correlations for the CRI Simple Reaction Time Index were

0.56 for Trail Making Test Part A, and 0.46 and 0.60 for the Grooved Pegboard Test dominant and nondominant hand, respectively (Erlanger et al., 2001).

In the previously mentioned study by Broglio and colleagues (2007), test-retest reliability was also examined for the CRI at baseline and at 45 and 50 days post baseline test. The CRI demonstrated extremely low intraclass correlations (0.03) for Simple Reaction Time Error score when days 45 and 50 were compared, and 0.15 for baseline to day 45. The correlations for simple reaction time were 0.65 (baseline to 45 days) and 0.36 (day 45 to 50) and for complex reaction time were 0.43 (baseline to 45 days) and 0.66 (day 45 to 50); the complex reaction time error score was 0.26 (baseline to 45 days) and 0.46 (day 45 to 50), and the processing speed index was 0.66 (baseline to 45 days) and 0.58 (day 45 to 50). These low correlations may be due to the three neuropsychological testing batteries being administered during one session and also to the lack of counterbalance of these three computerized test batteries.

Erlanger and colleagues (2003) reported that test-retest reliability for a 2-week interval was 0.82 for psychomotor speed, 0.70 for simple reaction time, and 0.68 for complex reaction time. Another study also examined the sensitivity of the CRI in detecting changes between baseline and post-injury testing, and it found that the CRI had a sensitivity of 77 percent in identifying a concussion (Erlanger et al., 2001). Thus, the CRI was found to be a valid method of identifying changes in psychomotor speed, reaction time, and processing speed after a sports-related concussion.

Immediate Post-Concussion Assessment and Cognitive Testing

ImPACT is an online computerized neuropsychological test battery composed of three general sections. First, athletes input their demographic and descriptive information by following instructions on a series of screens. The demographic section includes sport participation history, history of alcohol and drug use, learning disabilities, attention deficit hyperactive disorders, major neurological disorders, and history of previous concussion. Next, the athletes self-report any of 22 listed concussion symptoms, which they rate using a 7-point Likert scale. The third section consists of six neuropsychological test modules that evaluate the subject's attention processes, verbal recognition memory, visual working memory, visual processing speed, reaction time, numerical sequencing ability, and learning.

Schatz and colleagues (2006) examined the diagnostic utility of the composite scores and the PCSS of the ImPACT in a group of 72 concussed athletes and 66 non-concussed athletes. All athletes were administered a baseline test and all concussed athletes were tested within 72 hours of incurring a concussion. Approximately 82 percent of the participants in the concussion group and 89 percent of the participants in the control group were correctly classified. This indicates that the sensitivity of ImPACT was 81.9 percent and the specificity was 89.4 percent.

To examine the construct validity of ImPACT, Maerlender and colleagues (2010) compared the scores on the ImPACT test battery to a neuropsychological test battery and experimental cognitive measures in 54 healthy male athletes. The neuropsychological test battery included the California Verbal Learning test, the Brief Visual Memory Test, the Delis Kaplan Executive Function system, the Grooved Pegboard, the Paced Auditory Serial Attention Test, the Beck Depression Inventory, the Speilberger State-Trait Anxiety Questionnaire, and the Word Memory Test. The experimental cognitive measures included the N-back and the verbal continuous memory task. The following scores were generated: neuropsychological verbal memory score, neuropsychological working memory score, neuropsychological visual memory score, neuropsychological processing speed score, neuropsychological attention score, neuropsychological reaction time score, neuropsychological motor score, and neuropsychological impulse control score. The results indicated significant correlations between neuropsychological domains and all ImPACT domain scores except the impulse control factor. The ImPACT verbal memory correlated with neuropsychological verbal ($r=0.40$, $p=0.00$) and visual memory ($r=0.44$, $p=0.01$); the ImPACT visual memory correlated with neuropsychological visual memory ($r=0.59$, $p=0.00$); and the ImPACT visual motor processing speed and reaction time score correlated with neuropsychological working memory ($r=0.39$, $p=0.00$ and $r=-0.31$, $p=-.02$), neuropsychological process speed ($r=0.41$, $p=.00$ and $r=-0.37$, $p=0.01$), and neuropsychological reaction time score ($r=0.34$, $p=0.00$ and $r=-0.39$, $p=0.00$). It must be noted that the neuropsychological domain scores for motor, attention, and impulse control were not correlated with any ImPACT composite scores. Overall the results suggest that the cognitive domains represented by ImPACT have good construct validity with standard neuropsychological tests that are sensitive to cognitive functions associated with mTBI.

Allen and Gfeller (2011) also found good concurrent validity between ImPACT scores and a battery of paper-and-pencil neuropsychological tests. Specifically, 100 college students completed the traditional paper-and-pencil test battery used by the National Football League and the ImPACT test in a counterbalanced order. Five factors explained 69 percent of variance with the ImPACT test battery with the authors suggesting that ImPACT has good concurrent validity.

Although ImPACT has been reported to have good sensitivity, specificity, and construct validity, its test-retest reliability has been shown to be somewhat inconsistent. Iverson and colleagues (2003) examined the test-retest reliability over a 7-day time span using a sample of 56 non-concussed adolescent and young adults (29 males and 27 females with an average age of 17.6 years). The Pearson test-retest correlation coefficients and probable ranges of measurement effort for the composite scores were: verbal memory=0.70 (6.83 pts), visual memory=0.67 (10.59 pts), reaction time=0.79 (0.05 sec), processing speed=0.89 (3.89 pts), and post-concussion scale=0.65 (7.17 pts). There was a significant difference between the first and 7-day retest on the processing speed composite ($p < 0.003$) with 68 percent of the sample performing better on the 7-day retest than at the first test session.

In the 2007 study by Broglio and colleagues, the ImPACT intraclass correlations ranged from 0.28 to 0.38 (baseline to day 45) and 0.39 to 0.61 (day 45 to day 50) (Broglio et al., 2007). The correlations for each composite score were: verbal memory (0.23 for baseline to day 45, and 0.40 for day 45 to day 50), visual memory (0.32 and 0.39, respectively), motor processing speed (0.38 and 0.61, respectively), and reaction time (0.39 and 0.51, respectively). However, it must be pointed out that this study was flawed by methodological errors which contributed to the low intraclass correlation values.

Miller and colleagues (2007) conducted a test-retest study over a longer time period (4 months) with in-season athletes. The researchers administered a series of ImPACT tests to 58 non-concussed Division III football players during pre-season (before the first full-pads practice), at midseason (6 weeks into the season), and during post-season (within 2 weeks of the last game). The results indicated no significant differences in verbal memory ($p=0.06$) or in processing speed ($p=0.05$) over the three testing occasions. However, the scores for visual memory ($p=0.04$) and reaction time showed significant improvement as the season progressed ($p=0.04$). Even though the statistical difference was found at the P level of 0.05, when an 80 percent confidence interval was used, the ImPACT results could be interpreted as stable over a 4-month time period in football players. The test-retest reliability of ImPACT has been examined with even longer time periods.

In response, Elbin and colleagues (2011) investigated a 1-year test-retest reliability of the online version of ImPACT using baseline data from 369 high school varsity athletes. The researchers administered the two ImPACT tests approximately 1 year apart, as required by the participants' respective athletic programs. Results indicated that motor processing speed was the most stable composite score with an intraclass correlation of 0.85, followed by reaction time (0.76), visual memory (0.70), verbal memory (0.62), and PCSS (0.57).

The test-retest study of ImPACT with the longest elapsed time was conducted by Schatz (2010), who tested 95 college athletes over a 2-year interval. Motor processing speed was the most stable composite score over those 2 years with an intraclass correlation of 0.74, followed by reaction time (0.68), visual memory (0.65), and verbal memory (0.46). Even though the correlation for verbal memory did not reach the "acceptable" threshold (0.60), with the use of regression-based methods none of the participants' scores showed significant change. Furthermore, reliable change indices revealed that only a small percentage of participants (0 to 3 percent) showed significant change. This study suggests that college athletes' cognitive performance remains stable over a 2-year time period. In addition, the ImPACT test battery has been shown to have good psychometric properties.

In a small sample of non-athlete college students (n=30), Schatz and Putz (2006) administered three computerized batteries along with select paper-and-pencil tests, counterbalanced over three 40-minute testing sessions. The results showed shared correlations between all the computer-based tests in the domain of processing speed, and between select tests in the domains of simple and choice reaction time. Little shared variance was seen in the domain of memory, although external criterion measures were lacking in this area. Of the test measures used, ImPACT shared the most consistent correlations with the other two computer-based measures as well as with all external criteria except for internal correlations in the domain of memory. However, the authors were clear about the limitations in sample size and the lack of a clinical population as well as the other limitations of the study, and they cautioned against considering this a complete evaluative study. The study does, however, provide some framework for understanding the concurrent validity of these tools.

Previous concurrent validity studies indicated good validity when compared to individual tests. The convergent construct validity of ImPACT was good compared to a full battery of neuropsychological tests (Maerlender et al., 2010). Using a factor analytic approach, Allen and Gfeller (2011) also found good concurrent validity between ImPACT scores and a battery of paper-and-pencil neuropsychological tests. However, there were differences in factor structure between the paper-and-pencil battery and the ImPACT battery, suggesting differences in "coverage" of neuropsychological constructs.

REFERENCES

Allen, B. J., and J. D. Gfeller. 2011. The Immediate Post-Concussion Assessment and Cognitive Testing battery and traditional neuropsychological measures: A construct and concurrent validity study. *Brain Injury* 25(2):179-191.

Ayr, L. K., K. O. Yeates, H. G. Taylor, and M. Browne. 2009. Dimensions of postconcussive symptoms in children with mild traumatic brain injuries. *Journal of the International Neuropsychological Society* 15(1):19-30.

Barr, W. B. 2003. Neuropsychological testing of high school athletes: Preliminary norms and test-retest indices. *Archives of Clinical Neuropsychology* 18:91-101.

Barr, W. B., and M. McCrea. 2001. Sensitivity and specificity of standardized neurocognitive testing immediately following sports concussion. *Journal of the International Neuropsychological Society* 7(6):693-702.

Blake, T. A., K. A. Taylor, K. Y. Woollings, K. J. Schneider, J. Kang, W. H. Meeuwisse, and C. A. Emery. 2012. Sport Concussion Assessment Tool, Version 2, normative values and test-retest reliability in elite youth ice hockey. [Abstract.] *Clinical Journal of Sport Medicine* 22(3):307.

Bleiberg, J., R. L. Kane, D. L. Reeves, W. S. Garmoe, and E. Halpern. 2000. Factor analysis of computerized and traditional tests used in mild brain injury research. *Clinical Neuropsychologist* 14(3):287-294.

Broglio, S. P., M. S. Ferrara, S. N. Macciocchi, T. A. Baumgartner, and R. Elliott. 2007. Test-retest reliability of computerized concussion assessment programs. *Journal of Athletic Training* 42(4):509-514.

Broglio, S. P., M. S. Ferrara, K. Sopiarz, and M. S. Kelly. 2008. Reliable change of the Sensory Organization Test. *Clinical Journal of Sport Medicine* 18(2):148-154.

Bryan, C., and A. M. Hernandez. 2012. Magnitudes of decline on Automated Neuropsychological Assessment Metrics subtest scores relative to predeployment baseline performance among service members evaluated for traumatic brain injury in Iraq. *Journal of Head Trauma Rehabilitation* 27(1):45-54.

Cernich, A., D. Reeves, W. Y. Sun, and J. Bleiberg. 2007. Automated Neuropsychological Assessment Metrics sports medicine battery. *Archives of Clinical Neuropsychology* 22(1):S101-S114.

Coldren, R. L., M. P. Kelly, R. V. Parish, M. Dretsch, and M. L. Russell. 2010. Evaluation of the Military Acute Concussion Evaluation for use in combat operations more than 12 hours after injury. *Military Medicine* 175(7):477-481.

Coldren, R. L., M. L. Russell, R. V. Parish, M. Dretsch, and M. P. Kelly. 2012. The ANAM lacks utility as a diagnostic or screening tool for concussion more than 10 days following injury. *Military Medicine* 177(2):179-183.

Collie, A., P. Maruff, M. Makdissi, P. McCrory, M. McStephen, and D. Darby. 2003. CogSport: Reliability and correlation with conventional cognitive tests used in postconcussion medical evaluations. *Clinical Journal of Sport Medicine* 13(1):28-32.

Collins, M. W., S. H. Grindel, M. R. Lovell, D. E. Dede, D. J. Moser, B. R. Phalin, S. Nogle, M. Wasik, D. Cordry, K. M. Daugherty, S. F. Sears, G. Nicolette, P. Indelicato, and D. B. McKeag. 1999. Relationship between concussion and neuropsychological performance in college football players. *JAMA* 282(10):964-970.

Collins, M. W., G. L. Iverson, M. R. Lovell, D. B. McKeag, J. Norwig, and J. Maroon. 2003. On-field predictors of neuropsychological and symptom deficit following sports-related concussion. *Clinical Journal of Sport Medicine* 13(4):222-229.

Diver, T., G. Gioia, and S. Anderson. 2007. Discordance of symptom report across clinical and control groups with respect to parent and child. *Journal of the International Neuropsychological Society* 13(Suppl 1):63. [Poster presentation to the Annual Meeting of the International Neuropsychological Society, Portland, OR.]

DVBIC (Defense and Veterans Brain Injury Center). 2012. *Military Acute Concussion Evaluation.* https://www.jsomonline.org/TBI/MACE_Revised_2012.pdf (accessed August 23, 2013).

Dziemianowicz, M., M. P. Kirschen, B. A. Pukenas, E. Laudano, L. J. Balcer, and S. L. Galetta. 2012. Sports-related concussion testing. *Current Neurology and Neuroscience Reports* 12(5):547-559.

Echemendia, R. J., M. Putukian, R. S. Mackin, L. Julian, and N. Shoss. 2001. Neuropsychological test performance prior to and following sports-related mild traumatic brain injury. *Clinical Journal of Sport Medicine* 11(1):23-31.

Eckner, J. T., J. S. Kutcher, and J. K. Richardson. 2010. Pilot evaluation of a novel clinical test of reaction time in National Collegiate Athletic Association Division I football players. *Journal of Athletic Training* 45(4):327-332.

Eckner, J. T., J. S. Kutcher, and J. K. Richardson. 2011a. Between-seasons test-retest reliability of clinically measured reaction time in National Collegiate Athletic Association Division I athletes. *Journal of Athletic Training* 46(4):409-414.

Eckner, J. T., J. S. Kutcher, and J. K. Richardson. 2011b. Effect of concussion on clinically measured reaction time in nine NCAA Division I collegiate athletes: A preliminary study. *PM & R* 3(3): 212-218.

Eckner, J. T., J. S. Kutcher, S. P. Broglio, and J. K. Richardson. 2013. Effect of sport-related concussion on clinically measured simple reaction time. *British Journal of Sports Medicine*. Published online first: January 11, doi:10.1136/bjsports-2012-0915792013.

Elbin, R. J., P. Schatz, and T. Covassin. 2011. One-year test-retest reliability of the on-line version of ImPACT in high school athletes. *American Journal of Sports Medicine* 39(11):2319-2324.

Eonta, S. E., W. Carr, J. J. McArdle, J. M. Kain, C. Tate, N. J. Wesensten, J. N. Norris, T. J. Balkin, and G. H. Kamimori. 2011. Automated Neuropsychological Assessment Metrics: Repeated assessment with two military samples. *Aviation, Space, and Environmental Medicine* 82(1):34-39.

Erlanger, D., E. Saliba, J. Barth, J. Almquist, W. Webright, and J. Freeman. 2001. Monitoring resolution of postconcussion symptoms in athletes: Preliminary results of a Web-based neuropsychological test protocol. *Journal of Athletic Training* 36(3):280-287.

Erlanger, D., D. Feldman, K. Kutner, T. Kaushik, H. Kroger, J. Festa, J. Barth, J. Freeman, and D. Broshek. 2003. Development and validation of a web-based neuropsychological test protocol for sports-related return-to-play decision-making. *Archives of Clinical Neuropsychology* 18(3):293-316.

Falleti, M. G., P. Maruff, A. Collie, and D. G. Darby. 2006. Practice effects associated with the repeated assessment of cognitive function using the CogState battery at 10-minute, one week and one month test-retest intervals. *Journal of Clinical and Experimental Neuropsychology* 28(7):1095-1112.

Fazio, V. C., M. R. Lovell, J. E. Pardini, and M. W. Collins. 2007. The relation between post concussion symptoms and neurocognitive performance in concussed athletes. *NeuroRehabilitation* 22:207-216.

Field, M., M. W. Collins, M. R. Lovell, and J. Maroon. 2003. Does age play a role in recovery from sports-related concussion? A comparison of high school and collegiate athletes. *Journal of Pediatrics* 142(5):546-553.

French, L., M. McCrea, and M. Baggett. 2008. The Military Acute Concussion Evaluation (MACE). *Journal of Special Operations Medicine* 8(1):68-77.

Gagnon, I., B. Swaine, D. Friedman, and R. Forget. 2005. Exploring children's self-efficacy related to physical activity performance after a mild traumatic brain injury. *Journal of Head Trauma Rehabilitation* 20(5):436-449.

Galetta, K. M., J. Barrett, M. Allen, F. Madda, D. Delicata, A. T. Tennant, C. C. Branas, M. G. Maguire, L. V. Messner, S. Devick, S. L. Galetta, and L. J. Balcer. 2011a. The King-Devick test as a determinant of head trauma and concussion in boxers and MMA fighters. *Neurology* 76(17):1456-1462.

Galetta, K. M., L. E. Brandes, K. Maki, M. S. Dziemianowicz, E. Laudano, M. Allen, K. Lawler, B. Sennett, D. Wiebe, S. Devick, L. V. Messner, S. L. Galetta, and L. J. Balcer. 2011b. The King-Devick test and sports-related concussion: Study of a rapid visual screening tool in a collegiate cohort. *Journal of the Neurological Sciences* 309(1-2):34-39.

Galetta, M. S., K. M. Galetta, J. McCrossin, J. A. Wilson, S. Moster, S. L. Galetta, L. J. Balcer, G. W. Dorshimer, and C. L. Master. 2013. Saccades and memory: Baseline associations of the King-Devick and SCAT2 SAC tests in professional ice hockey players. *Journal of the Neurological Sciences* 328(1-2):28-31.

Gioia, G., and M. Collins. 2006. *Acute Concussion Evaluation (ACE): Physician/Clinician Office Version.* http://www.cdc.gov/concussion/headsup/pdf/ace-a.pdf (accessed August 23, 2013).

Gioia, G., M. Collins, and P. K. Isquith. 2008a. Improving identification and diagnosis of mild traumatic brain injury with evidence: Psychometric support for the Acute Concussion Evaluation. *Journal of Head Trauma Rehabilitation* 23(4):230-242.

Gioia, G., J. Janusz, P. Isquith, and D. Vincent. 2008b. Psychometric properties of the parent and teacher Post-Concussion Symptom Inventory (PCSI) for children and adolescents. [Abstract.] *Journal of the International Neuropsychological Society* 14(Suppl 1):204.

Gioia, G. A., J. C. Schneider, C. G. Vaughan, and P. K. Isquith. 2009. Which symptom assessments and approaches are uniquely appropriate for paediatric concussion? *British Journal of Sports Medicine* 43(Suppl 1):i13-i22.

Giza, C. C., J. S. Kutcher, S. Ashwal, J. Barth, T. S. D. Getchius, G. A. Gioia, G. S. Gronseth, K. Guskiewicz, S. Mandel, G. Manley, D. B. McKeag, D. J. Thurman, and R. Zafonte. 2013. *Evidence-Based Guideline Update: Evaluation and Management of Concussion in Sports.* Report of the Guideline Development Subcommittee of the American Academy of Neurology. American Academy of Neurology.

Guskiewicz, K. M. 2001. Postural stability assessment following concussion: One piece of the puzzle. *Clinical Journal of Sport Medicine* 11(3):182-189.

Guskiewicz, K. M., S. L. Bruce, R. C. Cantu, M. S. Ferrara, J. P. Kelly, M. McCrea, M. Putukian, and T. C. Valovich McLeod. 2004. National Athletic Trainers' Association position statement: Management of sport-related concussion. *Journal of Athletic Training* 39(3):280-297.

Iverson, G. L., and M. Gaetz. 2004. Practical consideration for interpreting change following brain injury. In *Traumatic Brain Injury in Sports: An International Neuropsychological Perspective,* edited by M. R. Lovell, R. J. Echemendia, J. T. Barth, and M. W. Collins. Exton, PA: Swets & Zeitlinger. Pp. 323-356.

Iverson, G. L., M. R. Lovell, and M. W. Collins. 2003. Interpreting change in ImPACT following sport concussion. *Clinical Neuropsychology* 17(4):460-467.

Janusz, J. A., M. D. Sady, and G. A. Gioia. 2012. Postconcussion symptom assessment. In *Mild Traumatic Brain Injury in Children and Adolescents: From Basic Science to Clinical Management,* edited by M. W. Kirkwood and K. O. Yeates. New York: Guilford Press. Pp. 241-263.

Jinguji, T. M., V. Bompadre, K. G. Harmon, E. K. Satchell, K. Gilbert, J. Wild, and J. F. Eary. 2012. Sport Concussion Assessment Tool-2: Baseline values for high school athletes. *British Journal of Sports Medicine* 46(5):365-370.

Kennedy, C., E. J. Porter, S. Chee, J. Moore, J. Barth, and K. Stuessi. 2012. Return to combat duty after concussive blast injury. *Archives of Clinical Neuropsychology* 27(8):817-827.

King, D., T., Clark, and C. Gissane. 2012. Use of a rapid visual screening tool for the assessment of concussion in amateur rugby league: A pilot study. *Journal of the Neurological Sciences* 320(1-2):16-21.

King, D., M. Brughelli, P. Hume, and C. Gissane. 2013. Concussions in amateur rugby union identified with the use of a rapid visual screening tool. *Journal of the Neurological Sciences* 326(1):59-63.

King-Devick. 2013. *King-Devick Test.* http://kingdevicktest.com (accessed August 23, 2013).

Kontos, A. P., R. J. Elbin, P. Schatz, T. Covassin, L. Henry, J. Pardini, and M. W. Collins. 2012. A revised factor structure for the Post-Concussion Symptom Scale: Baseline and postconcussion factors. *American Journal of Sports Medicine* 40(10):2375-2384.

Levinson, D. M., and D. L. Reeves. 1997. Monitoring recovery from traumatic brain injury using Automated Neuropsychological Assessment Metrics (ANAM V1.0). *Archives of Clinical Neuropsychology* 12(2):155-166.

Lovell, M. R., and M. W. Collins. 1998. Neuropsychological assessment of the college football player. *Head Trauma Rehabilitation* 13(2):9-26.

Lovell, M. R., G. L. Iverson, M. W. Collins, K. Podell, K. M. Johnston, D. Pardini, J. Pardini, J. Norwig, and J. C. Maroon. 2006. Measurement of symptoms following sports-related concussion: Reliability and normative data for the Post-Concussion Scale. *Applied Neuropsychology* 13(3):166-174.

Maddocks, D. L., G. D. Dicker, and M. M. Saling. 1995. The assessment of orientation following concussion in athletes. *Clinical Journal of Sport Medicine* 5(1):32-33.

Maerlender, A., L. Flashman, A. Kessler, S. Kumbhani, R. Greenwald, T. Tosteson, and T. McAllister. 2010. Examination of the construct validity of ImPACT™ computerized test, traditional, and experimental neuropsychological measures. *Clinical Neuropsychologist* 24(8):1309-1325.

Makdissi, M., D. Darby, P. Maruff, A. Ugoni, P. Brukner, and P. R. McCrory. 2010. Natural history of concussion in sport: Markers of severity and implications for management. *American Journal of Sports Medicine* 38(3):464-471.

McCaffrey, M. A., J. P. Mihalik, D. H. Crowell, E. W. Shields, and K. M. Guskiewicz. 2007. Measurement of head impacts in collegiate football players: Clinical measures of concussion after high- and low-magnitude impacts. *Neurosurgery* 61(6):1236-1243.

McCrea, M. 2001. Standardized mental status testing on the sideline after sport-related concussion. *Journal of Athletic Training* 36(3):274-279.

McCrea, M., J. Kelly, and C. Randolph. 1996. *Standardized Assessment of Concussion (SAC): Manual for Administration, Scoring and Interpretation.* Waukesha, WI: CNS Inc.

McCrea, M., J. P. Kelly, C. Randolph, J. Kluge, E. Bartolic, G. Finn, and B. Baxter. 1998. Standardized Assessment of Concussion (SAC): On-site mental status evaluation of the athlete. *Journal of Head Trauma Rehabilitation* 13(2):27-35.

McCrea, M., J. P. Kelly, and C. Randolph. 2000. *Standardized Assessment of Concussion (SAC): Manual for Administration, Scoring and Interpretation,* Second edition. Waukesha, WI: CNS Inc.

McCrea, M., K. M. Guskiewicz, S. W. Marshall, W. Barr, C. Randolph, R. C. Cantu, J. A. Onate, J. Yang, and J. P. Kelly. 2003. Acute effects and recovery time following concussion in collegiate football players: The NCAA Concussion Study. *JAMA* 290(19):2556-2563.

McCrory, P., W. Meeuwisse, K. Johnston, J. Dvořák, M. Aubry, M. Molloy, and R. Cantu. 2009. Consensus statement on concussion in sport: The 3rd International Conference on Concussion in Sport held in Zurich, November 2008. *British Journal of Sports Medicine* 43(Suppl 1):i76-i84.

McCrory, P., W. H. Meeuwisse, M. Aubry, B. Cantu, J. Dvořák, R. J. Echemendia, L. Engebretsen, K. Johnston, J. S. Kutcher, M. Raftery, A. Sills, B. W. Benson, G. A. Davis, R. G. Ellenbogen, K. Guskiewicz, S. A. Herring, G. L. Iverson, B. D. Jordan, J. Kissick, M. McCrea, A. S. McIntosh, D. Maddocks, M. Makdissi, L. Purcell, M. Putukian, K. Schneider, C. H. Tator, and M. Turner. 2013a. Child-SCAT3. *British Journal of Sports Medicine* 47(5):263-266.

McCrory, P., W. H. Meeuwisse, M. Aubry, B. Cantu, J. Dvořák, R. J. Echemendia, L. Engebretsen, K. Johnston, J. S. Kutcher, M. Raftery, A. Sills, B. W. Benson, G. A. Davis, R. G. Ellenbogen, K. Guskiewicz, S. A. Herring, G. L. Iverson, B. D. Jordan, J. Kissick, M. McCrea, A. S. McIntosh, D. Maddocks, M. Makdissi, L. Purcell, M. Putukian, K. Schneider, C. H. Tator, and M. Turner. 2013b. Consensus statement on concussion in sport: The 4th International Conference on Concussion in Sport held in Zurich, November 2012. *British Journal of Sports Medicine* 47(5):250-258.

McCrory, P., W. H. Meeuwisse, M. Aubry, B. Cantu, J. Dvořák, R. J. Echemendia, L. Engebretsen, K. Johnston, J. S. Kutcher, M. Raftery, A. Sills, B. W. Benson, G. A. Davis, R. G. Ellenbogen, K. Guskiewicz, S. A. Herring, G. L. Iverson, B. D. Jordan, J. Kissick, M. McCrea, A. S. McIntosh, D. Maddocks, M. Makdissi, L. Purcell, M. Putukian, K. Schneider, C. H. Tator, and M. Turner. 2013c. SCAT3. *British Journal of Sports Medicine* 47(5):259-262.

Miller, J. R., G. J. Adamson, M. M. Pink, and J. C. Sweet. 2007. Comparison of preseason, midseason, and postseason neurocognitive scores in uninjured collegiate football players. *American Journal of Sports Medicine* 35(8):1284-1288.

NeuroCom. 2013. *Sensory Organizing Test.* http://www.resourcesonbalance.com/neurocom/protocols/sensoryImpairment/SOT.aspx (accessed August 23, 2013).

Pardini, J. E., D. A. Pardini, J. T. Becker, K. L. Dunfee, W. F. Eddy, M. R. Lovell, and J. S. Welling. 2010. Postconcussive symptoms are associated with compensatory cortical recruitment during a working memory task. *Neurosurgery* 67(4):1020-1027; discussion 1027-1028.

Piland, S. G., R. W. Motl, K. M. Guskiewicz, M. McCrea, and M. S. Ferrara. 2006. Structural validity of a self-report concussion-related symptom scale. *Medicine and Science in Sports and Exercise* 38(1):27-32.

Randolph, C., S. Millis, W. B. Barr, M. McCrea, K. M. Guskiewicz, T. A. Hammeke, and J. P. Kelly. 2009. Concussion Symptom Inventory: An empirically-derived scale for monitoring resolution of symptoms following sports-related concussion. *Archives of Clinical Neuropsychology* 24(3):219-229.

Reeves, D. L., K. P. Winter, J. Bleiberg, and R. L. Kane. 2007. ANAM® genogram: Historical perspectives, description, and current endeavors. *Archives of Clinical Neuropsychology* 22(Suppl 1):S15-S37.

Register-Mihalik, J., K. M. Guskiewicz, J. D. Mann, and E. W. Shields. 2007. The effects of headache on clinical measures of neurocognitive function. *Clinical Journal of Sport Medicine* 17(4):282-288.

Riemann, B. L., K. M. Guskiewicz, and E. W. Shields. 1999. Relationship between clinical and forceplate measures of postural stability. *Journal of Sport Rehabilitation* 8(2):71-82.

Schatz, P. 2010. Long-term test-retest reliability of baseline cognitive assessments using ImPACT. *American Journal of Sports Medicine* 38(1):47-53.

Schatz, P., and B. O. Putz. 2006. Cross-validation of measures used for computer-based assessment of concussion. *Applied Neuropsychology* 13(3):151-159.

Schatz, P., J. Pardini, M. R. Lovell, M. W. Collins, and K. Podell. 2006. Sensitivity and specificity of the ImPACT Test Battery for concussion in athletes. *Archives of Clinical Neuropsychology* 21(1):91-99.

Schneider, J., and G. Gioia. 2007. Psychometric properties of the Post-Concussion Symptom Inventory (PCSI) in school age children. [Abstract.] *Developmental Neurorehabilitation* 10(4):282.

Schneider, K. J., C. A. Emery, J. Kang, G. M. Schneider, and W. H. Meeuwisse. 2010. Examining Sport Concussion Assessment Tool ratings for male and female youth hockey players with and without a history of concussion. *British Journal of Sports Medicine* 44(15):1112-1117.

Segalowitz, S., P. Mahaney, D. Santesso, L. MacGregor, J. Dywan, and B. Willer. 2007. Retest reliability in adolescents of a computerized neuropsychological battery used to assess recovery from concussion. *NeuroRehabilitation* 22(3):243-251.

Teasdale, G., and B. Jennett. 1974. Assessment of coma and impaired consciousness: A practical scale. *Lancet* 2(7872):81-84.

Valovich McLeod, T. C., W. B. Barr, M. McCrea, and K. M. Guskiewicz. 2006. Psychometric and measurement properties of concussion assessment tools in youth sports. *Journal of Athletic Training* 41(4):399-408.

Valovich McLeod, T. C., R. C. Bay, K. C. Lam, and A. Chhabra. 2012. Representative baseline values on the Sport Concussion Assessment Tool 2 (SCAT2) in adolescent athletes vary by gender, grade, and concussion history. *American Journal of Sports Medicine* 40(4):927-933.

Vaughan, C., G. A. Gioia, and D. Vincent. 2008. Initial examination of self-reported postconcussion symptoms in normal and mTBI children ages 5 to 12. [Abstract.] *Journal of the International Neuropsychological Society* 14(Suppl 1):207.

Vincent, A. S., T. Roebuck-Spencer, K. Gilliland, and R. Schlegel. 2012. Automated Neuropsychological Assessment Metrics (v4) Traumatic Brain Injury Battery: Military normative data. *Military Medicine* 177(3):256-269.

Wilde, E. A., S. R. McCauley, J. V. Hunter, E. D. Bigler, Z. Chu, Z. J. Wang, G. R. Hanten, M. Troyanskaya, R. Yallampalli, X. Li, J. Chia, and H. S. Levin. 2008. Diffusion tensor imaging of acute mild traumatic brain injury in adolescents. *Neurology* 70(12):948-955.

Yeates, K. O., E. Kaizar, J. Rusin, B. Bangert, A. Dietrich, K. Nuss, M. Wright, and H. G. Taylor. 2012. Reliable change in postconcussive symptoms and its functional consequences among children with mild traumatic brain injury. *Archives of Pediatrics and Adolescent Medicine* 166(7):615-622.